Handbook of Climate Psychiatry and Psychotherapy

A Manual for Clinicians

Handbook of Climate Psychiatry and Psychotherapy

A Manual for Clinicians

by

Elizabeth Haase, M.D.

Clinical Professor of Psychiatry, University of Nevada School of Medicine,
and Medical Director of Psychiatry, Carson Tahoe Regional Medical Center,
Carson City, Nevada

Note: The author has worked to ensure that all information in this book is accurate at the time of publication and consistent with general psychiatric and medical standards, and that information concerning drug dosages, schedules, and routes of administration is accurate at the time of publication and consistent with standards set by the U.S. Food and Drug Administration and the general medical community. As medical research and practice continue to advance, however, therapeutic standards may change. Moreover, specific situations may require a specific therapeutic response not included in this book. For these reasons and because human and mechanical errors sometimes occur, we recommend that readers follow the advice of physicians directly involved in their care or the care of a member of their family.

The author has indicated that she has no financial interests or other affiliations that represent or could appear to represent a competing interest with her work on this book.

Books published by American Psychiatric Association Publishing represent the findings, conclusions, and views of the individual authors and do not necessarily represent the policies and opinions of American Psychiatric Association Publishing or the American Psychiatric Association.

If you wish to buy 50 or more copies of the same title, please go to www.appi.org/specialdiscounts for more information.

Copyright © 2025 American Psychiatric Association

ALL RIGHTS RESERVED

First Edition

Manufactured in the United States of America on acid-free paper

29 28 27 26 25   5 4 3 2 1

American Psychiatric Association Publishing
800 Maine Avenue SW, Suite 900
Washington, D.C. 20024–2812
www.appi.org

Library of Congress Cataloging-in-Publication Data

Library of Congress Cataloging-in-Publication Data

Names: Haase, Elizabeth, 1963– author.

Title: Handbook of climate psychiatry and psychotherapy : a manual for clinicians / Elizabeth Haase.

Description: First edition. | Washington, DC : American Psychiatric Association Publishing, [2025] | Includes bibliographical references and index.

Identifiers: LCCN 2024051080 (print) | LCCN 2024051081 (ebook) | ISBN 9798894550831 (paperback ; alk. paper) | ISBN 9798894550848 (ebook)

Subjects: MESH: Climate Change | Psychological Distress | Psychotherapy—methods | Mental Health Services Classification: LCC RC480.5 (print) | LCC RC480.5 (ebook) | NLM WM 31 | DDC 616.89/14—dc23/eng/20250107

LC record available at https://lccn.loc.gov/2024051080

LC ebook record available at https://lccn.loc.gov/2024051081

British Library Cataloguing in Publication Data

A CIP record is available from the British Library.

For Maddie and Rennie

Contents

Acknowledgments xi

Part I   Introduction and Overview

1 Introduction 3

2 History of Climate Psychiatry 9

3 Psychiatric Ethics, Climate Justice,
and Climate Advocacy and Activism 17

Part II   Neuropsychiatric and Biological Effects
of Climate Change

4 Extreme Heat and Its Implications for
Psychiatry..37

5 Air Pollution Impacts on the Brain 75

6 Nutrition, Food and Water Insecurity,
and Mental Health..93

7 Climate-Related Shifts in Infectious
Diseases, Neuropsychiatric
Symptoms, and Associated Issues in
the Human-Microbiome Relationship 121

8 Climate Change, Extreme Weather, Natural Disasters, and Human Displacement 139

Part III Psychological Responses to Climate Change, Assessment, and Psychotherapeutic Response

9 Obstacles to Rational and Adequate Responses to Climate Change..................171

10 Emotional Reactions and Syndromes Associated With Climate Change 199

11 Assessment of the Patient: Climate-Related Vulnerabilities and Psychology....221

12 Psychotherapy Considerations and Approaches for Climate-Related Distress 237

Part IV Community, Institutional, and Global Psychiatry for Climate Change

13 Coordinating the Climate Psychiatry Response: Global, Institutional, Educational, and Research Agendas........281

14 Community Psychiatry and Its Role in
Climate Mitigation and Adaptation 295

15 Sustainable Psychiatry: Reducing
the Carbon Footprint of Mental
Health Care 313

Appendix: Climate Mental Health
Organizations and Resources
for Professional Engagement
and Patient Support 333

Index..339

Acknowledgments

This book is the synthesis of the efforts of literally thousands of people, whose collective concern for our planet has led them to devote themselves to understanding how people think, feel, decide, and react to climate change. Every one of them is a teacher and is acknowledged by the fruition of this book about the field we have all found together. I personally offer particular gratitude to my writing partner, Janet Lewis, whose subtle and creative thoughts permeate this book; to my Raindog, whose love and Buddhist compassion for the smallest life forms have given me new eyes; to Carson Tahoe Regional Medical Center, for valuing this work enough to give me time off for it; to my colleagues of the Climate Psychiatry Alliance, Climate Psychology Alliance, GAP Climate Committee, and the APA Committee on Climate Change and Mental Health and APA Caucus on Climate Change and Mental Health; and to Jessica Haller, my partner from the beginning.

PART I

Introduction and Overview

1

Introduction

Why This Book

The climate crisis is rapidly destabilizing life-sustaining systems around the globe. At the same time, progress to lower greenhouse gas emissions is both advancing and significantly faltering because of political conflict and inaction, culturally bound inertia, and global energy needs. Hundreds of millions of people are already suffering from extreme heat and extreme weather (Li et al. 2020) and their associated socioeconomic and health consequences. The damage to ecosystems has become broadly visible, and the majority of Americans are expressing distress about these effects (American Psychiatric Association 2020). There is a clarion call to move from the Anthropocene, an era and way of life organized around fossil fuel–based sources of energy and exploitation of natural resources, to the Symbiocene, in which humans thrive in mutually caretaking (symbiotic) relationships with those species and resources on which they depend for life.

Core elements of global warming affect neurobiology, psychiatric symptoms, and psychiatric epidemiology at statistically and clinically relevant levels through air pollution, extreme heat, and changes to food supplies and infectious diseases. Knowledge of the neuropsychiatric impacts of these global trends has emerged outside the mental health literature and is thus underappreciated within the practicing psychiatric community. Climate-related distress, including ecological anxiety, grief, and rage, is affecting most people and therefore also most of those who seek mental health care, but psychiatric systems and procedures are not in place to support clinical recognition and treatment. Awareness of this distress has emerged mostly in the media and environmental movement until the last half-dozen years, when clinicians across the allied mental health fields began to call it out and consider how to intervene. It is timely and imperative that psychiatrists and other mental health professionals have adequate information to address the clinical aspects of these climate effects in their practice.

This book was conceived because, although many books cover management of the psychological effects of climate change, most are oriented toward the lay reader. Examples include *A Field Guide to Climate Anxiety* (Ray 2020), *Emotional Resiliency in the Era of Climate Change* (Davenport 2017), *Turn the Tide on Climate Anxiety: Sustainable Action for Your Mental Health and the Planet* (Kennedy-Woodard and Kennedy-Williams 2022), *Taking the Heat: How Climate Change Is Affecting Your Mind, Body, and Spirit and What You Can Do About It* (Schneider 2022), *A Guide to Eco-Anxiety: How to Protect the Planet and Your Mental Health* (Grose 2020), and *Generation Dread: Finding Purpose in an Age of Climate Crisis* (Wray 2023). Others, exploring nature-based therapies, are oriented toward therapists, including *Ecotherapy: Healing Ourselves, Healing the Earth: A Guide to Ecologically Grounded Personality Theory, Spirituality, Therapy, and Education* (Clinebell 1996), *Nature and Therapy: Understanding Counselling and Psychotherapy in Outdoor Spaces* (Jordan 2014), *Wild Therapy: Rewilding Our Inner and Outer Worlds* (Totton 2021), and *Towards an Ecopsychotherapy* (Rust 2020).

Among books for professionals are *Climate Change and Human Well-Being* (Weissbecker 2011), *Global Climate Change and Human Health: From Science to Practice* (Luber and Lemery 2015), *Psychology and Climate Change: Human Perceptions, Impacts, and Responses* (Clayton and Manning 2018), *Climate Crisis, Psychoanalysis, and Radical Ethics* (Orange 2017), *Climate Change and Youth Mental Health* (Haase and Hudson 2024), *Engaging With Climate Change: Psychoanalytic and Interdisciplinary Perspectives* (Weintrobe 2013), and *Psychological Roots of the Climate Crisis: Neoliberal Exceptionalism and the Culture of Uncare* (Weintrobe 2021). Many more books have been published recently or are in development and will become excellent resources.

Despite the richness of this literature, none of these works has been tailored to address the day-to-day work that psychiatrists do in their offices, institutions, and communities. The goal of this book is therefore to lay out the range of issues inherent in the psychiatric and psychological response to climate change in a format that is accessible to office-based or clinic-based mental health clinicians, including

Introduction

physicians, physician assistants, nurse practitioners, and allied mental health professionals. To ensure utility on busy clinical days, the writing has been kept relatively informal, often formatted or bulleted, in hopes that clear subheadings, multiple tables, case vignettes, and a consistent format across chapters will allow the reader to easily find and label a climate-related experience identified by a patient and quickly read about various ways to understand and respond to the patient's need.

This book is divided into four parts. Part I includes this introduction and chapters providing an orientation to climate justice and the ethics, advocacy, and activism of engaging with climate change as a psychiatrist. Part II provides a review of the neurobiological impacts of climate effects on the brain. Part III includes chapters on how to perform a climate-informed patient assessment and make practical and psychotherapeutic interventions for climate adaptation and distress at the individual and group levels. Part IV provides discussion of the community, global, institutional, research, and educational aspects of climate psychiatry. The book also includes an appendix with some of the rapidly evolving resources for climate mental health and climate-related community involvement for both young people and adults.

A Mindset for Reading

Most psychiatrists already balance the enormous needs of providing expertise and care for all the aspects of psychiatry and keeping abreast of evolving topic areas. Although many psychiatrists are impressed by the impact of climate disasters, stresses, and future threats on their patients, they must also contend with responding to the whole life and psyche of the patient in a patient-centered way. Many have little knowledge of climate psychiatry as a topic area. They need a general primer that can be easily integrated into other aspects of delivering care, as well as a psychological framework with which to approach the patient adjusting to new climate-related stress.

The climate crisis presents each individual with a complex set of psychological tasks. On the one hand is the task of preventing climate progression through rapid personal transition to a sustainable way of living and active involvement in the social changes necessary to reach this goal. This transition requires a profound intrapsychic reassessment of personal assumptions, beliefs, values, and activities; rapid change away from long-held and culturally syntonic narratives, values, and actions; and a realignment of lifestyle to reflect an understanding of human society's interdependent relationship with nature.

The personal transition required by the climate crisis is difficult if not impossible to achieve without emotional support for deep psychic change, aspects of which psychiatrists and other mental health professionals can particularly, and sometimes uniquely, facilitate. However, this realignment also requires significant shifts not only in the individual psyche but also in a wide range of social and practical behaviors. For most people, both significant learning and participation in a community working toward this new way of life are essential for sustaining this needed adaptation.

Next, responding to the climate crisis requires that each individual be aware of and prepare for substantial physical and neurophysiological threats to brain and body, including the threat of death. The psychiatric response to this part of climate mental health falls more cleanly into the category of primary preventative health measures— advising on how to avoid heat illness, reduce adverse effects of air pollution, practice safety skills for extreme weather events, and prepare for coming scarcities of resources and threats to one's home habitat— both within individual patient interactions and at the community and national level. The existential anxieties linked to these threats must also be addressed.

The dual challenge of acting to prevent climate change while also adapting to its inevitable progression is complex. It requires oscillation between positions of acceptance and resistance. The psychological positions involved similarly oscillate between deep internal psychic work and civic engagement with an external focus. All of this must be done while coping with the increasing traumas of what has been variously termed the *metacrisis*, *permacrisis*, or *polycrisis* of compounding climate disasters. The qualities of uncertainty and unknowability combined with its global scale also make climate change a hyperobject: an object so vast and complex it is impossible to conceive of within a single human psyche. The psychic demands of managing practical and emotional responses to the combination of global uncertainties, ongoing climate trauma, internal realignments, actions to change one's community and country, and disruptions of one's relationship to the dominant American economic model and to the natural world lead easily to the collapse of psychic functions, to emotional overwhelm, and to the numbing of any capacity to cope creatively.

For these reasons, it is recommended that the reader approach clinical responsiveness to climate issues as the proverbial elephant in the room, taking it from a variety of angles one step at a time, with a humility to what cannot yet be seen. Some points of access can be understood

Introduction

by approaching the patient from each element of a bio-psycho-socio-environmental model. But the multifaceted need to support the patient from all of these perspectives also invites frequent shifts in the psychiatrist's activities. The psychiatrist may need to provide preventative medicine, prescribe climate-sensitive psychopharmacology, conduct motivational interviewing, and explore ecological, existential, and exploratory psychotherapies and cognitive science, as well as participate as a fellow traveler on a climate journey for which spiritual and Indigenous traditions provide some of the more relevant wisdom. Take the material in short snippets, organizing interventions not by diagnosis but by the symptoms or psychological problem that may be presented on a given day.

Despite the significant hurdles described here, the attitudes conducive to their response represent innate, positive, and relatively easily accessed qualities of the human psyche and can thus be expected and cultivated in the patient with excitement and optimism by the therapist. We are waking up to the new and exciting world required by the climate crisis together, much as an alert infant attunes itself to and learns quickly about its new reality. We are naturally symbiotic creatures, attaching to and cultivating the well-being of the beings around us. Development and change are our natural conditions across the life span. Regression of the kind we see now—immature, narcissistic, and paranoid retreats in response to climate demands—is not the norm. All animals have their defenses, which we are currently deploying in response to fearsome challenges. But this is what the human mind would be expected to do as it succors and protects itself in approaching a monumental task. Soon the schemas that have governed the old way of thinking will become outmoded, and we will move forward. We are in a phase of tremendous growth and innovation, of emergence and flow into a new reality. Psychiatric clinicians must lead by applying our knowledge to facilitate more rapid psychological change and prevent the public health and individual neuropsychiatric damage that is happening; by applying our souls to the empathic understanding of what we are losing and transforming that experience in ourselves and our patients into a new relationship with the planet, each other, and all beings.

References

American Psychiatric Association: APA Public Opinion Poll—Annual Meeting 2020. Washington, DC, American Psychiatric Association, 2020.

Available at: www.psychiatry.org/newsroom/apa-public-opinion-poll-2020. Accessed November 20, 2024.

Clayton S, Manning C (eds): Psychology and Climate Change: Human Perceptions, Impacts, and Responses. London, Academic Press, 2018

Clinebell H: Ecotherapy: Healing Ourselves, Healing the Earth: A Guide to Ecologically Grounded Personality Theory, Spirituality, Therapy, and Education. Minneapolis, MN, Fortress Press, 1996

Davenport L: Emotional Resiliency in the Era of Climate Change: A Clinician's Guide. London, Jessica Kingsley, 2017

Grose A: A Guide to Eco-Anxiety: How to Protect the Planet and Your Mental Health. London, Watkins, 2020

Haase E, Hudson K (eds): Climate Change and Youth Mental Health: Multidisciplinary Perspectives. Cambridge University Press, 2024

Jordan M: Nature and Therapy: Understanding Counselling and Psychotherapy in Outdoor Spaces. Hove, UK, Routledge, 2014

Kennedy-Woodard M, Kennedy-Williams P: Turn the Tide on Climate Anxiety: Sustainable Action for Your Mental Health and the Planet. London, Jessica Kingsley, 2022

Li D, Yuan J, Kopp RE: Escalating global exposure to compound heat-humidity extremes with warming. Environ Res Lett 15(6):64003, 2020

Luber G, Lemery J (eds): Global Climate Change and Human Health: From Science to Practice, 1st Edition. San Francisco, CA, Jossey-Bass, 2015

Orange DM: Climate Crisis, Psychoanalysis, and Radical Ethics. New York, Routledge, 2017

Ray SJ: A Field Guide to Climate Anxiety: How to Keep Your Cool on a Warming Planet. Oakland, University of California Press, 2020

Rust MJ: Towards an Ecopsychotherapy. London, Confer, 2020

Schneider B: Taking the Heat: How Climate Change Is Affecting Your Mind, Body, and Spirit and What You Can Do About It. New York, Simon & Schuster, 2022

Totton N: Wild Therapy: Rewilding Our Inner and Outer Worlds, 2nd Edition. Monmouth, UK, PCCS Books, 2021

Weintrobe S (ed): Engaging With Climate Change: Psychoanalytic and Interdisciplinary Perspectives. New York, Routledge, 2013

Weintrobe S: Psychological Roots of the Climate Crisis: Neoliberal Exceptionalism and the Culture of Uncare. New York, Bloomsbury Academic, 2021

Weissbecker I (ed): Climate Change and Human Well-Being: Global Challenges and Opportunities. New York, Springer, 2011

Wray B: Generation Dread: Finding Purpose in an Age of Climate Crisis. New York, The Experiment, 2023

2

History of Climate Psychiatry

Historical Origins

Historically, as well as philosophically, climate psychiatry and psychotherapy are embedded in understandings of our relationship with the Earth and the natural world. These perceptions owe their origins to the Indigenous and shamanistic practices of the earliest societies, the classical Greek and later philosophers, the Romantic poets and Transcendentalists of the nineteenth century, and the ecopsychology movement that began in the 1960s and even earlier. The core of this tradition is biophilia (Wilson 1984), the awareness of the psychological importance of our relationship with nature and the need to enhance reverence for nature and address distress and health problems that result from an imbalanced relationship to it to live properly and well.

The formal origins of what is termed *ecopsychology* can be traced to Robert Greenway, who coined the term *psychoecology* in 1963 (Reser 1995). Paul Shepard in 1982, Theodore Roszak in 1996, Ralph Metzner, and Harold Searles are also considered to be early founders of the ecopsychology field, and Howard Clinebell is credited with the first use of the term *ecotherapy* (Clinebell 1996). The ecopsychological perspective is about understanding human consciousness to be in nonhierarchical continuity with the larger ecological and cosmic consciousness(es) of Nature. It therefore understands human appreciation for and responsive codependency within this relationship as the source of mental health and its disruption as a source of insanity. The therapeutic goals of ecopsychology are to enhance the *ecological ego* by reducing tendencies to dominate and extract from nature, cultivating animism, and increasing responsibility to and reciprocity with nature in the ways humans interact with the world. Techniques of ecopsychology include animal therapies, gardening and horticulture therapies, nature and wilderness-based experiences, and others that are associated with a large literature on the centrality of engagement with nature for mental health (see Chapter 11, "Assessment of the Patient").

Mental Health Inclusion by the IPCC

Appreciation for how climate change–based disruption of natural systems adversely affects mental health and health in general has been slower to materialize outside of this movement. In general, broad global assessments about climate change are issued by the United Nations through the Intergovernmental Panel on Climate Change (IPCC). The IPCC is made up of scientist experts from 195 nations organized into three working groups and has issued reports every few years since 1990. It assesses climate risks using four Representative Concentration Pathways (RCPs) that reflect radiative forcing values (warming) in response to different greenhouse gas emission levels by 2100, with more emissions generating more climate change and related damage. The IPCC issued its first reports in 1990 and 1992; these reports covered human health in a short paragraph mentioning only ultraviolet radiation and changes in infectious diseases. The third report of the IPCC began to mention "socioeconomic threats," but only in tropical and subtropical countries, and again without explicit mention of mental health. By the IPCC's Fourth Assessment in 2007, coverage of the health threats of climate change reached 42 pages, but mental health received only five sentences on the psychiatric effects of natural disasters, with relevant concern sounded about increased encephalitis, more human suffering, and the adverse effects of poor physical health on the capacity of populations to adapt (Confalonieri et al. 2007). By the Fifth Assessment of the IPCC in 2014, mental health appeared as a half-page assessment, covering impacts of extreme weather, drought, and solastalgia (Smith et al. 2014). This report added health impacts of climate-altering air pollutants but not their neuropsychiatric sequelae. It was, however, the first appearance of the idea that large-scale, long-term, irreversible mental health impacts would result from climate change, in a graph that highlighted the irreversible health and mental health toll of climate change as this century progresses, regardless of mitigation and adaptation efforts (Figure 2.1).

Early Professional Efforts

The field of climate change and mental health received a significant boost from the United Nations Department of Public Information and Non-Governmental Organizations (UN DPI-NGO), which, between 2007 and 2009, organized two conferences that brought together 1,726 individuals from 500 organizations and 62 countries to discuss climate challenges. The resulting report to the Secretary General included a chapter on climate change and mental health. The group that produced this chapter, led by Inka Weissbecker and including psychiatrist Mindy Fullilove, found only one article on climate change and mental health in PsycINFO at the time of their initial work in 2008. They went on to produce a book, *Climate Change and Human Well-Being: Global Challenges and Opportunities* (Weissbecker 2011), that explored the topic of climate mental health through chapters authored by experts in relevant related literature on natural disasters, drought, conflict, gender vulnerability, place-based attachment, humanitarian crises, solastalgia, and posttraumatic growth. At the same time, the American Psychological Association, which has been a leader in the climate mental health field, started a task force on climate mental health and produced an important report (Swim et al. 2011), and psychoanalysts in the United Kingdom and other countries began to consider the psychological states associated with climate distress more deeply, culminating in *Engaging With Climate Change: Psychoanalytic and Interdisciplinary Perspectives* (Weintrobe 2013). These publications formed the entry point for many mental health professionals becoming aware of the ramifications of climate change for their fields.

Over these and the ensuing years, thousands of studies in environmental and public health, anthropology, and other nonpsychiatric fields significantly increased our understanding of the impacts of climate change on violence, conflict, suicide, involuntary migration, spiritual and cultural disruption, stress disorders, psychiatric conditions, and markers of mental distress such as hospitalizations. They made connections between malnutrition, heat, wildfires, drought, and other climate impacts that had previously not been appreciated to have

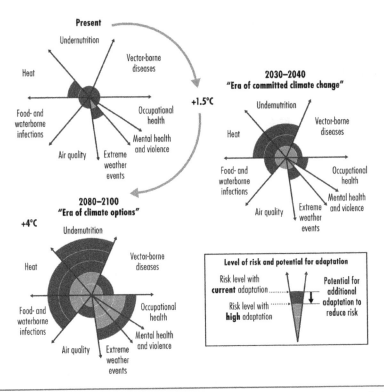

Figure 2.1 Projected health impacts from climate change and the potential for impact reduction through adaptation for global mean temperature increases of 1.5°C and 4°C above preindustrial levels at time points 2030–2040 and 2080–2100.

Impacts are identified in eight health-related sectors on the basis of the assessment of the literature and expert judgments of the authors of the 2014 IPCC Health Report. The width of the slices indicates in a qualitative way the relative importance in terms of the burden of ill health globally. Shading shows the current state of adaptation (*dark gray*) and a hypothetical highly adapted state (*light gray*), with maximal adaptive and mitigative efforts.

Source. Figure 11.6 in Smith et al. 2014. Use of IPCC figure(s) is at the User's sole risk. Under no circumstances shall the IPCC, WMO, or UNEP be liable for any loss, damage, liability, or expense incurred or suffered that is claimed to have resulted from the use of any IPCC figure(s), without limitation, any fault, error, omission, interruption, or delay with respect thereto. Nothing herein shall constitute or be considered to be a limitation upon or a waiver of the privileges and immunities of WMO or UNEP, which are specifically reserved.

significant mental health morbidity. By the time of the most recent 2022 IPCC Sixth Assessment on health and climate change, human well-being and mental health began to make a significant appearance. The concept of well-being was elevated to the title of the report, defining it as a state of predominantly positive emotions and moods associated with a life that is satisfying, meaningful, cognitively unimpaired, and productive and including qualities of freedom, agency, self-actualization, dignity, and relatedness both to the self and to the natural world, as well as the need for an adequate environment for mental health, including food, water, and economic and physical health (Cissé et al. 2022). There remains, however, little to no research by psychiatrists contributing to these assessments, and the number of firmly established quantitative effects of climate factors on mental health remains limited (Radua et al. 2024).

Beginnings of U.S. Federal Funding and Tracking of Climate Health

In the United States, the first work on climate change and health emerged via the National Climate Assessment, based on the Global Change Research Program (GCRP) legislation established by presidential initiative by George H.W. Bush in 1990. The first report was eventually issued in 2000 (National Assessment Synthesis Team 2000) and importantly included air pollution effects, with steadily increasing attention to mental health, such that by the fourth assessment, issued in 2018, mental health impacts were reported in every sector of climate health concern. The GCRP has been an important source of funding for knowledge on climate and health. It was supplemented by funding provided by the Biden administration's Inflation Reduction Act, which included the CDC's Climate and Health Program as well as the establishment of the federal Office of Climate Change and Health Equity. Although funding for climate mental health research and emotional resilience programs has not been formally included in the mission of these efforts, the programs provided for grants for health impacts of all kinds. Other legislation proposed to target climate mental health specifically, including the Community Mental Wellness and Resilience Act (CMWRA) and Green New Deal for Health Act, also received increasing congressional attention during these administrations.

Arrival of Psychiatry on the Scene

Within this larger context, early psychiatrists to raise the alarm about the scope of climate impacts on mental health were Lise Van Susteren, in a monograph published for the National Wildlife Federation (Coyle and Van Susteren 2012), and Steven Moffic, appearing with Dr. Van Susteren in an article in *Psychiatric News* (Moran 2011). Within a few years, they and other psychiatrists concerned about climate change began to meet and interact, banding together officially in 2016 to form the Climate Psychiatry Alliance (CPA) with the mission of raising awareness about the mental health implications of climate change and advocating for their mitigation. The CPA, led by its president Robin Cooper, obtained formal nonprofit status in 2018. This group worked in collaboration with and parallel to a related group of psychologists, the Climate Psychology Alliance, to raise media awareness and to work within their respective organizations to advance knowledge in the mental health professions about climate health impacts. Interest in the media was high because youth expressions of climate distress had exploded, and CPA members gave hundreds of interviews and talks at professional and community forums and in the national and international media over the subsequent four years. This led the American Psychiatric Association to form a Caucus on Climate Change and Mental Health, which lobbied successfully, along with the CPA, to form a Committee on Climate Change and Mental Health in 2020, for which I served as its inaugural chair.

Emergence of National and Global Climate Health and Mental Health Coalitions

From 2016 to 2020, representatives from various health and mental health professions and academic centers organized national initiatives in the United States and abroad. These efforts coalesced in the United States around the Medical Society Consortium on Climate and Health, ecoAmerica, Yale Program on Climate Change Communication, Social Climate Leadership Group, and other collaborative efforts. Recognition of the importance of behavioral change and mental resilience to advance global climate response strategies increased steadily in the first two decades of the millennium, as did appreciation of the central role of the medical community in communicating climate impacts to individuals. On the global stage, the 2022 establishment of COP², or Care of People and Planet, was supported by the United Nations Race to Resilience campaign after being introduced at COP26 in 2021. COP² has initiated a critical component of the international climate effort to support mental resilience, creating six global hubs for those providing mental wellness in community organizations and climate resilience efforts around the world. Numerous organizations are now devoted to the mental health implications of climate change (see the Appendix), providing many points of entry for those interested and a further rich history in evolution.

Key Points

- Climate psychiatry draws on centuries- and decades-old sources that include Indigenous and shamanistic traditions, classical Greek and philosophical understandings of Nature, Transcendentalism, the field of ecopsychology, and biophilia.
- The importance of climate mental health was only recently recognized by the IPCC but is among the most significant and irreversible health impacts of climate change.
- Climate psychiatry and climate mental health as a topic area have undergone explosive growth and evolution since 2015, alongside the growth of other climate and health national and global coalitions.

References

Cissé G, McLeman R, Adams H, et al: Health, wellbeing, and the changing structure of communities, in Climate Change 2022: Impacts, Adaptation and Vulnerability. Contribution of Working Group II to the Sixth Assessment Report of the Intergovernmental Panel on Climate Change. Edited by Pörtner H-O, Roberts DC, Tignor M, et al. Cambridge, UK, Cambridge University Press, 2022, pp 1041–1170

Clinebell H: Ecotherapy: Healing Ourselves, Healing the Earth: A Guide to Ecologically Grounded Personality Theory, Spirituality, Therapy, and Education. Minneapolis, MN, Fortress Press, 1996

Confalonieri U, Menne B, Akhtar R, et al: Human health, in Climate Change 2007: Impacts, Adaptation and Vulnerability. Contribution of Working Group II to the Fourth Assessment Report of the Intergovernmental

Panel on Climate Change. Edited by Parry ML, Canziani OF, Palutikof JP, et al. Cambridge, UK, Cambridge University Press, 2007, pp 391–431

Coyle KJ, Van Susteren L: The Psychological Effects of Global Warming on the United States: And Why the U.S. Mental Health System Is Not Adequately Prepared. National Forum and Research Report. Washington, DC, National Wildlife Federation Climate Education Program, 2012

Moran M: Psychiatry needs eyes wide open about environmental issues. Psychiatr News 46(5), 2011. Available at: https://psychiatryonline.org/doi/full/10.1176/pn.46.5.psychnews_46_5_17_1. Accessed October 30, 2023.

National Assessment Synthesis Team: Climate Change Impacts on the United States: The Potential Consequences of Climate Variability and Change. Washington, DC, U.S. Global Change Research Program, 2000. Available at: https://downloads.globalchange.gov/nca/nca-2000-report-overview.pdf. Accessed May 5, 2014.

Radua J, De Prisco M, Oliva V, et al: Impact of air pollution and climate change on mental health outcomes: an umbrella review of global evidence. World Psychiatry 23(2):244–256, 2024 38727076

Reser JP: Whither environmental psychology? The transpersonal ecopsychology crossroads. J Environ Psychol 15:235–257, 1995

Smith KR, Woodward A, Campbell-Lendrum D, et al: Human health: impacts, adaptation, and co-benefits, in Climate Change 2014: Impacts, Adaptation, and Vulnerability. Part A: Global and Sectoral Aspects. Contribution of Working Group II to the Fifth Assessment Report of the Intergovernmental Panel on Climate Change. Edited by Field CB, Barros VR, Dokken DJ, et al. Cambridge, UK, Cambridge University Press, 2014, pp 709–754

Swim JK, Stern PC, Doherty TJ, et al: Psychology's contributions to understanding and addressing global climate change. Am Psychol 66(4):241–250, 2011 21553950

Weintrobe S (ed): Engaging With Climate Change: Psychoanalytic and Interdisciplinary Perspectives. New York, Routledge, 2013

Weissbecker I (ed): Climate Change and Human Well-Being: Global Challenges and Opportunities. New York, Springer, 2011

Wilson EO: Biophilia: The Human Bond With Other Species. Cambridge, MA, Harvard University Press, 1984

3

Psychiatric Ethics, Climate Justice, and Climate Advocacy and Activism

Climate Justice

The most severe and deadly climate changes will be felt in great disproportion in the Global South and in disadvantaged populations worldwide, which already experience hardship, prejudice, and discrimination (Ebi et al. 2016). The World Health Organization conservatively predicts 250,000 more deaths per year due to climate change between 2030 and 2050 (World Health Organization 2023), and myriad examples exist of unequal climate impacts on the billions of people worldwide who have inadequate access to clean air, water, food, and electricity and who are at risk of mass death from extreme heat and other horrific outcomes. For example, the impact of extreme weather in vulnerable regions is fifteenfold greater than in less vulnerable areas, and food insecurity was experienced by 98 million more people in 2020 than in previous years. In this chapter, therefore, I cover climate justice, the medical ethics that underlie it, and advocacy actions that psychiatrists can take to mitigate this suffering.

Although all predictions are uncertain and can be modified by the tremendous adaptive potential of humanity, the Intergovernmental Panel on Climate Change (Cissé et al. 2022) has highlighted manifold outsized risks to vulnerable groups. These risks include waterborne illness, food scarcity, excess heat illness, cardiovascular and pulmonary illness, and poor mental health, combined with a lesser capacity to adapt to rapidly changing climate conditions due to social factors (Benevolenza and DeRigne 2019). Poverty, in particular, is both a risk factor for and consequence of climate effects, with elevated rates in areas of droughts, after natural disasters, and after health events that are common with heat illness (Hallegatte et al. 2016). Economic losses from climate impacts are already measured in the tens of trillions of dollars per year and are predicted to depress global average income by 20% permanently by 2050 (Kotz et al. 2024), affecting impoverished populations inequitably. All these impacts will fall on areas that already carry the environmental legacy of decades of exposure to greater levels of toxic contaminants, radiation, poor-quality environments, air pollution, and other environmental injustices.

Wealthy nations, particularly the United States, exceed others in per capita greenhouse gas emissions, and the emissions of the U.S. health care sector contribute significantly in fueling negative climate health impacts on its citizens (see Chapter 15, "Sustainable Psychiatry"). Although the disproportionate emissions of wealthy countries are commonly appreciated, the magnitude of the difference is not. In the United States, 2020 per capita emissions of 13.68 $tCO_2/cap/yr$ exceeded those of many African nations (0.07–0.54 $tCO_2/cap/yr$) by more than 26-fold and of India (1.74 $tCO_2/cap/yr$) by eightfold. Other countries that depend heavily on fossil fuels have a significantly disproportionate impact on global warming (Russia, 11.64 $tCO_2/cap/yr$), but excess emissions are not necessary for developed societies in the Northern Hemisphere, as demonstrated by the per capita emissions of Sweden (4.18 $tCO_2/cap/yr$) and the United Kingdom (4.66 $tCO_2/cap/yr$) (Crippa et al. 2021).

The vulnerable populations that will be most affected by these emissions (detailed in Chapter 14, "Community Psychiatry and Its Role in Climate Mitigation and Adaptation") have already suffered at the hands of exploitative colonial practices. Worldwide, these practices include extraction of their resources, harsh labor conditions, enslavement, subjugation, and genocide by imperialist governments allied with militarized dictatorships; destruction of their cultures and heritage; pollution of their lands; population decimation by pandemics and genocide; and other abusive and deadly assaults. In the recent history of the United States, unjust practices include inequities in housing, medical, and social service practices; racism; denial of historical fact; and disproportionate criminalization and violent victimization. Participants in this society and health professionals who have sworn to do no harm have an ethical imperative to rectify climate injustice and repay our ecological debt (Steele and Patel 2020) to affected people by slowing the progression of climate change and mitigating its impacts on those disproportionately affected. Ambivalence toward climate action passively facilitates continued harm to health and to the natural resources that sustain health, with particular infliction of such bystander injustice on those populations most affected.

The Ethical Imperative of Climate Action

Climate change has been called a perfect storm for human immoral behavior because it is global and intergenerational, crosses species boundaries, disperses cause and effect, occurs in a setting where our theories and institutions are weak, and undermines the belief that personal agency is effective, all of which tempt unethical action (Gardiner and Weisbach 2016). It can be difficult to maintain focus on the centrality of planetary health to individual patient well-being and to move flexibly between proactive actions that prevent climate change itself and reactive medical responses that help patients mitigate or recover from the health problems connected to climate effects. In individualistic, materialistic cultures particularly, it can be difficult for patients to understand that changing behavior to support planetary systems is good for them.

A review of the medical ethics that underlie the moral imperative to address climate change can help orient the psychiatrist to their role and responsibilities. The ethical concept of "tragedy of the commons" (Hardin 1968) may also be helpful as a mantra to return to: the idea that depleting shared systems will ultimately lead to negative feedback loops on resource sustainability that will deprive everyone. Contrary to the argument that developing countries should have access to the same fossil fuel–based resources that have fueled the advancement of postindustrial nations, evidence suggests that leapfrogging to clean energy strategies for wealth enhancement (Intergovernmental Panel on Climate Change 2012) will produce more sustainable economic models (Steele and Patel 2020).

As Singh (2012) has argued, however, the most unifying ethical stance for climate responsiveness for health professionals is, in fact, health ethics (Table 3.1). The ethics that shape pro-planetary behavior—the duties of care, stewardship, and rescue—overlap with identical medical obligations. Similarly, the principles of solidarity, beneficence, nonmaleficence, respect for life, accountability in relationships, and humanitarianism apply both in medical and mental health care and in human relationships to other living beings, including the natural systems that give us life and those that are disproportionately harmed by climate effects. These overarching values are supported by *The Principles of Medical Ethics* (American Psychiatric Association 2013), the document on professional ethical behavior referenced by the American Medical Association and the American Psychiatric Association.

These documents additionally require psychiatrists and other physicians to stay informed of new health risks, to share professional knowledge by educating their patients and speaking to the general public and the media about new health risks, and to improve public and community health. Physicians thus have a clear ethical responsibility to educate themselves about and work to mitigate adverse climate health and mental health impacts. As experts in psychological defenses, psychiatrists and other mental health professionals may be particularly effective at helping people appreciate how the fearful and diffuse topic of global climate threats is relevant to an individual's health and dis-ease. They can also use their relational skills to promote the interpersonal ethics of nonmaleficence, beneficence, respect for life, and accountability by cultivating mindful awareness of other types of

Table 3.1 Shared moral principles of medical and climate ethics

Respect for life

Beneficence

Nonmaleficence

Accountability in relationships

Humanitarianism

Duty of care

Duty of stewardship

Duty of rescue

human interdependence (e.g., with nature) and encouraging empathy, not only with other humans but also with nonhuman life-forms whose capacities for cognition, language, self-reflection, empathy, play, and cognition are increasingly being recognized.

Legal Remedies for Climate-Related Damage to Mental Health and Well-Being

The Principles of Medical Ethics further requires that physicians seek changes in laws that do not protect the health interests of their patients, including protecting physicians who take ethical actions with legal consequences (e.g., civil disobedience) from excess censure for unprofessional behavior (American Psychiatric Association 2013, Section 3.1). For this reason, a brief overview of climate law is provided. Environmental law (summarized from Cima 2022) has decades of precedent establishing the clear effect of environmental protection on the enjoyment of codified human rights, including life, property free of toxic damage, health, and water. This work has succeeded by proving that environmental damage has been caused by human action and prevents the execution of other, previously established human rights. It has not, however, until recently, recognized a healthy environment as a fundamental human right separate from environmental impacts on other rights. Applying this area of law to climate change has so far largely required proof that human action or inaction has been responsible for climate changes, and then further causality that these climate changes have harmed legally recognized human rights. This chain of proof for climate-related harm has placed a heavy burden on applicants for damages for the following reasons:

- Climate infringement on basic human rights involves multiple steps, adding room for alternative causal arguments
- Climate change has been defined as a process in and with impacts on nature, negating its human causes and effects
- The relationship between cause and human rights violations is often extraterritorial, where jurisprudence is more complex
- The law in general has typically supported past actions that cause current demonstrable individual harm, rather than current actions that cause harm to a group now or in the future

Since 2008, it has been accepted that climate change, specifically, alongside other environmental issues, is affecting other human rights, but it was not until 2015 that *State of the Netherlands v. Urgenda Foundation* (2019) established that government failure to meet carbon emission goals was causally linked to this harmful climate change and, therefore, that failing emission targets violated the human rights of Dutch citizens under national and European Union law. This view was upheld in *Juliana v. United States* (2016), in which the court upheld precedents that "a causal chain does not fail simply because it has several links, provided those links are not hypothetical or tenuous." Medical harm that infringes on the right to life is perhaps among the easiest damage to demonstrate, given the clear connection between climate-warming pollutants and medical illness, dementia, suicide, depression, autism, and other childhood disorders (Fann et al. 2021; Perera 2017; Radua et al. 2024). These cases, however, still do not establish a healthy environment as a fundamental human right.

Over the first two decades of the twenty-first century, however, more than 100 nations and states had enshrined the right to a healthy environment in their constitutions, creating momentum that culminated in the 2021 adoption of HRC Resolution 48/13 by the United Nations (U.N. Human Rights Council 2021), which recognized "the right to a clean, healthy and sustainable environment as a human right that is important for the enjoyment of human rights" and that it "requires the full implementation of the multilateral environmental agreements under the principles of international environmental law," thus supporting legal action on this basis. A number of countries limited their endorsement in legal terms (Tang and Spijkers 2022), and it is somewhat difficult to define legally how a healthy environment is a stand-alone human right. Nonetheless, the human right to a healthy environment is increasingly being given legal merit under a variety of legal banners (reviewed in de Vilchez and Savaresi 2021), including common good law (Cima 2022), which defines human rights, such as liberty and equality, as things governments are obligated to protect for the group because the individual rights of citizens cannot be protected without this community protection as well.

Climate inaction is also increasingly seen to have created conditions injurious enough to children's well-being as to be conceptualized as intergenerational injustice. Children are protected against such abuse by the Convention on the Rights of the Child (Gibbons 2014), which delineates rights that include survival, health, freedom from abuse and exploitation, and nondiscrimination, referring to the ability to develop a child's potential within a facilitatory context. Within this context, as described by the Ninth Circuit Court of Appeal's majority opinion in the groundbreaking, youth-led climate change case, *Juliana v. United States* (2020), these children's rights have been violated by governments: "A substantial evidentiary record documents the federal government has long promoted fossil fuel use despite knowing that it can cause catastrophic climate change." The term *tyranny of the contemporary* is sometimes used to describe actions against future well-being by governments and companies. In addition to their illegality vis-à-vis the rights of the child, they are a significant assault on children's mental health because the intentionality of corporate and governmental action to block climate progress robs young people of trust in adult protection and hope for the future, burdening them with feelings of rage, powerlessness, and fear that encumber maturation and emotional health (Hickman et al. 2021) and with the health consequences of fossil fuel pollutants. Failure to provide for the health and mental health needs of children constitutes child neglect. Although not professionally or legally obligated to report this form of child neglect as with other mistreatment of children, psychiatrists can be considered to have a duty to protect young people from such adverse climate effects through the courts.

The implications of climate law for forensic psychiatry have not been fully considered. Psychiatrist Lise Van Susteren testified in *Held v. Montana* (2023) about the impacts of climate change on the ability of youth to reach developmental potential and about their current climate distress. It is likely, however, that the scope of forensic psychiatry could come to include the impacts of heat waves on a person's violence or psychosis, the responsibility of governments for dementia care in an area with heavy air pollution, the mental health impacts of heat-related stillbirth on a young mother, and other as yet undefined dimensions. It is clear that the ethical and legal support for climate change gives psychiatrists multiple points of entry to advocate for their patients and communities, as discussed in the next section.

Activism and Advocacy for Climate Justice and Climate Rights

In responding to the mental health impacts and ethical imperatives of the climate crisis, many roles are available to mental health professionals, including clinician, advocate, activist, researcher, and educator, as summarized by the acronym CA^{2}RE (Table 3.2). The roles of activist and

Table 3.2 Climate-related roles for the psychiatrist

Acronym	Role
C	Clinician
A	Advocate
A	Activist
R	Researcher
E	Educator

advocate, however, may allow the climate-aware clinician the greatest freedom in expressing their passion about the climate crisis and the decline of the natural world.

Any act that challenges dominant narratives and power structures or moves toward environmental change is a form of activism, whether personal or professional. In response to climate-based social injustice and an increase in inequitable and conflictual conditions worldwide, social justice training and skills must be actively cultivated to best promote the welfare of all. These skills are also critical to improving health inequity and awareness of social determinants of health in the practice of medicine, particularly in the education of trainees (Tsai et al. 2021). They can be cultivated through practices such as critical pedagogy (Freire 2000) and critical race theory (Ansell 2008), theoretical approaches that teach skills including the following (Flores et al. 2014):

- Self-examination of biased, stereotyped attitudes and concepts of superiority and inferiority
- Awareness of intersectionality
- Education in cultural, institutional, and structural forms of oppression
- Giving voice and power to those less fortunate
- Consciousness-raising
- Appreciation for the doing, thinking, and being of other groups
- Engagement with cultural, intergroup, and intragroup conflict
- Gathering skills to transform institutions and create societal change

In these approaches, it is the responsibility of the privileged individual to inform themself about, incite, and support action within less privileged groups.

Psychiatric Ethics, Climate Justice, and Climate Advocacy

Personal advocacy and activism can include the following:

- A large range of reforming activities, including artivism, hacktivism, guerrilla tactics, nonviolent and violent civil disobedience, vigils, culture jamming, boycotts, consumer choice campaigns, shareholder activity, and alternative community building
- Participation in environmental and climate-related groups such as Citizens' Climate Lobby, Greenpeace, the Natural Resources Defense Council, and Sierra Club
- Participation in professional groups such as Physicians for Social Responsibility
- Political activities, including voting, running for office, and development and promotion of legislation
- Education-oriented activities within and outside one's profession, writing, and media representation of issues
- Activities oriented toward legal reform
- Work within personal institutions such as churches and schools to promote paradigm and power shifts

These activities can be loosely organized conceptually under the roles of the Citizen, the Reformer, the Rebel, and the Agents of Change (Moyer 2001). Terry Patten and others have also highlighted the spiritual aspects of activism, coupling inner psychological and spiritual work to activist activity. These practices result in cultural as well as personal evolution of new forms of more deeply connected human consciousness. These roles are characterized as follows:

- Citizen—Advocates for actions to correct problems in line with existing national ideals through established civic actions such as lobbying, voting, and community action (e.g., ensuring all citizens have equal access to housing)
- Reformer—Advocates to change existing institutions, laws, and policies to make social change (e.g., passing new laws to ensure gender equality)
- Rebel—Acts to disobey or challenge the status quo with the goal of disrupting existing power structures and bringing in new structures and ideas (e.g., Extinction Rebellion, a global environmental movement based on nonviolent civil disobedience)
- Agents of Change—Work with relationships and grassroots efforts within existing institutions to effect new social structures and mores

Individuals should engage with whichever model fits their personal strengths and style best because each strategy contributes value to civic life.

Ethical and just activity regarding climate change is also a form of meaning-based coping that can have positive mental health benefits (Ojala 2024), not just for clinicians but for patients as well. Although activists can experience significant harm if they are too isolated or demoralized by inadequate or hostile responses such as attacks on social media, verbal or physical harassment, or shunning, studies have generally shown improvements in positive affect, self-actualization, vitality, hope, and meaning (Klar and Kasser 2009) associated with activist activity. Ballard and Ozer (2016) described a number of ways activism can support youth mental health and well-being: improved social capital, improved connections to others, increased sense of personal identity and purpose, lessened stress through empowerment, and improved coping. Research has shown that activism can also support emotional regulation in young people, who become better able to decenter from and observe their own emotions (Fernandez and Watts 2022). Harré (2007) explored the role of activism as an *identity project*, a term that unifies four important areas of successful identity formation: belonging, growth/stimulation, efficacy/agency, and integrity. Activism can also buffer depression and burnout during prolonged struggles (Bandura 2000) and is thus an important part of the climate mental health toolbox. Tips for being a successful activist are included in Table 3.3. Whether advocating as an individual or a professional or helping patients act on causes meaningful to them, these pointers support effective activism.

Patient-oriented professional advocacy actions that psychiatrists and other mental health professionals can take include the following:

- Lobbying policymakers for fossil-fuel reduction through organizational and established channels
- Lobbying policymakers to include the needs of the mentally ill in climate adaptation plans
- Educating the public through lectures, op-eds, public health messaging, and health care marketing about the health and mental health impacts of climate change
- Adopting and advocating for carbon-reduction measures in psychiatric practice and institutions in line with international health care targets, including incentivizing sustainability through reimbursement metrics (Salas et al. 2020)

Table 3.3 Tips for effective climate activism

Know what you want and why you want it.

Be on the side of the angels: Frame your position as the moral high ground to appeal to the best in both sides.

Make your opposition uncomfortable. People are biased not to act. Frame your position as the best solution, one that it is heartless to ignore.

Think about why your opponents might want to do what you ask. Appeal to this reasoning in them.

Come with constructive proposals to solve the problem.

Carefully select and groom your presenters.

Be polite and respectful, no matter what.

Stay on message: Ask for one thing, only one thing, and be content when you succeed.

Be a gracious loser.

- Collaborating with labor unions and policymakers to ensure that no workers are left behind during the transition from current dirty energy to clean energy jobs and to a regenerative economy by virtue of elimination of the sources of their livelihood, a process sometimes referred to as making a *just transition*
- Lobbying that climate investments and programs target for support persons who are most affected
- Rectifying research that underestimates mortality among marginalized racial and ethnic groups and other underrepresented populations (Spiller et al. 2021)
- Ensuring that mental health impacts of climate change are prioritized in national and local climate legislation, policy, and strategy, such as the National Health Security Strategy in the United States
- Leading on community preparation for climate-related health risks

Activism for climate justice, particularly in planning climate investments for large programs, can be supported by incorporating the Environmental Protection Agency's Environmental Justice Screening and Mapping Tool, EJScreen (Environmental Protection Agency 2024), in state and local planning.

Communicating About Climate Change in Advocacy, Activist, and Community Work

Climate concern expressed by a trusted physician has been shown to be one of the most important predictors of climate concern and action (ecoAmerica et al. 2015). In a small study (Lindemer 2023), climate activism by medical professionals was shown to come with some costs, however, including being seen as overly political, offending the patient, abusing professional power, losing patient trust, and lowering of professional reputation. It has even been associated with creating workplace disagreement, a deteriorated workplace environment, social exclusion, blame, and loss of employment. Lindemer recommended the following ways that clinicians can mitigate these difficulties:

- Being conscious of who, what, where, and when in having these conversations
- Creating opportunities for others to ask, rather than offering information
- Practicing health advocacy for, rather than at, the patient
- Advocating for climate action implicitly by promoting actions with climate co-benefits, such as biking and walking
- Positing climate change as a medical concern
- Actively delineating the medical responsibilities that mandate climate activism
- Creating and engaging with professional support networks in this area
- Supporting climate activists who may have less restrictive roles

Organizations that conduct significant advocacy around climate and health or mental health issues and can support these efforts are available in the Appendix. Psychiatrists also need to practice self-examination and be attentive to their own biases, blind spots, and competing roles and priorities. A discussion of climate health may be validating for some patients and invalidating or irrelevant for others. Psychotherapeutic attention to tact, dosage, and timing can help deliver such information without personal bias, being mindful of the patient's individual situation and needs as well as the need to expand awareness of the larger systems that must be supported for the needs of those with mental health problems to survive and thrive.

Psychiatric Ethics, Climate Justice, and Climate Advocacy

Relevant and low-risk climate-adaptive advice from any physician includes education about the health impacts of climate change and support for climate-friendly policies and behaviors that improve patient health, including time in nature; keeping pets; community gardening; and initiatives for clean energy, green space, resilience, and carbon mitigation at the local, national, and global levels to support air quality. Social prescribing programs, such as for nature and arts therapies, cultural activity, and social services, are supported by insurance and government benefits and can be coordinated by a trained individual known as a link worker, community navigator, or similar title (Drinkwater et al. 2019).

What works in effective climate communication has been extensively studied. The data-driven skills for effective climate communication are presented in Table 3.4.

It is reasonable to expect that groups will struggle with the uncertainty of climate information, demonstrating skepticism and distrust. Additional communication techniques that have been shown to be helpful for framing climate issues to groups include the following:

- Describing the broader context of data variation and consensus (e.g., "Although some variation exists in the data, studies overwhelmingly trend toward...")
- Sharing a warning about the potential political polarization of accurate climate messages
- Using range-based communication (e.g., "Warming in the range of 3°C–5°C will...")

Table 3.4 Communication skills for talking about climate change

Address local climate impacts

Speak the language and values of the group addressed (farming, religion, business)

Discuss health impacts

Talk about family and the moral obligation to future generations

Discuss costs of inaction and savings from action rather than jobs

Pivot immediately to talking about solutions

Source. ecoAmerica et al. 2015.

- Describing likely climate events by the chances they will not occur (e.g., "There is a 20% chance the polar ice sheets will not fully melt" rather than "It is 80% likely they will," which can lead to demoralization and inaction)
- Describing the chance of events as "as high as" rather than "unlikely to be higher than"
- Using "likely" rather than "unlikely" statements
- Presenting material visually
- Using anecdotes and personal stories
- Using analogies about uncertainty from other disciplines, such as medicine:

    - "We don't know exactly what it is, but because it is a concerning finding, like any mass or tumor, we want to act on it."
    - "As with any disease, the longer treatment is postponed, the worse it gets."

Armed with knowledge of climate and health ethics, legal remedies, communication, advocacy, and activism skills and the motivation to redress the tremendous unjust burdens posed by the climate crisis described in this chapter, psychiatrists and other mental health professionals can lean into addressing the compelling issues of our time in a way that provides inspiration, hope, and benefit to the populations we serve.

Key Points

- Climate injustice refers to the grossly disproportionate harm from global warming for vulnerable populations.
- The carbon emissions of the United States vastly outstrip those of other postindustrial nations, creating an ecological debt to those who increasingly suffer as a result of these excess emissions.
- Historical and social injustices from racism and colonialist abuses of peoples and resources add to the impacts of climate change on mental health and demand redress.
- Climate ethics and medical ethics overlap significantly and provide guidance for psychiatric climate action.
- International recognition concerning the legal right to a healthy environment is on the rise, and psychiatrists can expect to

participate in lawsuits arguing for climate mitigation based on health and mental health harms.

- Privileged groups, such as health professionals, have an ethical obligation to combat health injustices perpetuated by inequitable power structures through critical pedagogy, advocacy, and activism.
- Roles for the clinician in climate activism and advocacy include participation in national and international policy, public health, community preparation, patient care, education, workplace support, health care sustainability, advocacy for youth and minority groups, and other activities.
- Best practice climate and clinical communication skills are critical for effective advocacy and activism and can help overcome skepticism, distrust, and other obstacles to climate progress.

References

American Psychiatric Association: The Principles of Medical Ethics: With Annotations Especially Applicable to Psychiatry. Arlington, VA, American Psychiatric Association, 2013

Ansell A: Critical race theory, in Encyclopedia of Race, Ethnicity, and Society, Volume 1. Edited by Schaefer RT. Thousand Oaks, CA, SAGE, 2008, pp 344–347

Ballard PJ, Ozer EJ: The implications of youth activism for health and well-being, in Contemporary Youth Activism: Advancing Social Justice in the United States. Edited by Conner J, Rosen SM. Santa Barbara, CA, Praeger, 2016, pp 223–244

Bandura A: Exercise of human agency through collective efficacy. Curr Dir Psychol Sci 9(3):75–78, 2000

Benevolenza MA, DeRigne LA: The impact of climate change and natural disasters on vulnerable populations: a systematic review of literature. J Hum Behav Soc Environ 29(2):266–281, 2019

Cima E: The right to a healthy environment: reconceptualizing human rights in the face of climate change. Rev Eur Comp Int Environ Law 31(1):38–49, 2022

Cissé G, McLeman R, Adams H, et al: Health, wellbeing, and the changing structure of communities, in Climate Change 2022: Impacts, Adaptation and Vulnerability. Contribution of Working Group II to the Sixth Assessment Report of the Intergovernmental Panel on Climate Change. Edited by Pörtner H-O, Roberts DC, Tignor M, et al. Cambridge, UK, Cambridge University Press, 2022, pp 1050–1058

Crippa M, Guizzardi D, Solazzo E, et al: GHG emissions of all world countries, EUR 30831 EN. Luxembourg, Publications Office of the European Union, 2021. Available at: https://edgar.jrc.ec.europa.eu/booklet/GHG_emissions_of_all_world_countries_booklet_2021report.pdf. Accessed November 21, 2024.

de Vilchez P, Savaresi A: The right to a healthy environment and climate litigation: a game changer? Yearbook of International Environmental Law 32(1):3–19, 2021

Drinkwater C, Wildman J, Moffatt S: Social prescribing. BMJ (Online), 364:l1285, 2019

Ebi KL, Fawcett SB, Spiegel J, et al: Carbon pollution increases health inequities: lessons in resilience from the most vulnerable. Rev Panam Salud Publica 40(3):181–185, 2016 27991976

ecoAmerica, Lake Research Partners; Krygsman K, Speiser M, et al: Let's Talk Climate: Messages to Motivate Americans. Washington, DC, ecoAmerica, 2015

Environmental Protection Agency: EJScreen: Environmental Justice Screening and Mapping Tool. Washington, DC, Environmental Protection Agency, 2024. Available at: www.epa.gov/ejscreen. Accessed November 21, 2024.

Fann NL, Nolte CG, Sarofim MC, et al: Associations between simulated future changes in climate, air quality, and human health. JAMA Netw Open 4(1):e2032064, 2021 33394002

Fernandez JS, Watts RJ: Sociopolitical development as emotional work: how young organizers engage emotions to support community organizing for transformative racial justice. J Adolesc Res 38(4): 697–725, 2022

Flores MP, De La Rue L, Neville HA, et al: Developing social justice competencies: a consultation training approach. The Counseling Psychologist 42(7):998–1020, 2014

Freire P: Pedagogy of the Oppressed, 30th Anniversary Edition. New York, Bloomsbury, 2000

Gardiner SM, Weisbach DA: Debating Climate Ethics. New York, Oxford University Press, 2016

Gibbons ED: Climate change, children's rights, and the pursuit of intergenerational climate justice. Health Hum Rights 16(1):19–31, 2014

Hallegatte S, Bangalore M, Bonzanigo L, et al: Shock Waves: Managing the Impacts of Climate Change on Poverty. Climate Change and Development Series. Washington, DC, World Bank, 2016

Hardin G: The tragedy of the commons: the population problem has no technical solution; it requires a fundamental extension in morality. Science 162(3859):1243–1248, 1968 5699198

Harré N: Community service or activism as an identity project for youth. J Community Psychol 35(6):711–724, 2007

Held v Montana, No. CDV-2020-307 (Mont. 1st Dist. Ct. August 14, 2023)

Hickman C, Marks E, Pihkala P, et al: Climate anxiety in children and young people and their beliefs about government responses to climate change: a global survey. Lancet Planet Health 5(12):e863–e873, 2021 34895496

Intergovernmental Panel on Climate Change: Summary for policymakers, in Renewable Energy Sources and Climate Change Mitigation: Special Report of the Intergovernmental Panel on Climate Change. Edited by Edenhofer O, Pichs-Madruga R, Sokona Y, et al. New York, Cambridge University Press, 2012, pp 3–26

Juliana v United States, 217 F. Supp. 3d 1224 (D. Or. 2016), pp 1248–1268

Juliana v United States, 947 F. Supp. 3d 1159 (9th Cir. 2020)

Klar M, Kasser T: Some benefits of being an activist: measuring activism and its role in psychological well-being. Polit Psychol 30(5):755–777, 2009

Kotz M, Levermann A, Wenz L: The economic commitment of climate change. Nature 628(8008):551–557, 2024 38632481

Lindemer A: The costs of climate activism for medical professionals: a case study of the USA, the UK, and Germany. Lancet Planet Health 7(9): e770–e776, 2023 37673547

Moyer B: The four roles of social activism by Bill Moyer. Brunswick, Australia, The Commons Library, 2001. Available at: https://commonslibrary.org/the-four-roles-of-social-activism. Accessed May 28, 2023.

Ojala M: Coping with climate change among young people: meaning-focused coping and constructive hope, in Climate Change and Youth Mental Health: Multidisciplinary Perspectives. Edited by Haase E, Hudson K. Cambridge, UK, Cambridge University Press, 2024, pp 269–286

Perera FP: Multiple threats to child health from fossil fuel combustion: impacts of air pollution and climate change. Environ Health Perspect 125(2):141–148, 2017 27323709

Radua J, De Prisco M, Oliva V, et al: Impact of air pollution and climate change on mental health outcomes: an umbrella review of global evidence. World Psychiatry 23(2):244–256, 2024 38727076

Salas RN, Friend TH, Bernstein A, et al: Adding a climate lens to health policy in the United States. Health Aff (Millwood) 39(12):2063–2070, 2020 33284694

Singh JA: Why human health and health ethics must be central to climate change deliberations. PLoS Med 9(6):e1001229, 2012 22679396

Spiller E, Proville J, Roy A, et al: Mortality risk from PM2.5: a comparison of modeling approaches to identify disparities across racial/ethnic groups in policy outcomes. Environ Health Perspect 129(12):127004, 2021 34878311

State of the Netherlands v Urgenda Foundation, ECLI:NL:HR:2019:2007 (December 20, 2019)

Steele P, Patel S: Tackling the triple crisis: using debt swaps to address debt, climate and nature loss post-COVID-19. London, International Institute for Environment and Development, 2020

Tang K, Spijkers O: The human right to a clean, healthy and sustainable environment. Chin J Environ Law 6(1):87–107, 2022

Tsai J, Lindo E, Bridges K: Seeing the window, finding the spider: applying critical race theory to medical education to make up where biomedical models and social determinants of health curricula fall short. Front Public Health 9:653643, 2021 34327185

U.N. Human Rights Council: Resolution 48/13: The Human Right to a Clean, Healthy and Sustainable Environment. U.N. Doc A/HRC/RES/48/13. Geneva, Switzerland, U.N. Human Rights Council, October 18, 2021

World Health Organization: Climate change fact sheets. Geneva, Switzerland, World Health Organization, October 12, 2023. Available at: www.who.int/news-room/fact-sheets/detail/climate-change-and-health. Accessed November 21, 2024.

PART II

Neuropsychiatric and Biological Effects of Climate Change

4

Extreme Heat and Its Implications for Psychiatry

Increasing Global Temperatures Due to Climate Change

Rising environmental temperatures are the defining element of global warming. The understanding of their broad and diverse impacts on human physiology and psychology is therefore core to climate psychiatry. As summarized by the Intergovernmental Panel on Climate Change (IPCC; Hoegh-Guldberg et al. 2018), it is estimated that global temperatures will rise by 2°F–10°F in this century, depending on greenhouse gas reduction. Temperature increases are higher over land, particularly in urban areas, and are disproportionately higher in the midlatitudes of the Earth during the warm season and in the Arctic over the cold season. Large areas of the southern United States, Africa, India, and the Middle East have therefore seen a quadrupling of heat waves and an expansion of the hot season by a quarter of a year in the past few decades. How fast global temperatures continue to climb going forward will make dramatic differences in impact: a difference of between 2.7°F and 3.6°F is predicted to make a 22% difference in the number of people frequently exposed to extreme heat, with a great deal of the globe experiencing daily temperatures over 90°F for a third of the year by the end of this century.

In this chapter, I go into substantial detail about thermoregulation and heat illness, focusing particularly on aspects of physiology and pathophysiology that are controlled by psychiatrically relevant neurotransmitters and impacted by psychiatric illnesses and medications. The level of detail is provided to highlight the pervasive and subtle effects higher temperatures will have on all aspects of our patients' neurophysiology and lives. It may also suggest more avenues for psychiatric engagement, such as the following:

- Educating patients about heat effects and how to protect themselves
- Developing protocols for monitoring and mitigating heat risks for communities and medical institutions
- Changing which medications we prescribe and how we tell patients to take them
- Researching new and existing adrenergic, GABAergic, dopaminergic, and serotonergic modifiers of thermoregulation that might be manipulated to mitigate the increased heat-related risks for patients with mental illness
- Inspiring climate justice work to increase protections for those at greatest risk

Defining High Temperatures

Definitions of heat events vary and are presented in Table 4.1. The National Weather Service in the United States also issues heat-related warnings that include heat advisories and excessive heat warnings. The related terms *heat watch* and *heat outlook* are used for anticipated high temperatures about which we have more uncertainty regarding timing and degree. In contrast to raw thermometer temperatures, experienced temperature is also highly dependent on both human adaptation to heat and environmental variables. The comfortable temperature range for inhabitants of different regions can vary dramatically (Figure 4.1). For example, those acclimatized to a hot, humid climate may find temperatures up to 82°F in humid environments and 105°F in dry environments perfectly comfortable, whereas peers living in a temperate climate would feel uncomfortable and struggle physiologically at temperatures greater than approximately 65°F (humid) and 93°F (dry) (Folk 1974).

Extreme Heat and Its Implications for Psychiatry

Table 4.1 Defining heat events

Term	Definition
Heat wave (World Meteorological Association)	5 or more days greater than 9°F over seasonal norms
Heat wave (United States)	3 or more days greater than 90°F (± a few degrees by region)
Heat advisory	Predicted temperatures greater than 100°F for at least 2 days
Excessive heat warning	2 or more days of predicted temperatures greater than 105°F
Heat index	A measure of temperature that accounts for heat and humidity
Wet bulb globe temperature[a]	A sophisticated measure of effective temperature that incorporates humidity, sun angle, wind speed, and cloud cover, often used for sports, outdoor work, and military operations

[a]*Wet bulb globe temperature* has effectively replaced the older term *wet bulb temperature*.

Human Heat Physiology

Human thermoregulation is a remarkable, complex physiological system that manages the dual challenges of keeping tissues viable despite extreme external temperature swings and regulating normal core temperatures so that vital organs are exposed to variations of no more than several degrees around 37°C or 98.6°F. The thermoregulatory system can be conceptually organized by thinking of it as an external shell and an internal core. The external shell sends signals about surface temperature to the brain, which initiates compensatory mechanisms in the internal core through both feed-forward and feedback loops. The human temperature set point of approximately 98.6°F is only 9°F from our heat tolerance limit and 18°F from our cold tolerance limit; thus, humankind is relatively more vulnerable to heat stress than to cold.

Surface skin temperatures can vary remarkably, over 77°F, with frostbite occurring only below freezing and burns starting only when skin has contact with surfaces with temperatures greater than 109.5°F. The

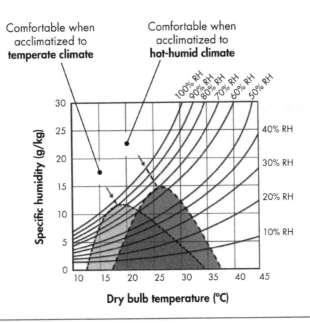

Figure 4.1 Adjustment in thermal comfort with acclimatization to a tropical (hot and humid) climate in resting subjects. Comfort level is altered in relation to specific humidity (i.e., grams of water per kilogram of air), dry bulb temperature, and relative humidity.

RH=relative humidity.
Source. Adapted from Folk 1974.

first 2–3 cm of surface tissues of our bodies, up to 54% of body mass, frequently vary by up to 36°F (Dubois 1951; Greenleaf and Kaciuba-Uscilko 1989). Exercising skeletal muscle can be hotter by 18°F than the rest of the body. Humans have survived core temperatures from 56.7°F to 114°F (Tansey and Johnson 2015). Maintaining optimal tissue temperature across these extremes is one of our most important bodily functions, consuming upward of 75% of our energy and engaging almost every hormonal and neurotransmitter system of importance to psychiatry.

There are five predominant ways the body can heat up and cool down (reviewed in Almeida et al. 2015). The major mechanisms of heat production in response to cold stress are

- Brown fat thermogenesis
- Shivering
- Exercise

Extreme Heat and Its Implications for Psychiatry

Heat is generated in brown fat when adenosine triphosphate (ATP) levels drop, leading to the release of noradrenaline from sympathetic nerve fibers. This activates an uncoupling protein 1 (UCP1) that releases fatty acids and glucose from fat, which are distributed within the mitochondria-rich cells of brown fat and are broken down, with the release of ATP and thermal energy. Shivering starts automatically as temperatures drop as a result of multiple receptor and neurotransmitter interactions on warm- and cold-sensitive neurons in the preoptic area (POA; see section "Human Heat Neurophysiology"). Shivering can increase metabolic rate two- to fivefold (Gagnon and Crandall 2018), although this pales in comparison to exercising, which can increase metabolic rate up to a hundredfold, 80% of which is released as heat (Hargreaves and Spriet 2020). The body retains the heat it generates through vasoconstriction and also through behavioral changes such as heat-seeking behavior, postural change, and cuddling close with others. Vasoconstriction, which is the primary mechanism for preserving body heat, can drop local tissue temperatures about tenfold to keep heat in the core. It is mediated mostly by norepinephrine and secondarily by neuropeptide Y and other factors via central α_1-adrenergic receptors and peripheral α_2-adrenergic receptors.

The mechanisms of heat release (cooling) include sweating and vasodilation, which lead to convective (movement of warmer fluids or gases), conductive (transfer of heat through direct contact), or radiant (through electromagnetic wave effects) heat loss, as well as behavioral adaptations such as fanning oneself or exposing skin. Sweating is our most efficient way of releasing heat; every liter of sweat that evaporates reflects the release of approximately 580 kilocalories of heat energy from the body through evaporative heat loss. Conditioning and acclimatization can increase sweating capacity to upward of 6 L per hour, releasing up to 1,700 watts (*very* approximately 1,500 calories) of energy. Sweating is mediated primarily by M1 postganglionic cholinergic neurons that act on eccrine sweat glands (Gagnon and Crandall 2018). Vasodilation releases heat in the periphery through special arteriovenous (AV) shunts, which are physiologically distinct from capillaries, which also carry nutrition. These shunts have a dramatic capacity to expand blood flow up to a hundredfold, whereas vasoconstriction can decrease flow only by tenfold (Kurz 2008). These AV shunts are tonically shut down by local catechols except during heat stress, when they dilate rapidly and dramatically to achieve blood flows of 6 L/ minute under the influence of undefined neurotransmitter actions that involve several cotransmitters. Putative candidates include vasoactive intestinal peptide, acetylcholine, substance P, prostaglandins, histamine, and potentially others (Smith and Johnson 2016). Heat release requires significant increases in cardiac output, up to 7 L/minute, to keep up with vasodilation, and involves significant fluid loss and renal adjustment.

Human Heat Neurophysiology

Thermoregulatory adjustments are coordinated by the neurons, receptors, and neurotransmitters that are at the core of biological psychiatry, modulated by a host of psychoactive hormones and other factors. Understanding this system, which so many of our medications would be expected to affect, is thus of critical importance for psychiatrists as extreme temperatures become more frequent. In the periphery, adjustments to temperature are largely dependent on thermal-sensitive transient receptor potential (TRP) channels, including vanilloid (TRPV) and melastatin (TRPM) subfamilies. This remarkable family of ion channels each shows a greater activation at a particular temperature range or threshold, allowing the body to coordinate a nuanced response to a changing temperature milieu as cells are exposed to it. For example, TRPM8 is most sensitive below approximately 25°C, TRPV4 from 25°C–34°C, TRPV3 from 33°C–39°C, and TRPV1 above 42°C (Almeida et al. 2015). TRPV1 receptor knockout has also been implicated in stress and depressive responses in animals through actions affected by fluoxetine as well as modulation of 5-HT$_{1A}$, GABA$_A$, and N-methyl-D-aspartate receptors (Sartim et al. 2017; You et al. 2012). These findings suggest that the role of these TRPV receptors in the negative emotions, violence, and suicidality elicited by higher temperatures, as well as their interactions with psychiatric medications, deserve greater attention and research.

Warm-sensitive neurons can be found predominantly in four tissues: the skin, the deep abdominal viscera, the spinal cord, and the brain, although they are also located diffusely elsewhere in the body. Neurons in the skin send signals via those in the dorsal horn of the spinal cord to those in the POA of the anterior hypothalamus, which acts as the central coordinator of the heat response, "the brain's thermostat," along with the nearby periventricular nucleus. A subset of the neurons in the POA is sensitive to both peripheral and central changes in temperature; these appear to contain special sensory units that compare actual with target temperature values (Siemens and Kamm 2018).

Extreme Heat and Its Implications for Psychiatry

The predominant action of the POA is to adjust the tonic baseline of thermoregulation, which is sympathetic vasoconstriction through GABAergic signaling. Input to the POA is mediated by opposing actions of TRPM2 receptors, which activate cooling responses, and prostaglandin EP_3 receptors, which activate heat production, although other candidate receptors are likely involved as well. GABAergic output from the POA acts on two sites: the nucleus raphe dorsalis (NRD) and the dorsomedial hypothalamus (DMH). These act on serotonergic tracts (in the NRD) and glutamatergic and dopaminergic tracts (in the DMH). The net effect of these actions is summated in the nucleus raphe pallidus (NRP), which generates a sympathetic response generally favoring heat generation through multiple actions, including increased shivering, coordination of cardiac sympathetic neurons that increase heart rate, brown fat thermogenesis, and actions on antidiuretic hormone and renin (Petroianu 2022; Tan and Knight 2018).

These roles of serotonin, glutamate, and dopamine through the POA-NRP-DMH interneurons are not yet well understood. It is generally accepted that

- Systemic dopamine agonists decrease body temperature
- Excess dopamine blockade, or dopamine depletion, leads to hyperthermia, as in neuroleptic malignant syndrome (NMS), probably through D_2 receptors
- Increased brain serotonin concentrations are generally hyperthermic, as in serotonin syndrome and the fever sometimes associated with use of citalopram

This understanding is made more complicated because the important POA GABAergic neuronal system acts in opposite ways, to increase or decrease heat, depending on whether the external environment is warm or cold. These neurotransmitters also have other effects on body temperature beyond their direct effects modifying vascular tone. The information currently available about this includes the following:

- Peripheral dopamine administration can raise or lower peripheral temperature depending on the agent and whether it acts on D_2 or D_1 receptors, whereas central D_2 blockade can contribute to NMS.
- Peripheral actions on TRPM receptors are also involved: for example, duloxetine inhibits TRPM2 independent of its serotonin and dopamine reuptake actions, and thus may contribute to hyperthermia (Toda et al. 2019).

- 5-HT$_{1A}$, 5-HT$_3$, and 5-HT$_7$ agonism appears to lower body temperature (Voronova 2021).
- Contradictorily, the 5-HT$_3$ receptor antagonist ondansetron (Zofran) seems to be effective in reversing postoperative shivering (Zhou et al. 2016), an unwanted pro-thermic behavior in that setting that causes dangerous cellular oxygen consumption and lactic acidosis (Tie et al. 2014).
- 5-HT$_{2A}$, 5-HT$_{2B}$, 5-HT$_{2C}$, and 5-HT$_6$ agonism favors hyperthermia.
- 5-HT$_4$ agonism favors cholinergic activation, with unknown temperature effects.
- A role for 5-HT$_5$ has not been found at this time (Petroianu 2022).

Animal models are still unclear about basic processes involved with all of these effects, and the opposing effects of GABA actions in different environmental temperatures (see discussion in Chang et al. 2022). Their clear relationship to psychiatric work, however, highlights how important it is to improve awareness of heat neurophysiology, to sensitize practitioners to the temperature-related symptoms of patients on different psychiatric medications during heat exposure, and to attune them to research developments. The goal of progressing this area of knowledge is for practitioners to be able to tailor medication practices to local weather stressors in a way that reduces heat risk to patients with mental illness, whose heat morbidity is extremely high, as described in the section "Mental Illness and Heat."

Hormonal Influences on Thermoregulation Relevant to Heat Illness

The thermoregulatory system is also modified by various hormones relevant to psychiatry, including those involved in fluid homeostasis. At the level of the POA, different subsets of warm-sensitive neurons can be separated by their sensitivity to leptin, production of brain-derived neurotrophic factor (BDNF), and other less delineated influences (Tan and Knight 2018). The roles of androgens, orexins, and other compounds involved in hypothalamic regulation of fluid homeostasis, sleep, mating, metabolism, and other physiology associated with thermoregulation are not elucidated clearly, but are relevant for psychiatrists, for example, coordinating the relationship between high temperatures and sleep disturbance, which may mediate heat-related suicide. Estrogen has a wide variety of both warming and cooling effects, and women are more vulnerable to heat stress than are men, starting by the age of 40 (Leach et al. 2024). The actions of estrogen include both central actions via ERα and possibly ERβ receptors as well as rapid actions of 17β-estradiol on endothelial nitric oxide synthase (eNOS) to rapidly produce NO from L-arginine in peripheral vascular beds. Progesterone appears to be active mostly in the periphery and to be predominantly vasoconstrictive (Uchida and Izumizaki 2021). Thyroid hormones have significant and well-recognized thermogenic effects on brown and white fat metabolism via UCP1 expression and induction (Yau and Yen 2020). Hyperthyroid states elevate body temperature 1°C–2°C by mechanisms independent of UCP1 and can increase to 106°F during thyroid storms (Dittner et al. 2019). In conjunction with increased hyperthyroid cardiac demand, elevated body temperature increases vulnerability to heat illness.

Group Differences in Physiological Heat Tolerance

Differences in heat physiology confer individual and group variability as well as probable increased mortality risk for warmer individuals independent of global warming (Obermeyer et al. 2017). A summary of somatic factors influencing heat tolerance is provided in Table 4.2.

Heat Tolerance in Children

Differences among groups in heat tolerance are most evident in relation to age, with children and older people having dramatically less capacity to withstand heat stress. According to Vanos (2015), poor heat tolerance in children is related to comparative differences in the following:

- Higher metabolic rate due to growth and activity levels
- Smaller body surface area, so that with higher metabolism, more heat needs to be released per unit surface area (often double that of adults)
- Greater percentage of body water, so greater relative need for hydration
- Lower rate of sweating per sweat gland, leading to greater reliance on convective heat loss

Table 4.2 Somatic influences on heat responsiveness

Cardiovascular disease

Hypertension

Renal insufficiency

Obesity

Age (young or old)

Sex

Conditioning

Genetic differences (*RYR1, CACNA1S*)

Hormonal effects (thyroid, menopause)

Sleep disorders (bidirectional effects)

Medical medication effects (see Table 4.4)

Psychiatric medication effects (see Table 4.4)

Neurological illness with autonomic dysfunction

Psychiatric disorders

Substance use (alcohol, cocaine, stimulants, methamphetamine, MDMA, hallucinogens)

Note. MDMA=3,4-methylenedioxymethamphetamine.

- Slower capacity to acclimatize to heat
- Reliance on adults to signal appropriate caution in high temperatures

Heat Tolerance in Older Adults

Older adults have double the heat mortality of other groups, much of which is due to comorbid illness and social and behavioral factors related to isolation, mobility, and cognition. Physiologically, however, they also have significantly less heat responsiveness. Heat vulnerability in older adults is due to the following factors (Meade et al. 2020):

- Less sensitive thermoreceptors in the skin, leading to less activation of central heat response
- Less vasodilation with heat, connected to lower local NO bioavailability

Extreme Heat and Its Implications for Psychiatry

- Reduced cardiac reserve, limiting the ability to increase compensatory cardiac output during vasodilation and contributing to cardiovascular collapse
- Lower percentage body water, increasing sensitivity to dehydration
- Arterial stiffening, lessening vascular responsiveness
- Reduced renal function, including less fluid conservation during dehydration
- Less sensitivity to fluid regulatory hormones:

  - Dysregulation of the renin-angiotensin-aldosterone system
  - Blunted sensitivity to thirst signals mediated by carotid receptors sensitive to osmolality and blood pressure
  - Blunted sensitivity to vasopressin, resulting in less renal water conservation
  - Greater angiotensin II release, reducing renal and small arteriole blood flow and increasing central antidiuretic hormone and vasopressin secretion, sodium retention, and blood pressure
  - Adrenal aldosterone release, promoting renal sodium resorption

- Reduced autonomic regulation of peripheral, splanchnic, and cerebral vascular flow
- Reduced sweat rate due to less sweat production per gland for releasing heat than in middle-aged adults

These factors in sum lead to lesser ability to vasodilate in response to heat stress and dramatically less flexible adaptation to higher temperatures in older adults, with core temperatures remaining elevated for hours despite normalization of ambient temperature after heat stress. Because the population is aging alongside an increase in temperatures, an understanding of these factors is essential for physicians, particularly when treating patients taking medications that influence or interact with these effects.

Vignette

Jeff is a 67-year-old construction worker with a history of alcohol and cocaine use who is receiving antipsychotic treatment for amphetamine psychosis, with recent complaint of sexual side effects of his medications. After a summer heat wave, he came to an appointment distraught and more depressed. He reported that he had overheated during sexual intercourse, landing him in the emergency department with heatstroke, blood pressure of 220/120, and transient stroke symptoms. He had been embarrassed by his sexual underperformance, and had punched the wall in his frustration, even taking out his gun with the thought it was time to end his life. The psychiatrist was suspicious—Jeff's hypertension did not match the heatstroke diagnosis, and the mood exacerbation seemed greater than expected from heat alone, even accounting for the effects of heat on violent and suicidal behavior. She queried substance relapse. Jeff confessed he had purchased a little cocaine to boost his libido. He also had been camping in the desert, "like the good old days," but he had been a bit low on water. The stimulant effects of cocaine on thermoregulation as well as the dehydration additionally contributed to the rapid increase in Jeff's body temperature. Jeff had also felt paranoid while taking the cocaine, so he had taken a double dose of his antipsychotic medications to cut the high, which further affected his heat tolerance and stroke risk. Jeff was educated about his heat risks and protective measures, and the psychiatrist became more vigilant in preventative patient education about heat effects.

Racial and Sex Differences in Heat Tolerance

Although it would seem intuitive that genetic and racial differences in heat physiology might exist, research is limited and, in the case of race, distorted by racist historical stereotyping that has portrayed African Americans, Asians, Mexicans, and Hawaiians as better able to tolerate heat to justify abusive work conditions and has compared these groups to animals in grotesquely denigrating ways (Derickson 2019). Genetic differences between individuals clearly do exist, as suggested by cases of persons who develop exertional heat illness at much lower temperatures than others and by *RYR1* and *CACNA1S* mutations common in persons susceptible to exertional heat illness and malignant hyperthermia, but research is inconclusive (van den Bersselaar et al. 2022). Further investigation of genetic differences in heat tolerance is essential, particularly in those with mental disorders who are shown to have the highest risk of heat death.

Sex differences also play a role in thermoregulation. Females are different in their heat response because they

- Are smaller with lower body mass
- Typically have higher body fat

Extreme Heat and Its Implications for Psychiatry 49

- Are less fit than men overall in most cultures
- Sweat less than men, particularly at high work rates and in humid environments
- Have a greater surface-to-mass ratio
- Have different hormonal influences on thermoregulation than men

Each of the factors above conveys advantages and disadvantages in terms of heat vulnerability. For example, reduced sweating helps prevent dehydration but decreases evaporative heat loss. Females have the disadvantage of a smaller surface for heat release overall and a smaller *heat sink* (core body mass) into which to distribute heat with exertion or temperature extremes, but they have a potentially larger capacity to release heat proportionally by virtue of surface area to body size. In military settings, women have equal heat illness but half the heatstroke of men yet, using a standard heat tolerance test, are 3.7 times more likely to be heat intolerant (Corbett et al. 2023; Giersch et al. 2022). Differences in core temperature during phases of the menstrual cycle or when taking oral contraceptives can be 1.8°F–3.6°F but do not appear to be associated with significant physiological differences. The available literature suggests that gendered role factors (e.g., the settings that women are more likely to spend time in, access to air conditioning, access to water, cultural practices such as required heavy clothing) play a more important role in heat vulnerability for women than sex itself, particularly in societies where women have more traditional roles.

Heat Illness and Mortality

Symptoms of Heat Illness

The World Health Organization recognizes a number of heat illnesses (Table 4.3). Patients can experience sunburn, prickly heat, heat cramps, and heat edema, defined as edema or anasarca, after 10–14 days in a hot, moist environment.

Heatstroke and Heat Exhaustion

Heat exhaustion and heatstroke are the two most common and important heat illnesses. Heat exhaustion is defined by its symptoms, whereas heatstroke can be defined as occurring when core body temperature increases 4.5°F from its resting value or when changes in consciousness

Table 4.3 Heat-related illnesses

Heat edema

Prickly heat

Sunburn

Heat cramps

Classic heatstroke

Exertional heatstroke

Heat exhaustion

occur (Garcia et al. 2022). Heat exhaustion typically occurs as core temperature reaches approximately 100°F–101°F. To dissipate the heat, peripheral vessels dilate, blood pressure drops, vessels to the gut and brain contract to divert blood to the surface to cool, and heart rate increases to keep pace with the increased vascular demand. Cardiac output must increase significantly: from a typical value of 4.7 L up to 7 L/minute. Pupils dilate because of the increased adrenergic tone needed to maintain blood pressure to the increased vascular bed. The poor blood supply to the brain from vascular contraction is associated with nausea and a pounding headache. Profuse sweating occurs, up to several liters in an hour, and can rapidly lead to dehydration; by the time a person feels thirsty, the average fluid deficit is 3 L. Dehydration itself then further raises body temperature, possibly because the need to maintain central blood volume and pressure through peripheral vasoconstriction and fluid retention begins to compete with the ability to release heat with vasodilation and sweating. The increasing ratio of sodium to calcium in the POA may contribute to this vasoconstriction as dehydration continues (Myers et al. 1976).

Heatstroke is the endgame of heat exhaustion and carries a potential mortality of 80%. It is divided into classic heatstroke (from heat exposure or poor heat tolerance in unhealthy sedentary individuals) and exertional heatstroke (from exercise), with different physiologies. Athletes show individual variation in the external temperatures connected to exertional heatstroke. As heat exhaustion progresses, core temperatures continue to rise, approaching 105°F and above, and sweating capacity is lost. Skin becomes hot and dry, heart rate increases, and hypotension worsens. Changes in cognition are considered a tipping point defining heatstroke. Interleukin 6 rises, along with anti-inflammatory acute phase reactants and heat shock proteins, especially HSP72, which accumulates in the brain. These heat-protective molecules are likely adaptive at lower levels to prevent the unfolding and denaturing of proteins, but they may exacerbate inflammatory toxicity at high levels (Dehbi et al. 2010). In the brain and the gut, tight junction barriers break down, leading to leakage of endotoxins in the gut and to cerebral edema, with attendant seizures, confusion, and eventually coma. Gut endotoxins may rise particularly when the liver is functioning poorly or in conditions associated with chronic inflammation such as obesity and metabolic disease. As these processes continue, cellular enzymes begin to denature, cells function abnormally, and cells die. In the brain, cerebellar damage and central pontine myelinolysis are most common. Morbidity and mortality increase, with signs including hyponatremia, acidosis, disseminated intravascular coagulation, and diffuse organ failure (Garcia et al. 2022; Horseman et al. 2013). CNS imaging studies show cytotoxic, microembolic, and hypoxic damage to the brain most commonly in a pattern that resembles posterior reversible encephalopathy syndrome, with marked cerebellar atrophy and ataxia in survivors most common clinically (Shimada et al. 2020).

Risk Factors for Heat-Related Morbidity and Mortality

The established risk factors for heat-related death include overexposure to high temperatures, being very young or very elderly, being obese, having medical conditions that increase cardiovascular (OR 2.48, 95% CI [1.3–4.8]) and pulmonary risks (OR 1.61, 95% CI [1.2–2.1]), being unable to care for oneself (OR 2.97, 95% CI [1.8–4.8]), not leaving home daily (OR 3.35, 95% CI [1.6–6.9]), being bedbound (OR 6.44, 95% CI [4.5–9.2]) (Bouchama et al. 2007; Semenza et al. 1999), or having neurological conditions that impair autonomic function such as diabetes or Parkinson's disease. Additional risk factors include urban residence, poverty, low education, homelessness, substance use and abuse, and, very significantly, just having a mental illness itself (Bouchama et al. 2007; Harlan et al. 2013). Stroke risk rises because of a 25% increase in blood viscosity as well as the inflammatory changes associated with heatstroke discussed in the previous subsection, "Heat Stroke and Heat Exhaustion" (Meade et al. 2020). Poor ability to care for oneself and lack of adequate social activity and networks to access help underlie several of the previously mentioned risks and are common in patients with psychiatric illness. Risk of heat-related death dropped by two-thirds in the Bouchama meta-analysis when individuals had access to a cool shower, air conditioning, or a cooling shelter. Merely owning a working fan reduces heat illness by 30% (Semenza et al. 1999), and air conditioning reduces it by 80% (Naughton et al. 2002).

Occupational workers also face much higher heat risks, including heat illness, kidney disease, and mental distress. Those who work in hot environments, such as farm workers and those working with furnaces or other heat-generating equipment, are most at risk. Sex, youth, dehydration, inappropriate clothing, workload, piece rate payment, and job decision latitude are associated with more heat-related illness in workers; protective actions are provided in the section "Managing and Mitigating Heat Risk for Individuals, Patients, and Communities" in this chapter (Amoadu et al. 2023; El Khayat et al. 2022).

Mental Illness and Heat

Mental Illness Increases Risk of Heat-Related Morbidity and Mortality

The risks for heat morbidity and mortality associated with mental illness and substance abuse are of special importance for psychiatrists and all mental health clinicians. It has been known since the 1970s that patients with mental illnesses have very high rates of heat-related death. These findings were first published in a study from the New York State Psychiatric Institute, showing a relative risk of death of 1.52–1.74 for hospitalized psychiatric patients during a heat wave, defined as temperatures higher than only 89°F (Bark 1998). Semenza et al. (1996), writing in *The New England Journal of Medicine,* found that persons with mental illness had 3.5 times the odds of dying in a July heat wave in Chicago than did nonpsychiatric patients. Page et al. (2012) looked at 22,562 deaths in England and found a 4.9% increase in mortality for every 1.8°F increase in temperatures in the top 7% of normal for persons with schizophrenia, dementia, or substance use diagnoses compared with mortality in primary care control subjects. Young people with alcohol use also taking antipsychotics and anxiolytics were particularly vulnerable. Hansen et al. (2008) noted similar risks overall and a mortality risk of 12.7 times average in men with early-onset dementia during the Australian heat waves of 1996–2003, as well as a 7.3% increase in admissions for mental illness with temperatures higher than 82°F. In a more recent study in Canada, Lee et al. (2023) found that people with schizophrenia had the highest death rate of any group with chronic illness during a heat wave, with an OR of mortality of 3.07 (95% CI [2.39–3.94]).

Patients With Mental Illness Handle Heat Differently

It is likely that social factors and medical comorbidities that contribute to heat mortality overall also contribute significantly to elevated heat illness and death in persons with mental disorders. Among their risks, however, are unique physiological differences in thermoregulation. Clinically, it can be observed that patients with schizophrenia often wear excess warming clothing even in hotter seasons, and patients with schizophrenia have decreased body temperature compared with control subjects. They have lesser ability to raise skin temperature in the heat but greater heat preservation in the cold, as well as abnormal diurnal timing and range of body temperature and excess heat production with exercise (Chong and Castle 2004; Shiloh et al. 2001). Depressed patients had long ago been found to have increased nocturnal body temperature (Avery et al. 1982), and youth with bipolar disorder have recently been shown to have an increase in brain temperature compared with control subjects that correlated with depression severity (Zou et al. 2023). Patients with depression, bipolar disorder, panic disorder, and prior suicide attempts have all been shown to have abnormalities of total electrodermal activity or skin conductance, a measure that includes sympathetic tone, sweating, and emotional effects, suggesting that their ability to sweat to release heat may be affected, particularly when they are stressed (Sarchiapone et al. 2018). Although these findings taken together do not offer clarity, they do support further study of these groups under heat duress.

Mental Symptoms and Illness Are Affected by Higher Temperatures and Heat Events

The different processing of temperature in persons with mental disorders has clinical relevance. Patients with bipolar disorder have been found to have up to a sixfold rate of elevated hospital admissions for mania in warmer months (Amr and Volpe 2012), whereas those with PTSD are up to two times more likely to be admitted (Solt et al. 1996).

Temperature can also have positive effects on psychiatric illnesses: rates of both nonseasonal depression (Amr and Volpe 2012) and bingeing and purging behavior (Lam et al. 1996) have been found to be lower in summer months. When considering the comfortable physiological range 32°F–75°F, Kessler et al. (2007) showed a positive correlation between warmer temperatures and lower lifetime prevalence of mood disorders, whereas colder temperatures were associated with more selective serotonin reuptake inhibitor use in a study by Wortzel et al. (2019).

Higher temperature extremes, however, have a consistently and significantly deleterious effect on mental symptoms, including general mental symptoms (Obradovich et al. 2018), negative emotions (Noelke et al. 2016), affective markers on internet posts (Baylis et al. 2018), number of days rated as poor mental health days (Obradovich et al. 2018), and overall visits to emergency departments for suicide attempts, violence, homicide, or other mental health reasons (Basu et al. 2012; Mullins and White 2019). These increases in negative mental health impacts are defined variously as over 20°C/70°F or over 30°C/86°F, as increments over upper warm means, or as swings of temperature. They can occur acutely in response to a heat event or chronic heat increases, and they are likely mediated in part by poor sleep (Obradovich et al. 2017).

Higher Temperatures Increase Suicide, Violent Behavior, and Violent Conflict

Rates of suicide and violence, in particular, increase with temperatures outside the range of human comfort. Every 1.8°F increase in temperature over 98.6°F is associated with a 4% increase in interpersonal and 14% increase in intergroup violence (Hsiang et al. 2013) and a 0.7%–2.3% increase in population-wide suicides (Dumont et al. 2020). This heat-related suicide increase is independent of, and sometimes greater than, the impact of economic stress (Fountoulakis et al. 2016) and has been predicted to wipe out the gains of existing suicide prevention programs in the United States by 2050 (Burke et al. 2018).

High Temperatures Increase Rates of Violence

High temperatures in domestic, civic, and international settings have been shown to correlate with higher rates of all types of violence ranging from individual violent crime, domestic violence, rape, group-on-group

Extreme Heat and Its Implications for Psychiatry

violence, and others to civil and international conflicts (Hsiang et al. 2013). Projections indicate nine excess violent crimes per 100,000 people per 2°F temperature rise (Anderson 1989). Following on this data, by 2099, the United States alone will endure 22,000 murders, 180,000 rapes, 1.2 million aggravated assaults, 2.3 million simple assaults, 260,000 robberies, 1.3 million burglaries, 2.2 million larcenies, and 580,000 vehicle thefts in excess of those expected at current temperatures (Ranson 2014). Increased suicide, conflict, and aggression may be aggravated in agricultural areas affected by unfavorable climate conditions affecting crops, leading to greater economic stress and unemployment (Carleton 2017; Crost et al. 2018).

These increases in suicide and violence are increasingly being encountered by mental health workers and in mental health settings, even if their impact on psychiatric services has not been assessed. Suicides and violent crime also have broad secondary effects on families and communities, increasing grief, depression, PTSD, copycat suicidality, stress-related medical illness, and worsening societal and economic stability. One study estimated the economic cost of suicides due to climate heat effects alone at $2–$3 billion/year (Belova et al. 2022). Much can be done to prepare mental health workers and their delivery systems for heat-related surges in these events.

Medication and Substance Use Effects on Heat Tolerance

As is forecasted by the primary roles of serotonin, norepinephrine, dopamine, GABA, and glutamate in thermoregulation, medications and substance use add significantly to the already concerning risks of climate-related higher temperatures. Medications and substances impact heat tolerance in several categories:

- Medications and substances that directly affect core body temperature or thermoregulatory mechanisms such as sweating (e.g., antipsychotics, cocaine)
- Medications that affect downstream systems important in thermoregulation (e.g., antihypertensives acting on renin or angiotensin to change vascular responsiveness)
- Medications and substances that impair the behavioral ability to notice and respond to heat-related symptoms (e.g., benzodiazepines, alcohol)

- Medications and substances that raise temperature by increasing physical activity and agitation (e.g., cocaine)
- Medications that may change the behavioral response to heat, such as disrobing and thirst (e.g., antipsychotics, antidepressants, speculatively)
- Medications that are affected by heat-related changes in the body (e.g., lithium)

In some cases, a substance may both impair thermoregulation and have other effects, such as the way alcohol use causes vasodilation, increases the risk of dehydration through diuresis, and also impairs consciousness, impacting behavioral response. Medications may also interact with each other to potentiate their mutual adverse thermoregulatory and other effects. For example, anticoagulant medications such as dabigatran (Pradaxa) and rivaroxaban (Xarelto) used to reduce stroke risk are renally cleared, leading to higher blood levels when the patient is dehydrated and thus an increased risk of bleeding, which then exacerbates heat-related stroke risk. Impaired sleep during heat waves may lead patients to increase the use of hypnotics (Min et al. 2021) and further their thermal dysregulation (Echizenya et al. 2003).

There is evidence that psychiatric medications contribute more than other classes of medications to these adverse influences on heat tolerance. The risk of heat-related hospital admission has been reported to be highest for anticholinergic medications (OR 6.0, 95% CI [1.8–19.6]), antipsychotics (OR 4.6, 95% CI [1.9–11.2]), and anxiolytics (OR 2.4, 95% CI [1.3–4.4]) compared with other medications (Martin-Latry et al. 2007), although more studies are indicated (Meadows et al. 2024).

Classes of psychiatric medications and illicit substances that are likely to act through changes in peripheral cooling include the following:

- Sympathomimetics (e.g., medications for ADHD, cocaine, methamphetamine), through vasoconstriction
- Anticholinergic, antipsychotic, antidepressant, and antihistaminergic medications, through decreased sweating (Cheshire and Fealey 2008; Marcy and Britton 2005)
- Medications that alter heart rate or blood pressure, including α- and β-blockers, calcium channel blockers, and those that affect hydration, such as diuretics

Psychiatric medication classes that may act on the central POA to change core thermoregulation include the following:

Extreme Heat and Its Implications for Psychiatry 57

- Dopamine agonists given for Parkinson's disease or restless legs syndrome, which can precipitate hyperthermia when withdrawn suddenly
- Antipsychotics, which have been associated with both hypothermia and hyperthermia (Zonnenberg et al. 2019)
- Substances that increase central serotonin and are associated with serotonin syndrome, including antidepressants, meperidine, tramadol, linezolid, and dextromethorphan, which may increase set body temperature and also change sweating peripherally
- Tricyclic antidepressants, via multiple mechanisms, including cardiac conductance through quinidine-like properties, lower blood pressure through α_1 receptors, and decreased sweating through anticholinergic and antihistaminergic binding
- Benzodiazepines or other substances active at the GABA receptor

A summary of medications that have been associated with thermoregulation, particularly hyperthermia, and their putative potential impacts and mechanisms of action is provided in Table 4.4. Few specific data are available about the exact site and mechanism of activity (e.g., β-blockers) for most of these medications and how they will affect an individual's tolerance of climate-related heat extremes, an area where research would be significantly helpful.

Managing and Mitigating Heat Risk for Individuals, Patients, and Communities

Climate Justice Issues and Global Temperature Risk

Marginalized and disadvantaged groups are much more affected and need particular attention when heat risks are addressed programmatically. The increased risks that they face from heat include increases in episodes of heat illness, total mortality, cardiac events, strokes, and renal failure; exacerbations of asthma; and increases in mental health events, preterm births, sudden infant death syndrome, and emergency department and hospital stays. The risk of mortality in the United States is elevated for Black and Latinx people, particularly those who are not citizens, and for Native Americans. People who live in the

Table 4.4 Medications and illicit substances likely to affect thermoregulation

Class/agent	Effect	Proposed mechanisms
Amphetamines, cocaine, methamphetamine, sibutramine	Hyperthermia, risk stroke/MI	Peripheral vasoconstriction via α_2 receptors, agitation/exercise, central hyperthermia via increased DAT activity/ROS production, mobilization of thyroid/adrenal hormones, and increased central cytokines
PCP	Hyperthermia	Uncoupling oxidative phosphorylation
MDMA	Hyperthermia, skeletal muscle tension	Indirect serotonin agonism, monoamine release, and blockade of reuptake
MAOIs	Hypothermia overall, hyperthermia with serotonergic or adrenergic crisis	Inhibited breakdown of serotonin, dopamine, and norepinephrine
Dopamine agonists: carbidopa/levodopa (Sinemet), pramipexole, bromocriptine	Hyperthermia on withdrawal	Rare, unknown

Extreme Heat and Its Implications for Psychiatry

Table 4.4 Medications and illicit substances likely to affect thermoregulation (*continued*)

Class/agent	Effect	Proposed mechanisms
Anti-adrenergics (α- and β-blockers)	Impaired vasodilation and vasoconstriction, hypotension, impaired sweating, blunted chronotropic reserve	Blocking of α- and β-agonist contributions that increase sweating mediated by cholinergic actions α_1, α_{2A}, and α_{2C} agonists promote hypothermia and hypotension β-blockers: antagonize noradrenergic cutaneous vasodilation, decrease cardiac output via β_1, hypotension via β_1, decrease renin via β_1
Antipsychotics	Paradoxical/inflexible central thermoregulation, decreased sweating, baseline elevated core temperature	D_2 modulation of GABA-mediated vasodilation in the POA, anticholinergic and antihistaminergic binding, unknown effects on TRPV receptors
Anticholinergics	Hyperthermia, decreased sweating	Inhibition of cholinergic sweating, activation of skeletal muscle
SSRIs, SNRIs	Hyperthermia, changes in sweating	Variable central modulation of POA output by action at 5-HT_{1A} and 5-HT_{2C} receptors, peripheral modulation of sweating, and temperature feedback

Table 4.4 Medications and illicit substances likely to affect thermoregulation (*continued*)

Class/agent	Effect	Proposed mechanisms
Dextromethorphan	Hyperthermia, changes in sweating	Central modulation of POA output, peripheral modulation of sweating, and temperature feedback
Tricyclic antidepressants	Vascular instability, impaired cooling	Quinidine-like effects on cardiac output, α_2-mediated hypotension, anticholinergic binding
Antihistamines	Impaired sweating	Anticholinergic effects
General anesthetics	Shivering, central hyperthermia	Modulation of core temperature
Opioid analgesics, particularly tramadol, fentanyl, meperidine	Central hyperthermia, mixed peripheral actions	Central and peripheral serotonergic activity
Herbs: St. John's wort, Syrian rue, Panax ginseng, nutmeg, yohimbine	Poorly characterized potential effects	Effects on serotonergic action, MAO-A and COMT inhibition, nitric oxide secretion, anticholinergic effects, respectively
Benzodiazepines	Impaired behavioral response, heat loss, possible dehydration	Sleep-mediated decrease in core temperature, peripheral vasodilation
Pregabalin, gabapentin	Toxicity/impaired behavioral response during dehydration; variable overall effects	Interference with renal clearance during dehydration, action on POA thermoactive neurons promoting hyperthermia

Extreme Heat and Its Implications for Psychiatry

Table 4.4 Medications and illicit substances likely to affect thermoregulation (*continued*)

Class/agent	Effect	Proposed mechanisms
Lithium	Lithium toxicity	Dehydration
Topiramate, zonisamide	Loss of evaporative cooling	Impaired sweating
Diuretics	Dehydration, loss of evaporative cooling, electrolyte imbalances	Decreased peripheral blood flow, dehydration due to diuresis during heat events
ACE inhibitors, ARBs	Hypotension, dehydration, impaired thirst	Interference with regulation of vascular tone, thirst receptors, and renal fluid balance
Anti-arrhythmics: amiodarone, digoxin, quinidine	Dehydration due to diarrhea, cardiovascular failure, digoxin toxicity	Association with diarrhea; may limit inotropic and chronotropic reserve; dehydration
Calcium channel blockers	Hypotension, poor cardiac output	Direct effects, decreased chronotropic cardiac reserve

Note. ACE=angiotensin-converting-enzyme; ARBs=angiotensin-converting-enzyme blockers; COMT catechol-O-methyltransferase; DAT=dopamine transporter; MAOI=monoamine oxidase inhibitor; MAO-A=monoamine oxidase A; MDMA=3,4-methylenedioxymethamphetamine; MI=myocardial infarction; PCP=phencyclidine; POA=preoptic area; ROS=reactive oxygen species; SNRIs=serotonin-norepinephrine reuptake inhibitors; SSRIs=selective serotonin reuptake inhibitors; TRPV=transient receptor potential vanilloid.
Source. Bowyer and Hanig 2014; Maguire 2015; Meade et al. 2020; Texas Department of Criminal Justice 2023; U.S. Department of the Army and Air Force 2003; Walter and Carraretto 2015.

Global South and in the southwest United States, migrants, outdoor workers, those in urban and redlined areas, the homeless, those with mental illness, and those in poverty all have much greater exposure to temperature extremes and inability to cool off (reviewed in Berberian et al. 2022). Interventions must be particularly focused on helping them during temperature extremes.

Interventions to Protect the Individual From Climate-Related Heat Impacts

Heat illness can be dramatically curtailed by simple individual, workplace, and community measures. For the individual, these include acclimatization, avoiding heat extremes, and using protective devices to lessen heat impact.

Acclimatization is the most effective way to reduce patients' heat health risks. About 70%–80% of heat acclimatization occurs in the first 4–7 days and persists for 2–4 weeks, dropping off quickly after week 2 without reinforcement. Exercise has a large additive effect on acclimatization; simply being in a hot place is not sufficient for maximal acclimatization. In general, physically fit individuals become acclimatized about 50% faster than do individuals who are not physically fit. Heavy exercise for at least 30 minutes in the heat for 7–14 days is required for maximal heat adjustment. Such acclimatization significantly improves heat tolerance. Unacclimatized subjects at rest in a hot, humid environment of 108.5°F and 92% humidity with a rectal temperature of 101.3°F are near their heat limit. Yet in one study, 23 of 24 subjects were able to walk for 100 minutes in 120°F heat after 8 days of acclimatization training, although none could perform this task on the first day. Heat-acclimatized cyclists can bike 27 miles in 98.6°F heat and sustain a core temperature of 104°F through the entire course without collapse (Périard et al. 2015).

Physiological changes with acclimatization (Figure 4.2) include a 0.3°F reduction of core temperature; a reduced heart rate of 3–8 BPM; and increased sweating, onset of sweating, and resorption of sodium, which reduces sweat sodium by 22%–59%. This adaptation occurs by dramatic changes in sweat gland function, with greater sodium resorption, more dilated sweat glands, and earlier onset of sweating at the new acclimatized lower core temperature. The decrease in sodium per liter of sweat may drop from 60 to 10 mEq—only 16% of the original sodium content. Adaptive expression of aldosterone and vasopressin increases daily fluid retention by 2–3 L, expanding plasma volume protectively against cardiovascular collapse. Thirst sensitivity increases to an extent that voluntary dehydration (underhydration) decreases by 30%. For unclear reasons, heat also lowers blood and muscle lactate levels

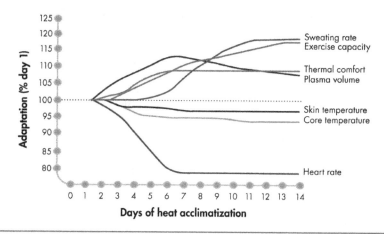

Figure 4.2 Time course of heat acclimatization adaptations with repeated training in the heat.

Source. Adapted from Racinais S, Casa D, Brocherie F, et al: Translating science into practice: the perspective of the Doha 2019 IAAF World Championships in the heat. Front Sports Act Living 1:39, 2019 33344962. Used with permission (see https://creativecommons.org/licenses/by/4.0).

induced by exercise. Heat shock proteins are protectively expressed. More than 130 genes are upregulated and 89 genes downregulated during the acclimatization process (summarized from Périard et al. 2015).

In sum, acclimatization is a powerful physiological process that dramatically increases heat tolerance. Since the remarkable early work of Aldo Dreosti (1935), dozens of effective heat acclimatization protocols have been tested, with demonstration of the positive effects described earlier in this section (Brown et al. 2022). The CDC recommends the following:

- Building up over several days to 2 hours a day of heat exposure, broken into 1-hour periods
- Daily outdoor exposure to 15 minutes of ambient heat for more vulnerable individuals
- Performing activities that the individual will need to do in the heat during exposure
- Starting new workers at 20% of the expected work duration, increasing by 20% per day
- Starting returning workers at 50% of exposure time and increasing to 60%, 80%, and 100% on days 2–4

Interventions should be highly tailored to an individual's conditioning and comorbid conditions, as well as the activity for which they are training, such as running track or serving in the military under extreme heat and humidity. Athletes can train for 60–90 minutes outdoors or indoors, including in rooms heated for this purpose. Various national agencies, however, recommend that sports practices for young people be canceled entirely at temperatures above 90°F. Acclimatization protocols can also be developed for older adults, who are at the highest heat risk, and might include passive warming in a sauna or bath, exercise in the home, or direct but passive exposures to external high temperatures of increasing duration (Cole et al. 2023).

Additional and common measures individuals can take to keep themselves safe during heat events are listed in Table 4.5.

If an individual does fall ill with heatstroke or heat exhaustion, the immediate interventions are as follows:

- Move them to a cool place
- Have them lie down
- Remove clothing
- Elevate the legs
- Push hydration; water and electrolyte-enriched drinks can both be safely offered
- Put them in a shower or tub of water or, if one is not available, apply wet clothes or spray with water to increase evaporative cooling
- Pack armpits, groin, and neck with ice
- Call 911 if any neurological symptom (e.g., refusal to drink, confusion, agitation, syncope, seizure) is present

Hospital-based care of heat exhaustion and stroke is focused on immediately decreasing core temperature through surface cooling with iced blankets and pads, infusion of IV cold saline, and, in the extreme, running the blood through a cold extracorporeal membrane oxygenation (ECMO) machine. In a recent review, no one method was found to be superior, but ice water or water cooling is generally preferred and effective unless the patient is unconscious (Rublee et al. 2021).

Patient Interventions to Mitigate Heat Effects

As a particularly vulnerable group, psychiatric patients require specific interventions to help them better manage extreme heat. These primarily involve education about their increased risks, the likely

Table 4.5. Personal, home, and work modifications to prevent heat illness

Limit time outdoors, especially midday

Save high-exertion work for the morning and evening

Wear light clothing and a hat

Eat lightly

Use a buddy system for emergency notification

Install air conditioning (70% lower mortality)

Use fans

Ventilate laundry and stove outside

Check heart rate on wearable devices, rest >120 BPM

Wear vests, neckbands, and hard hats with inserted frozen material

Have a cooler and an attached cooling blanket available at worksites

Increase ventilation

Block radiant heat from kilns and other hot machines with reflective surfaces

Insulate hot surfaces

Repair leaks from heat-producing appliances

Install shade awnings around the home

Wear dermal patches to monitor overheating

Note. BPM=beats per minute.

fluctuation of their symptoms with changes in temperature, and the risks associated with their medications. Patient and family education is also needed about anticipated increases in extreme violent and suicidal emotions with heat extremes and how to ride them out. For many patients, this will be adequate, but those with substance abuse or dementia may need particular emphasis on how to contact identified helpers and take shelter when cognition is impaired and temperatures are rising. Querying patients about their experiences with extreme heat may elicit complaints that suggest a need to lower doses of medications that particularly affect blood pressure, sweating, or other aspects of the heat response. Some patients (e.g., those with schizophrenia or dementia) may not accurately judge their body temperature and might benefit from a dermal patch that triggers this awareness.

Community Strategies for Mitigating Adverse Heat Effects

Communities can also take significant action to mitigate adverse heat effects. For instance, zoning and infrastructure regulations can include the following:

- Adequate tree canopy
- Reflective (white) or green roof requirements
- Reflective or permeable pavement requirements
- Smart growth practices
- Energy Star or other low-energy building requirements
- Identified cooling centers
- Phone trees to contact and triage isolated or less able residents during heat waves
- Provision of fans or air conditioners to those unable to afford them, including solar-powered devices for homeless groups
- Adequate access to fountains and drinking water during hot months

Psychiatrists have a public health role in advocating for these changes.

Heat Illness Mitigation in the Workplace

Persistent high temperatures and heat waves threaten all outdoor workers and those who work indoors in occupations requiring high physical activity or high-temperature infrastructure such as mining, smelting, kitchen work, and so on. On April 12, 2022, the federal Occupational Safety and Health Administration (OSHA) announced the launch of a National Emphasis Program (NEP) to protect millions of workers from heat illness and injuries, defining heat priority days as days when the heat index is expected to be greater than 80°F. The NEP created the first enforcement mechanism for inspecting workplaces for heat-related hazards, although it does not render any penalties. It authorized OSHA to inspect any alleged heat-related fatality, catastrophe, complaint, or referral regardless of whether the worksite falls within a targeted industry of the NEP and to engage in proactive outreach on heat priority days. It also called on employers to do the following:

Extreme Heat and Its Implications for Psychiatry   **67**

- Provide adequate breaks, shade, water, training, equipment, and acclimatization to protect workers from heat illness
- Engage in proactive technical and compliance efforts to help keep workers safe on the job
- Train employees and managers in the hazards of heat-related risk
- Attend to symptoms and signs of heat illness in workers
- Provide first aid for heat illness at the jobsite
- Establish an emergency action plan for the care of heat illness

This program represents a substantial step forward for workers in adverse heat conditions.

Key Points

- Higher and more extreme temperatures are associated with a range of heat illnesses, medical and psychiatric morbidities, and heat mortality that particularly affect those with poor social determinants of health, those with mental illness, and those taking psychiatric medication.
- Climate psychiatrists should be prepared to advise patients about heat-protective measures such as acclimatization and to provide basic treatment for life-threatening heat illness.
- Higher temperatures are significantly contributing to increasing suicide, violence, and violent conflict at the individual, community, and societal levels.
- The neurotransmitter, receptor, and brain systems involved in thermoregulation overlap with those central to neuropsychiatry, necessitating greater research into their mechanisms and effects.
- Greater understanding of the mechanisms and neurotransmitters involved in thermoregulation will allow psychiatrists to tailor treatments to improve safety and lower morbidity and mortality as heat extremes from global warming increase in duration and intensity.
- Roles for the climate psychiatrist in responding to extreme temperatures include education, advocacy, and implementation of systems for monitoring and treating heat illness at the level of the individual patient and for the community as a whole.

References

Almeida MC, Vizin RCL, Carrettiero DC: Current understanding on the neurophysiology of behavioral thermoregulation. Temperature (Austin) 2(4):483–490, 2015 27227068

Amoadu M, Ansah EW, Sarfo JO, et al: Impact of climate change and heat stress on workers' health and productivity: a scoping review. J Clim Change Health 12:100249, 2023

Amr M, Volpe FM: Seasonal influences on admissions for mood disorders and schizophrenia in a teaching psychiatric hospital in Egypt. J Affect Disord 137(1–3):56–60, 2012 22244374

Anderson CA: Temperature and aggression: ubiquitous effects of heat on occurrence of human violence. Psychol Bull 106(1):74–96, 1989 2667010

Avery DH, Wildschiødtz G, Rafaelsen OJ: Nocturnal temperature in affective disorder. J Affect Disord 4(1):61–71, 1982 6461688

Bark N: Deaths of psychiatric patients during heat waves. Psychiatr Serv 49(8):1088–1090, 1998 9712220

Basu R, Pearson D, Malig B, et al: The effect of high ambient temperature on emergency room visits. Epidemiology 23(6):813–820, 2012 23007039

Baylis P, Obradovich N, Kryvasheyeu Y, et al: Weather impacts expressed sentiment. PLoS One 13(4):e0195750, 2018 29694424

Belova A, Gould CA, Munson K, et al: Projecting the suicide burden of climate change in the United States. GeoHealth 6(5):e2021GH000580, 2022

Berberian AG, Gonzalez DJX, Cushing LJ: Racial disparities in climate change-related health effects in the United States. Curr Environ Health Rep 9(3):451–464, 2022 35633370

Bouchama A, Dehbi M, Mohamed G, et al: Prognostic factors in heat wave related deaths: a meta-analysis. Arch Intern Med 167(20):2170–2176, 2007 17698676

Bowyer JF, Hanig JP: Amphetamine- and methamphetamine-induced hyperthermia: implications of the effects produced in brain vasculature and peripheral organs to forebrain neurotoxicity. Temperature (Austin) 1(3):172–182, 2014 27626044

Brown HA, Topham TH, Clark B, et al: Seasonal heat acclimatisation in healthy adults: a systematic review. Sports Med 52(9):2111–2128, 2022 35460514

Burke M, González F, Baylis P, et al: Higher temperatures increase suicide rates in the United States and Mexico. Nat Clim Chang 8:723–729, 2018

Carleton TA: Crop-damaging temperatures increase suicide rates in India. Proc Natl Acad Sci USA 114(33):8746–8751, 2017 28760983

Chang S, Ryu Y, Bang SK, et al: An increase in peripheral temperature following cocaine administration is mediated through activation of dopamine D2 receptor in rats. Life (Basel) 12(2):143, 2022 35207431

Cheshire WP, Fealey RD: Drug-induced hyperhidrosis and hypohidrosis: incidence, prevention and management. Drug Saf 31(2):109–126, 2008 18217788

Chong TWH, Castle DJ: Layer upon layer: thermoregulation in schizophrenia. Schizophr Res 69(2–3):149–157, 2004 15469188

Cole E, Donnan KJ, Simpson AJ, et al: Short-term heat acclimation protocols for an aging population: systematic review. PLoS One 18(3):e0282038, 2023 36862716

Corbett J, Wright J, Tipton MJ: Sex differences in response to exercise heat stress in the context of the military environment. BMJ Mil Health 169(1):94–101, 2023 32094215

Crost B, Duquennois C, Felter JH, et al: Climate change, agricultural production and civil conflict: evidence from the Philippines. J Environ Econ Manage 88:379–395, 2018

Dehbi M, Baturcam E, Eldali A, et al: Hsp-72, a candidate prognostic indicator of heatstroke. Cell Stress Chaperones 15(5):593–603, 2010 20174993

Derickson A: "A widespread superstition": the purported invulnerability of workers of color to occupational heat stress. Am J Public Health 109(10):1329–1335, 2019 31415199

Dittner C, Lindsund E, Cannon B, et al: At thermoneutrality, acute thyroxine-induced thermogenesis and pyrexia are independent of UCP1. Mol Metab 25:20–34, 2019 31151797

Dreosti AO: Problems arising out of temperature and humidity in deep mining on the Witwatersrand. J Chem Metall Min Soc S Afr 36(5):102–129, 1935

Dubois EF: The many different temperatures of the human body and its parts. West J Surg, Obstet Gynecol 59(9):476–490, 1951 14867268

Dumont C, Haase E, Dolber T, et al: Climate change and risk of completed suicide. J Nerv Ment Dis 208(7):559–565, 2020 32205773

Echizenya M, Mishima K, Satoh K, et al: Heat loss, sleepiness, and impaired performance after diazepam administration in humans. Neuropsychopharmacology 28(6):1182–1206, 2003 12700718

El Khayat M, Halwani DA, Hneiny L, et al: Impacts of climate change and heat stress on farmworkers' health: a scoping review. Front Public Health 10:782811, 2022 35211437

Folk GE: Adaptation and heat loss: the past thirty years, in Heat Loss From Animals and Man. Edited by Monteith JL, Mount LE. London, Elsevier, 1974, pp 119–146

Fountoulakis KN, Savopoulos C, Zannis P, et al: Climate change but not unemployment explains the changing suicidality in Thessaloniki Greece (2000–2012). J Affect Dis 193:331–338, 2016 26796233

Gagnon D, Crandall CG: Sweating as a heat loss thermoeffector, in Handbook of Clinical Neurology, Vol 156. Edited by Romanovsky AA. New York, Elsevier, 2018, pp 211–232

Garcia CK, Renteria LI, Leite-Santos G, et al: Exertional heat stroke: pathophysiology and risk factors. BMJ Med 1(1):e000239, 2022 36936589

Giersch GEW, Garcia CK, Stachenfeld NS, et al: Are there sex differences in risk for exertional heat stroke? A translational approach. Exp Physiol 107(10):1136–1143, 2022 35598159

Greenleaf JE, Kaciuba-Uscilko H: Acclimatization to Heat in Humans, NASA Tech Memo 101011. Moffett Field, CA, National Aeronautics and Space Administration, 1989

Hansen A, Bi P, Nitschke M, et al: The effect of heat waves on mental health in a temperate Australian city. Environ Health Perspect 116(10):1369–1375, 2008 18941580

Hargreaves M, Spriet LL: Skeletal muscle energy metabolism during exercise. Nat Metab 2(9):817–828, 2020 32747792

Harlan SL, Declet-Barreto JH, Stefanov WL, et al: Neighborhood effects on heat deaths: social and environmental predictors of vulnerability in Maricopa County, Arizona. Environ Health Perspect 121(2):197–204, 2013 23164621

Hoegh-Guldberg O, Jacob D, Taylor M, et al: Impacts of 1.5°C global warming on natural and human systems, in Global Warming of 1.5°C. Edited by Masson-Delmotte V, Zhai P, Pörtner H-O, et al. Cambridge, UK, Cambridge University Press, 2018, pp 175–312

Horseman MA, Rather-Conally J, Saavedra C, et al: A case of severe heatstroke and review of pathophysiology, clinical presentation, and treatment. J Intensive Care Med 28(6):334–340, 2013 22232203

Hsiang SM, Burke M, Miguel E: Quantifying the influence of climate on human conflict. Science 341(6151), 1212–1212, 2013 24031020

Kessler RC, Angermeyer M, Anthony JC, et al: Lifetime prevalence and age-of-onset distributions of mental disorders in the World Health Organization's World Mental Health Survey Initiative. World Psychiatry 6(3):168–176, 2007 18188442

Kurz A: Physiology of thermoregulation. Best Pract Res Clin Anaesthesiol 22(4):627–644, 2008 19137807

Lam RW, Goldner EM, Grewal A: Seasonality of symptoms in anorexia and bulimia nervosa. Int J Eat Disord 19(1):35–44, 1996 8640200

Leach OK, Cottle RM, Fisher KG, et al: Sex differences in heat stress vulnerability among middle-aged and older adults (PSU HEAT Project). Am J Physiol Regul Integr Comp Physiol 327(3):R320–R327, 2024 39005081

Lee MJ, McLean KE, Kuo M, et al: Chronic diseases associated with mortality in British Columbia, Canada during the 2021 western North America extreme heat event. GeoHealth 7(3):e2022GH000729, 2023

Maguire LA: The Effects of Gabapentin on the Firing Rates of Thermoregulatory Neurons in the Preoptic Anterior Hypothalamus in Modulation of Hot Flashes. Paper 140, Undergraduate Honors Thesis. Williamsburg, VA, College of William and Mary, 2015

Marcy TR, Britton ML: Antidepressant-induced sweating. Ann Pharmacother 39(4):748–752, 2005 15728327

Martin-Latry K, Goumy MP, Latry P, et al: Psychotropic drugs use and risk of heat-related hospitalisation. Eur Psychiatry 22(6):335–338, 2007 17513091

Meade RD, Akerman AP, Notley SR, et al: Physiological factors characterizing heat-vulnerable older adults: a narrative review. Environ Int 144:105909, 2020 32919284

Meadows J, Mansour A, Gatto MR, et al: Mental illness and increased vulnerability to negative health effects from extreme heat events: a systematic review. Psychiatry Res 332:115678, 2024 38150812

Min KB, Lee S, Min JY: High and low ambient temperature at night and the prescription of hypnotics. Sleep 44(5):zsaa262, 2021 33442740

Mullins JT, White C: Temperature and mental health: evidence from the spectrum of mental health outcomes. J Health Econ 68:102240, 2019 31590065

Myers RD, Simpson CW, Higgins D, et al: Hypothalamic Na+ and Ca++ ions and temperature set-point: new mechanisms of action of a central or peripheral thermal challenge and intrahypothalamic 5-HT, NE, PGEi and pyrogen. Brain Res Bull 1(3):301–327, 1976 974810

Naughton MP, Henderson A, Mirabelli MC, et al: Heat-related mortality during a 1999 heat wave in Chicago. Am J Prev Med 22(4):221–227, 2002 11988377

Noelke C, McGovern M, Corsi DJ, et al: Increasing ambient temperature reduces emotional well-being. Environ Res 151:124–129, 2016 27475052

Obermeyer Z, Samra JK, Mullainathan S: Individual differences in normal body temperature: longitudinal big data analysis of patient records. BMJ 359:j5468, 2017 29237616

Obradovich N, Migliorini R, Mednick SC, et al: Nighttime temperature and human sleep loss in a changing climate. Sci Adv 3(5):e1601555, 2017 28560320

Obradovich N, Migliorini R, Paulus MP, et al: Empirical evidence of mental health risks posed by climate change. Proc Natl Acad Sci USA 115(43):10953–10958, 2018 30297424

Page LA, Hajat S, Kovats RS, et al: Temperature-related deaths in people with psychosis, dementia and substance misuse. Br J Psychiatry 200(6):485–490, 2012 22661680

Périard JD, Racinais S, Sawka MN: Adaptations and mechanisms of human heat acclimation: applications for competitive athletes and sports. Scand J Med Sci Sports 25(Suppl 1):20–38, 2015 25943654

Petroianu GA: Hyperthermia and serotonin: the quest for a "better cyproheptadine." Int J Mol Sci 23(6):3365, 2022 35328784

Ranson M: Crime, weather, and climate change. J Environ Econ Manage 67:274–302, 2014

Rublee C, Dresser C, Giudice C, et al: Evidence-based heatstroke management in the emergency department. West J Emerg Med 22(2):186–195, 2021 33856299

Sarchiapone M, Gramaglia C, Iosue M, et al: The association between electrodermal activity (EDA), depression and suicidal behaviour: a systematic review and narrative synthesis. BMC Psychiatry 18(1):22, 2018 29370787

Sartim AG, Moreira FA, Joca SRL: Involvement of CB1 and TRPV1 receptors located in the ventral medial prefrontal cortex in the modulation of stress coping behavior. Neuroscience 340:126–134, 2017 27771531

Semenza JC, Rubin CH, Falter WD, et al: Heat-related deaths during the July 1995 heat wave in Chicago. N Engl J Med 335(2):84–90, 1996 8649494

Semenza JC, McCullough JE, Flanders WD, et al: Excess hospital admissions during the July 1995 heat wave in Chicago. Am J Prev Med 16(4):269–277, 1999 10493281

Shiloh R, Weizman A, Epstein Y, et al: Abnormal thermoregulation in drug-free male schizophrenia patients. Eur Neuropsychopharmacol 11(4):285–288, 2001 11532382

Shimada T, Miyamoto N, Shimada Y, et al: Analysis of clinical symptoms and brain MRI of heat stroke: 2 case reports and a literature review. J Stroke Cerebrovasc Dis 29(2):104511–104511, 2020 31151838

Siemens J, Kamm GB: Cellular populations and thermosensing mechanisms of the hypothalamic thermoregulatory center. Pflugers Arch 470(5):809–822, 2018 29374307

Smith CJ, Johnson JM: Responses to hyperthermia: optimizing heat dissipation by convection and evaporation: neural control of skin blood flow and sweating in humans. Auton Neurosci 196:25–36, 2016 26830064

Solt V, Chen CJ, Roy A: Seasonal pattern of posttraumatic stress disorder admissions. Compr Psychiatry 37(1):40–42, 1996 8770525

Tan CL, Knight ZA: Regulation of body temperature by the nervous system. Neuron 98(1):31–48, 2018 29621489

Tansey EA, Johnson CD: Recent advances in thermoregulation. Adv Physiol Ed 39(3):139–148, 2015 26330029

Texas Department of Criminal Justice: Drugs Associated With Heat Stress. Correctional Managed Healthcare Policy No D-27.2, Attachment A. Austin, Texas Department of Criminal Justice, January 2023. Available at: www.tdcj.texas.gov/divisions/cmhc/docs/cmhc_policy_manual/D-27.02_Attachment_A.pdf. Accessed November 22, 2024.

Tie HT, Su GZ, He K, et al: Efficacy and safety of ondansetron in preventing postanesthesia shivering: a meta-analysis of randomized controlled trials. BMC Anesthesiol 14:12, 2014 24588846

Toda T, Yamamoto S, Umehara N, et al: Protective effects of duloxetine against cerebral ischemia-reperfusion injury via transient receptor potential melastatin 2 inhibition. J Pharmacol Exp Ther 368(2):246–254, 2019 30523061

Extreme Heat and Its Implications for Psychiatry

Uchida Y, Izumizaki M: Effect of menstrual cycle and female hormones on TRP and TREK channels in modifying thermosensitivity and physiological functions in women. J Therm Biol 100:103029, 2021 34503776

U.S. Department of the Army and Air Force: Heat Stress Control and Heat Casualty Management. Army Tech Bull TB-MED 507. Washington, DC, Department of the Army and Air Force, March 7, 2003. Available at: https://usariem.health.mil/assets/docs/partnering/tbmed507.pdf. Accessed November 21, 2024.

van den Bersselaar LR, Kruijt N, Bongers CCWG, et al: Comment on "Overlapping mechanisms of exertional heat stroke and malignant hyperthermia: evidence vs. conjecture." Sports Med 52(3):669–672, 2022 34626340

Vanos JK: Children's health and vulnerability in outdoor microclimates: a comprehensive review. Environ Int 76:1–15, 2015 25497108

Voronova IP: 5-HT receptors and temperature homeostasis. Biomolecules 11(12):1914, 2021 34944557

Walter E, Carraretto M: Drug-induced hyperthermia in critical care. J Intensive Care Soc 16(4):306–311, 2015 28979436

Wortzel JR, Norden JG, Turner BE, et al: Ambient temperature and solar insolation are associated with decreased prevalence of SSRI-treated psychiatric disorders. J Psychiatr Res 110:57–63, 2019 30594025

Yau WW, Yen PM: Thermogenesis in adipose tissue activated by thyroid hormone. Int J Mol Sci 21(8):3020, 2020 32344721

You IJ, Jung YH, Kim MJ, et al: Alterations in the emotional and memory behavioral phenotypes of transient receptor potential vanilloid type 1-deficient mice are mediated by changes in expression of 5-HT1A, GABA(A), and NMDA receptors. Neuropharmacology 62(2):1034–1043, 2012 22074644

Zhou C, Zhu Y, Liu Z, et al: 5-HT3 receptor antagonists for the prevention of postoperative shivering: a meta-analysis. J Int Med Res 44(6):1174–1181, 2016 27856931

Zonnenberg C, Bueno-de-Mesquita JM, Ramlal D, et al: Antipsychotic-related hypothermia: five new cases. Front Psychiatry 10:543, 2019 31417438

Zou Y, Heyn C, Grigorian A, et al: Measuring brain temperature in youth bipolar disorder using a novel magnetic resonance imaging approach: a proof-of-concept study. Curr Neuropharmacol 21(6):1355–1366, 2023 36946483

5

Air Pollution Impacts on the Brain

Understanding Air Pollution and Its Importance for Psychiatry

Climate change is associated with air pollution through the products released by burning fossil fuels and the effects of global warming on worsening air quality, including increased wildfires, ground ozone, pollens, dust, smog, and other contributors to poor-quality air. Air pollution is responsible for up to 9 million deaths per year (Lelieveld et al. 2019), primarily from strokes, heart attacks, and respiratory diseases, and it causes extensive morbidity and disability as well as billions of dollars in economic losses across the world (Owusu and Sarkodie 2020). Increasing awareness of these damages, which are now known to occur at even lower levels of air pollution than previously recognized as harmful, led the World Health Organization to revise their 2005 Global Air Quality Guidelines in 2021, reducing the threshold for pollutants considered safe. Still, more than 90% of the world lives regularly with air quality worse than these revised acceptable levels (World Health Organization 2023). These current acceptable standards for pollutants are as follows:

- $PM_{2.5}$: 5 μm^3
- PM_{10}: 15 μm^3
- NO_2: 25 μm^3

Air pollution is composed of particulate matter (classified by size as $PM_{2.5}$ μm, PM_{10} μm, and ultrafine particles, 0.1 μm), oxidative gases (ground ozone [O_3], carbon monoxide [CO], sulfur dioxide [SO_2], and nitrogen oxides [NO and NO_2]), and gaseous organic compounds (polycyclic aromatic hydrocarbons [PAHs], volatile organic compounds [VOCs], and others). It also contains heavy metals (iron, vanadium, nickel, copper, and manganese) and microplastics (O'Brien et al. 2023), as well as bacteria, fungi, viruses, and their endotoxins (He et al. 2023), including those that may distribute global antibiotic resistance (Zhou et al. 2023). The six criteria pollutants regulated in the United States are lead, nitric oxides, SO_2, CO, O_3, and particulate matter. Air pollution particles are formed when PAHs bind to organic carbon (carbon naturally in the air) and elemental carbon (resulting from dust, fires, ash, and fuels), then aggregate and pick up charged molecules (Figure 5.1).

Air pollution exposure is highly dependent on locale. For example, higher exposure to sulfur oxides occurs near shipping channels, soot and PAHs are concentrated near coal plants, and traffic-related

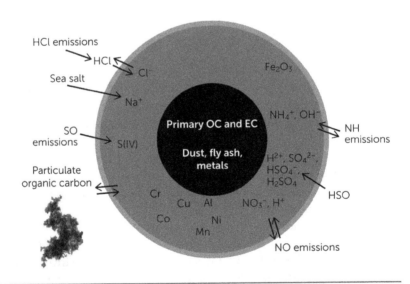

Figure 5.1 Structure of an air pollution particle.

Organic carbon (OC) and elemental carbon (EC) from dust, ash, and fires create a core that attracts heavy metals, nitrogen compounds, iron oxides, and water, which charge the particle and create oxidative radicals when interacting with enzymes on tissue surfaces.

Fe_2O_3=iron(III) oxide; HCl=hydrochloric acid; NH_4^+=ammonium; HSO_4^-=hydrogen sulfate; NOx=nitrogen oxides; SOx=sulfur oxides.

Air Pollution Impacts on the Brain 77

air pollution (TRAP) is concentrated near roads. Wind, heat, humidity, barometric inversions, and solar radiation are also important determinants of air quality. Air pollution arises from multiple sources, overwhelmingly those associated with the burning of fossil fuels: coal mining, coal plants, industrial processing, transportation (automotive, air, and ship), oil production, forest fires, agriculture, landfill, land and crop burning, petroleum coke extraction, and other sources.

When reading research papers on the physical and neuropsychiatric impacts of air pollution, therefore, the practitioner should bear in mind the type of pollutant studied, the source of this pollution, and the time frame and scale of the study. Positive findings occur with both acute air pollution events and chronic exposure to poor-quality air. Acute health effects often lag 1–7 days behind an abrupt worsening of air quality yet show clear associations. Results should also be considered for their significance relative to environmental conditions that frequently co-occur with air pollution, such as drought, extremes of temperature and humidity, as well as other etiologies for the psychiatric symptoms associated with air pollution, which include depression and dementia. The ability of neuropsychiatric pathology associated with air pollution to stand out with statistical significance against this background of confounding variables is remarkable.

Health and Mental Health Impacts of Air Pollution

Cardiovascular damage is the major source of mortality from air pollution and is thought to result in part from an imbalance between the formation and degradation of nitric oxide, contributing to inflammation of the vascular endothelium. This inflammation contributes to atherosclerotic plaque, leading to myocardial infarction, and disrupts the blood-brain barrier, contributing to stroke (Hahad et al. 2020). Inflammatory reactions also contribute to the pulmonary effects of air pollution, which include asthma, chronic obstructive pulmonary disease, pulmonary infections, and lung cancer (Kurt et al. 2016).

Brain impacts of air pollution exposure are also thought to arise primarily from inflammatory and oxidative cell damage. Particulate air pollution, particularly ultrafine particles, can translocate to the brain through endocytosis across the pulmonary epithelium into the vasculature, across the blood-brain barrier through retrograde neuronal transport via the olfactory and trigeminal nerves, and potentially through other mechanisms. Particles can be visualized in brain tissue. Exposure to particulate and other air pollution is associated with cytokine activation (e.g., interleukin 6 [IL-6], IL-2, IL-1β, tumor necrosis factor [TNF]), monoamine hyperfunction, mitochondrial dysfunction, changes in nitric oxide synthesis and endothelin-1, and cell damage and death, with accumulation of lipid membrane fragments, macrophages, amyloid-β42, α-synuclein, and other by-products around microglia and neurons (Calderón-Garcidueñas et al. 2016; Hahad et al. 2020).

Children are particularly vulnerable to the health impacts of air pollution because they are more active and respire more than adults, have less ability to break down airborne toxins, are more vulnerable to genetic and epigenetic damage during development (reviewed in Xu et al. 2012), and achieve 80% of their lung growth by age 6. As a result, their long-term lung capacity can be particularly limited if damaged by this age (Z. Chen et al. 2015). Poor air quality is also disproportionately experienced by racially and socioeconomically discriminated populations (Jbaily et al. 2022), a source of environmental injustice that can up to triple its mortality impacts for older Black Americans, among other adversity (Di et al. 2017; Spiller et al. 2021).

People who cook over open indoor fires (predominantly women globally), firefighters (see Chapter 8, "Climate Change, Extreme Weather, Natural Disasters, and Human Displacement"), and workers in occupations that produce smoke and toxic gases are also vulnerable groups. In addition to improving these conditions where possible in homes, workplace protections for these groups are needed, as shown in Table 5.3 in the section "Psychiatric Advocacy to Improve Air Quality."

Neuropsychiatric Impacts of Air Pollution

Air pollution is strongly associated with adverse neuropsychiatric consequences across the life span. These impacts are both directly causal and/or significantly contributory, increasing the risk of neuropsychiatric illnesses such as autism spectrum disorder, Parkinson's disease, dementia, and stroke up to fourfold (J.C. Chen et al. 2015; Fu et al. 2019). From the prenatal period through the end of life, air pollution exposure worsens fetal development, maternal mental health, child development, brain aging, and societal and individual well-being. It contributes to elevated rates of ADHD, intellectual disability, autism spectrum disorder, behavioral disorders, depression, suicide, psychosis, dementia, and other mental disorders, as reviewed in the next two sections of this chapter. Improved air quality results in rapid improvements in many of these outcomes in children (Perera 2017) and has also been demonstrated to improve attention and white matter integrity in older adults (Lin et al. 2024). Since the passage of the Clean Air Act of 1970 in the United States, the combined emissions for criteria pollutants have dropped 78%, with stunning impacts on health and productivity outcomes from 1970 to 2020. The benefit:cost ratio for the gains accruing from these federal policies has been estimated as greater than $30:$1 (Environmental Protection Agency 1997, 2011). Notably, psychiatric impacts had not been empirically identified in time to be included in these larger analyses.

Impacts on Children

Starting in utero, the development of children's brains is significantly affected by exposure to air pollution. As summarized in excellent reviews by Herting et al. (2024), Kim et al. (2020), and Perera (2017), this exposure is associated with a 5%–30% incidence of low birth weight, small size for gestational age, and preterm birth; fetal exposure to air pollution, particularly $PM_{2.5}$ and O_3, has been associated with developmental delay, poor psychological development at age 6 months, lower IQ in childhood, and cognitive impairment in old age. ADHD has been associated with $PM_{2.5}$ and NO_2 exposure (Donzelli et al. 2019; Kaur et al. 2023), and studies found a resulting increase in anxiety, depression, and behavioral disorders. Costs for lesser lifetime achievement and earnings and greater health spending measure in the billions of dollars annually. Maternal air pollution exposure during pregnancy has also now been convincingly associated with a 1.5- to twofold risk of autism spectrum disorder in children (Chun et al. 2020; Dutheil et al. 2021). In addition to these impacts on the fetus, second-trimester 10-μm increases in $PM_{2.5}$ exposure were associated with postpartum anhedonia and depression in a study of 557 predominantly Hispanic and Black women, with worsened Edinburgh Postnatal Depression Scale scores in Black mothers particularly (Sheffield et al. 2018). These maternal effects increase the primary air pollution risks to the fetus across the pregnancy, exposing these infants to the further adverse mental health impacts of maternal depression. Negative effects also occur in older youth, who show higher rates of depression and suicidal thinking with chronic air pollution exposure (Xie et al. 2023).

Vignette

James, age 9, was referred to a child psychiatrist for anxiety after several intubations for severe asthma. His mother reported behavior disruption, low grades, and attentional problems in school. Noting James's address near a major freeway, the psychiatrist determined that air pollution might be significantly exacerbating the child's medical illness. She recommended that the family move several blocks farther down the street near a small park (climate adaptation) and install an air filter in his bedroom (climate mitigation). Two years later, the psychiatrist received a postcard that James's grades had improved. He was spending time in the park without breathing difficulty. His anxiety and behavioral problems had subsided, demonstrating the reversible impacts of air pollution on mental health and behavioral disorders.

Impacts on Adults

In adolescence through middle years, air pollution exposure is associated with an increased risk of depression and suicide, as well as elevated risks of psychosis and bipolar disorder, although these latter two have been less studied. In terms of depression, acute worsening of air quality is associated with more new diagnoses of depression, more prescriptions for antidepressants, and more emergency department visits for depression, and long-term exposure carries the risk of depressive diagnoses in the top quartile of poor-quality air and with every 10-μm increase (Yang et al. 2023; reviewed also in Hahad et al. 2020). The increases in depression in these studies carry an OR that ranges from 1.01–1.06 (95% CI [0.99–1.13]) and are associated with $PM_{2.5}$ and NO_2 exposure, with lower associations for PM_{10} and no association with O_3 (Zeng et al. 2019). Some studies of long-term air pollution exposure show a more significantly elevated depression risk and associations with schizophrenia spectrum and anxiety disorders (Nobile et al. 2023).

Suicide is also elevated by air pollution exposure. In a systematic review and meta-analysis, Heo et al. (2021) found a relative increased risk of suicide per interquartile range worse-quality air of 1.02–1.03 (95% CI [1.0–1.05]), a similar conclusion to that drawn in a review by Dumont et al. (2020). As has been found across diagnoses, the types of air pollution most implicated are $PM_{2.5}$, PM_{10}, and NO_2. Given that temperature also increases the risk of suicide independent of air quality, the combination of air pollution and high temperatures on very hot days with poor air could increase the relative risk of suicide by up to 20%.

Studies have shown associations between a diagnosis of schizophrenia or psychotic exacerbation and exposure to benzene, CO, dust, and PM_{10} (Bakolis et al. 2021; Buoli et al. 2018). Psychotic experiences also increase after exposure to the top quartile of $PM_{2.5}$ or NO_2 concentrations (OR 1.4–1.7), explaining 60% of the association between adolescent psychotic experiences and urbanicity (Newbury et al. 2019). A heightened prevalence of schizophrenia is also found in areas of the United States that have, until recently, relied on coal plants for energy. More studies are needed in this area.

By far the most numerically significant impact of air pollution in adults, however, is on the incidence of dementia, which has been affirmed in multiple large high-quality studies including more than 12 million subjects older than age 50 years (Tsai et al. 2019), and is listed as a top epidemiological dementia risk (Livingston et al. 2020). Long-term exposure to $PM_{2.5}$ (in contrast to stroke, where the greater risk is associated with NO_2) confers a threefold risk for dementia, rising to almost fivefold for Alzheimer's disease (Tsai et al. 2019), perhaps particularly in women and those carrying the *APOE* ε4 allele (J.C. Chen et al. 2015).

Implications of the Effects of Air Pollution on Brain Pathology for Population Health

In considering the implications for clinical practice of these findings on exposure to air pollution, it is worth noting that the accumulating impacts of air pollution have been associated with additional nonsyndromal psychiatric symptoms. These include a 20%–40% increase in common mental health symptoms such as fatigue and irritability (assessed by the Clinical Interview Schedule—Revised CIS-R), a 20%–30% increase in physical complaints, and a 33% increase in psychotic experiences (Bakolis et al. 2021), as well as an increase in violent crime (Herrnstadt and Muehlegger 2015) and domestic violence (Kuo and Putra 2021). The mental health effects of air pollution also increase presentations for psychiatric care, including an increase in hospital outpatient visits, 0.5%–1.8% increases in hospital admissions for depression (Gu et al. 2020), more visits to the emergency department and use of emergency management services, and other system demands (Fang et al. 2023). Air pollution exposure leads to an increase in psychiatric emergency visits, even with exposure of only 1 day or small variations of the larger PM_{10} particles (Oudin et al. 2018).

Addressing Air Pollution in Clinical Settings

Air pollution can thus be expected in the acute setting to present clinicians and patients with a broad increase in symptoms and greater danger of psychiatric acuity and suicide. In areas with chronically poor air, clinicians can expect a mounting epidemiological toll of child psychiatric disorders, depression, and dementia in particular. For the working mental health practitioner, advocacy to improve air quality at the levels of the individual patient, the community, and national policy initiatives is a particularly effective and efficient way to reduce both global warming and adverse psychiatric consequences of the gases that produce it.

Patients can be educated about air pollution as part of routine preventative care and also when poor air quality provides an opportunity to address their concerns. Wildfires, smog, and pollen events may open a window to ask if they have noticed an increase in cardiopulmonary or psychiatric symptoms, inquire how they are protecting themselves from the adverse conditions, and also query their emotional impacts. Open-ended questions may include asking how the weather or air has been affecting them, whether they are doing anything to improve their air quality, and whether they are aware of the connections between air quality and mental health. The answers to these questions will suggest which of the interventions in Table 5.1 may be most helpful.

Cognitively, patients will be better equipped to take action to mitigate air pollution if they are able to appreciate its personal relevance in a meaningful way. To make more concrete the connection between microscopic particles, health, and brain pathology, the practitioner can review micrographs and graphics from internet sources showing the size and source of air pollution particles and compare their air pollution exposure to that of a number of cigarettes smoked (Muller and Muller 2015).

It is also essential to tackle the difficult task of connecting the dots between air pollution impacts, climate change, and social behavior by saying something such as "Air pollution can be reduced by lessening our use of fossil fuels, which means we need to work on it not only just for you but also at a community level if we are to make significant

Air Pollution Impacts on the Brain

Table 5.1 Individual actions to reduce personal exposure to indoor and outdoor air pollution

Actions to reduce exposure to outdoor air pollution

Track local air pollution levels at www.airnow.gov

Remain indoors on extreme air pollution days

Decrease exercise on high-pollution days

Avoid exercise near high-traffic areas

Install HEPA air filters in the home, particularly in sleeping areas[a]

Reduce commute time (significantly reduces TRAP)

Use an N95 or P100 respirator[b] on extreme air pollution days

Create a "clean zone" at home with few windows, no carpets, and high filtration

Actions to reduce exposure to indoor air pollution

Use a HEPA air filter (removes particles at least down to 3 µm and often 1 µm)

Clean and test HVAC systems regularly

Eliminate pet dander with regular shampooing of animals and beds; keep pets out of bedroom

Minimize clutter

Reduce carpeting

Test for radon

Seal windows and doors with weather stripping

Use carbon monoxide detectors

Cover trash

Adopt a shoes-off policy

Wash bedding weekly

Use microfiber dusters

Eliminate indoor smoking and vaping of tobacco, cannabis, and other substances

Use natural cleaners (and elbow grease)

Reduce use of candles, incense, and perfumes

Table 5.1 Individual actions to reduce personal exposure to indoor and outdoor air pollution (*continued*)

Ventilate the home regularly

Improve hood ventilation of gas stoves

Eliminate indoor wood-burning fireplaces

Test ceilings and paints for asbestos, lead, and formaldehyde

Note. HEPA=high-efficiency particulate air; HVAC=heating, ventilation, and air-conditioning; TRAP=traffic-related air pollution.
[a]Both the California Air Resources Board and the Association of Home Appliance Manufacturers maintain vetted lists of air filters that emit little to no ozone.
[b]For information on respirators, see www.cdc.gov/niosh/npptl/topics/respirators/disp_part/default.html.
Source. Summarized from Laumbach et al. 2015.

inroads for your health, just as we do by passing laws to regulate smoking or to stop people from dumping toxins in our rivers." This intervention is necessary to preserve psychiatric treatment principles of neutrality and reality testing. Air pollution is an example of a social problem in which "the political is personal." Disavowal of its societal etiologies has adverse consequences, colluding with a model of the psyche that ignores the macro-societal forces influencing patient well-being, and it disempowers the patient by suggesting there is nothing they can do relationally to shape these social and global forces, which may increase the patient's sense of vulnerability to them.

Patient Distress and Extreme Poor-Quality Air

Exposure to high air pollution is associated with physical discomfort, including irritation of the eyes, nose, and throat; chest tightness; coughing, wheezing, and shallow or short breath; increased phlegm; nausea; and fatigue. Breathlessness, dyspnea, and air hunger are unpleasant sensations associated with fears of suffocation, loss of control, and mortality terrors (Williams and Carel 2018), which are higher in individuals with high anxiety sensitivity (Alius et al. 2013).

Anxiety is both a heralding symptom of and a response to respiratory distress, and it can lead to dysfunctional breathing that worsens the sensation of breathlessness. Psychiatrists must be prepared to assist patients who are panicking about their responses to toxic air, particularly those who have had traumatic experiences of breathlessness due to asthma or other respiratory crises. During an air pollution event, patients need clinician help to differentiate panic from hypoxic distress, diaphoresis, chest pain, sudden lightheadedness, and weakness or numbness, which should prompt emergency evaluation for chronic obstructive pulmonary disease, myocardial infarction, or stroke. Panic will be equally if not more common (Manisalidis et al. 2020).

Poor-quality air is also highly distressing as an environmental experience. Hazy days have emotional impacts ranging from unpleasant, anxious moods to aggressiveness and agitation (Xu et al. 2020). This phenomenon has many possible explanations, including decreased sunlight. In Chinese studies, the number of symptoms experienced and the perceived (rather than actual) danger of the air pollution (Ho et al. 2014) and its chronicity may influence psychological distress (Rajper et al. 2018), although few studies have been done in this area. Giving patients a sense of control over their acute distress is helpful for decreasing excessive anxiety. Patients may respond well to intellectual explanations of the relationship between anxiety and overbreathing, as well as to learning breathing techniques. Techniques aimed at disidentification with distress, as well as the development of grit and persistence, may be helpful.

Psychiatric Advocacy to Improve Air Quality

The multiple impacts of air pollution on psychiatric disorders create an ethical imperative to mitigate its damage on the population and individual levels. We are tasked by our psychiatric code of ethics to educate ourselves and provide relevant information to the public about emerging scientific knowledge (American Psychiatric Association 2013, Section 5) and "to participate in activities contributing to the improvement of the community and the betterment of public health" (American Psychiatric Association 2013, Section 7). To fulfill this obligation, the psychiatric professional can take on the role of policy advocate and public health educator, supporting measures such as those in Table 5.2 and Table 5.3.

The legislation of air pollution has established policy that has had significant impacts on public health. Since the passage of the Clean Air Act Amendments in 1990, non-particle pollutants have dropped by up to 80%,

Table 5.2 Policy actions to reduce air pollution impacts on brain health

Support workplace protections for air pollution

Include neurodevelopmental impacts in the cost assessment of fuel standards

Enforce fuel efficiency standards

Promote clean energy policies

Advance free public transportation

Provide subsidies to switch household and transport fuel types

Target existing sources of combustion-related pollutants for urgent reduction

Restrict use of combustion air pollutants in dense residential areas, particularly in disadvantaged urban areas (e.g., through congestion pricing)

Expand air monitoring and decrease combustion fuel use in places where children spend time, such as schools and parks

Promote mitigating strategies such as vegetative barriers

Expand research on the health impacts of ultrafine particles

saving an estimated 230,000 lives and 2 trillion dollars of health-related costs annually. Until recent increases in wildfires, visibility in national parks had increased by 20–30 miles, improving views that are associated with feelings of affection, playfulness, and elation (Ulrich 1979).

Unfortunately, particulate matter and other greenhouse gases have continued to rise, making these the latest frontier for American clean air action (Ku and Haase 2023). Numerous organizations devoted to air quality improvement have active local chapters that can be readily accessed. In the United States and United Kingdom, these include Moms Clean Air Force, the American Lung Association's Healthy Air Campaign, the Coalition for Clean Air, Clean Air Fund, Citizens' Climate Lobby, Earthjustice, and Little Ninja. These groups educate communities and support local legislation to improve clean transport and meet emissions reduction targets. There is strong bipartisan public support for action on clean air (Baumann et al. 2024), including on fossil-fuel pollutants, and advocacy is therefore likely to have greater success than in other areas of environmental and climate concern.

Air Pollution Impacts on the Brain

Table 5.3 Workplace air quality protection

Ensure adequate ventilation

Create and follow maintenance protocols for ventilation and HVAC systems

Monitor and repair leaks and flooding

Mitigate humidity or dry air with (de)humidifiers

Minimize use of toxic disinfectants and other cleaners

Monitor industry or site-specific toxins (e.g., radon, mercury, benzene, asbestos, formaldehyde)

Use high-quality HVAC filters to remove fungal spores and particulate matter

Use CDC-approved respirators as indicated (Centers for Disease Control and Prevention 2021)

Follow OSHA standard of General Duty (a safe, nontoxic workplace)

Solicit NIOSH evaluation if health complaints arise

Note. HVAC=heating, ventilation, and air-conditioning; NIOSH=National Institute for Occupational Safety and Health; OSHA=Occupational Safety and Health Administration.

Key Points

- Air pollution causes high global mortality through strokes, heart attacks, pulmonary disease, and other medical illnesses.
- Air pollution causes significant neuropsychiatric damage across the life span that is well understood scientifically and has annual societal and personal costs of trillions of dollars.
- Psychiatrists need to attend particularly to the impact of air pollution on dementia, suicide risk, and child cognitive and behavioral disorders.
- The Clean Air Act has led to dramatic improvements in air quality and cost savings.
- Increases in dust, wildfires, microplastics, and pollens and associated effects of climate change and the Anthropocene are undermining existing progress on clean air.
- Because the public is broadly supportive of actions to regulate air quality, advocacy for better air pollution policy is a particularly

effective nonpartisan strategy with the double benefits of preventing both climate change and psychiatric illness.

References

Alius MG, Pané-Farré CA, Von Leupoldt A, et al: Induction of dyspnea evokes increased anxiety and maladaptive breathing in individuals with high anxiety sensitivity and suffocation fear. Psychophysiology 50(5):488–497, 2013 23421426

American Psychiatric Association: The Principles of Medical Ethics With Annotations Especially Applicable for Psychiatry. Arlington, VA, American Psychiatric Association, 2013

Bakolis I, Hammoud R, Stewart R, et al: Mental health consequences of urban air pollution: prospective population-based longitudinal survey. Soc Psychiatry Psychiatr Epidemiol 56(9):1587–1599, 2021 33097984

Baumann A, Farrell E, Stauffer C: American Lung Association poll. New York, Global Strategy Group, 2024

Buoli M, Grassi S, Caldiroli A, et al: Is there a link between air pollution and mental disorders? Environ Int 118:154–168, 2018 29883762

Calderón-Garcidueñas L, Leray E, Heydarpour P, et al: Air pollution, a rising environmental risk factor for cognition, neuroinflammation and neurodegeneration: the clinical impact on children and beyond. Rev Neurol (Paris) 172(1):69–80, 2016 26718591

Centers for Disease Control and Prevention: NIOSH-approved particulate filtering facepiece respirators, in The National Personal Protective Technology Laboratory (NPPTL). Atlanta, GA, Centers for Disease Control and Prevention, September 15, 2021. Available at: www.cdc.gov/niosh/npptl/topics/respirators/disp_part/default.html. Accessed December 12, 2024.

Chen JC, Wang X, Wellenius GA, et al: Ambient air pollution and neurotoxicity on brain structure: evidence from women's health initiative memory study. Ann Neurol 78(3):466–476, 2015

Chen Z, Salam MT, Eckel SP, et al: Chronic effects of air pollution on respiratory health in Southern California children: findings from the Southern California Children's Health Study. J Thorac Dis 7(1):46–58, 2015 25694817

Chun H, Leung C, Wen SW, et al: Maternal exposure to air pollution and risk of autism in children: a systematic review and meta-analysis. Environ Pollut 256:113307, 2020 31733973

Di Q, Wang Y, Zanobetti A, et al: Air pollution and mortality in the Medicare population. N Engl J Med 376(26):2513–2522, 2017 28657878

Donzelli G, Llopis-Gonzalez A, Llopis-Morales A, et al: Particulate matter exposure and attention-deficit/hyperactivity disorder in children: a systematic review of epidemiological studies. Int J Environ Res Public Health 17(1):67, 2019 31861799

Dumont C, Haase E, Dolber T, et al: Climate change and risk of completed suicide. J Nerv Ment Dis 208(7):559–565, 2020 32205773

Dutheil F, Comptour A, Morlon R, et al: Autism spectrum disorder and air pollution: a systematic review and meta-analysis. Environ Pollut 278:116856, 2021 33714060

Environmental Protection Agency: The Benefits and Costs of the Clean Air Act, 1970 to 1990: Report for U.S. Congress. Washington, DC, Environmental Protection Agency, 1997. Available at: www.epa.gov/ environmental-economics/benefits-and-costs-clean-air-act-1970-1990-1997. Accessed December 12, 2024.

Environmental Protection Agency: The Benefits and Costs of the Clean Air Act from 1990 to 2020: Summary Report. Washington, DC, Environmental Protection Agency, 2011. Available at: www.epa.gov/ clean-air-act-overview/benefits-and-costs-clean-air-act-1990-2020-second-prospective-study. Accessed December 12, 2024.

Fang D, Bing W, Yao-hui H, et al: The association of air pollutants with hospital outpatient visits for child and adolescence psychiatry in Shenzhen, China. Environ Res 216(Pt 2):114598, 2023

Fu P, Guo X, Cheung FMH, et al: The association between PM2.5 exposure and neurological disorders: a systematic review and meta-analysis. Sci Total Environ 655:1240–1248, 2019

Gu X, Guo T, Si Y, et al: Association between ambient air pollution and daily hospital admissions for depression in 75 Chinese cities. Am J Psychiatry 177(8):735–743, 2020 32312109

Hahad O, Lelieveld J, Birklein F, et al: Ambient air pollution increases the risk of cerebrovascular and neuropsychiatric disorders through induction of inflammation and oxidative stress. Int J Mol Sci 21(12):4306, 2020 32560306

He T, Jin L, Li X: On the triad of air PM pollution, pathogenic bioaerosols, and lower respiratory infection. Environ Geochem Health 45(4):1067–1077, 2023 34236582

Heo S, Lee W, Bell ML: Suicide and associations with air pollution and ambient temperature: a systematic review and meta-analysis. Int J Environ Res Public Health 18(14):7699, 2021 34300149

Herrnstadt E, Muehlegger E: Air Pollution and Criminal Activity: Evidence From Chicago Microdata (NBER Working Paper 21787). Cambridge, MA, National Bureau of Economic Research, 2015

Herting MM, Bottenhorn KL, Cotter DL: Outdoor air pollution and brain development in childhood and adolescence. Trends Neurosci 47(8):593–607, 2024 39054161

Ho RC, Zhang MW, Ho CS, et al: Impact of 2013 South Asian haze crisis: study of physical and psychological symptoms and perceived dangerousness of pollution level. BMC Psychiatry 14(1):81, 2014 24642046

Jbaily A, Zhou X, Liu J, et al: Air pollution exposure disparities across US population and income groups. Nature 601(7892):228–233, 2022 35022594

Kaur S, Morales-Hidalgo P, Arija V, et al: Prenatal exposure to air pollutants and attentional deficit hyperactivity disorder development in children: a systematic review. Int J Environ Res Public Health 20(8):5443, 2023 37107725

Kim Y, Manley J, Radoias V: Air pollution and long term mental health. Atmosphere (Basel) 11(12):1355, 2020

Ku BS, Haase E: Clearing the air for mental health: the Clean Air Act of 1963, in Struggle and Solidarity: Seven Stories of How Americans Fought for Their Mental Health Through Federal Legislation. Edited by Compton MT, Manseau MW. Washington, DC, American Psychiatric Association Publishing, 2023, pp 97–132

Kuo P-F, Putra IGB: Analyzing the relationship between air pollution and various types of crime. PLoS One 16(8):e0255653, 2021 34388188

Kurt OK, Zhang J, Pinkerton KE: Pulmonary health effects of air pollution. Curr Opin Pulm Med 22(2):138–143, 2016 26761628

Laumbach R, Meng Q, Kipen H: What can individuals do to reduce personal health risks from air pollution? J Thorac Dis 7(1):96–107, 2015 25694820

Lelieveld J, Klingmüller K, Pozzer A, et al: Cardiovascular disease burden from ambient air pollution in Europe reassessed using novel hazard ratio functions. Eur Heart J 40(20):1590–1596, 2019 30860255

Lin YC, Fan KC, Wu CD, et al: Yearly change in air pollution and brain aging among older adults: a community-based study in Taiwan. Environ Int 190:108876, 2024 39002330

Livingston G, Huntley J, Sommerlad A, et al: Dementia prevention, intervention, and care: 2020 report of the Lancet Commission. Lancet 396(10248):413–446, 2020 32738937

Manisalidis I, Stavropoulou E, Stavropoulos A, et al: Environmental and health impacts of air pollution: a review. Front Public Health 8:14, 2020 32154200

Muller RA, Muller EA: Air pollution and cigarette equivalence. Berkeley, CA, Berkeley Earth, December 17, 2015. Available at: https://berkeleyearth.org/air-pollution-and-cigarette-equivalence. Accessed December 12, 2024.

Newbury JB, Arseneault L, Beevers S, et al: Association of air pollution exposure with psychotic experiences during adolescence. JAMA Psychiatry 76(6):614–623, 2019 30916743

Nobile F, Forastiere A, Michelozzi P, et al: Long-term exposure to air pollution and incidence of mental disorders: a large longitudinal cohort study of adults within an urban area. Environ Int 181:108302, 2023 37944432

O'Brien S, Rauert C, Ribeiro F, et al: There's something in the air: a review of sources, prevalence and behaviour of microplastics in the atmosphere. Sci Total Environ 874:162193, 2023 36828069

Oudin A, Åström DO, Asplund P, et al: The association between daily concentrations of air pollution and visits to a psychiatric emergency unit: a case-crossover study. Environ Health 17(1):4, 2018 29321054

Owusu PA, Sarkodie SA: Global estimation of mortality, disability-adjusted life years and welfare cost from exposure to ambient air pollution. Sci Total Environ 742:140636, 2020 32721745

Perera FP: Multiple threats to child health from fossil fuel combustion: impacts of air pollution and climate change. Environ Health Perspect 125(2):141–148, 2017

Rajper SA, Ullah S, Li Z: Exposure to air pollution and self-reported effects on Chinese students: a case study of 13 megacities. PLoS One 13(3):e0194364, 2018 29547657

Sheffield PE, Speranza R, Chiu YM, et al: Association between particulate air pollution exposure during pregnancy and postpartum maternal psychological functioning. PLoS One 13(4):e0195267, 2018 29668689

Spiller E, Proville J, Roy A, et al: Mortality risk from PM2.5: a comparison of modeling approaches to identify disparities across racial/ethnic groups in policy outcomes. Environ Health Perspect 129(12):127004, 2021 34878311

Tsai TL, Lin YT, Hwang BF, et al: Fine particulate matter is a potential determinant of Alzheimer's disease: a systemic review and meta-analysis. Environ Res 177:108638, 2019 31421449

Ulrich RS: Visual landscapes and psychological well-being. Landsc Res 4(1):17–23, 1979

Williams T, Carel H: Breathlessness: from bodily symptom to existential experience, in Existential Medicine: Essays on Health and Illness. Edited by Aho K. Lanham, MD, Rowman and Littlefield International, 2018, pp 145–160

World Health Organization: Ambient Air Quality Database, 2022 Update: Status Report. Geneva, Switzerland, World Health Organization, 2023. Available at: www.who.int/publications/i/item/9789240047693. Accessed November 9, 2023.

Xie H, Cao Y, Li J, et al: Affective disorder and brain alterations in children and adolescents exposed to outdoor air pollution. J Affect Disord 331:413–424, 2023 36997124

Xu W, Ding X, Zhuang Y, et al: Perceived haze, stress, and negative emotions: an ecological momentary assessment study of the affective responses to haze. J Health Psychol 25(4):450–458, 2020 28810492

Xu Z, Sheffield PE, Hu W, et al: Climate change and children's health—a call for research on what works to protect children. Int J Environ Res Public Health 9(9):3298–3316, 2012 23202687

Yang T, Wang J, Huang J, et al: Long-term exposure to multiple ambient air pollutants and association with incident depression and anxiety. JAMA Psychiatry 80(4):305–313, 2023 36723924

Zeng Y, Lin R, Liu L, et al: Ambient air pollution exposure and risk of depression: a systematic review and meta-analysis of observational studies. Psychiatry Res 276:69–78, 2019 31029037

Zhou Z, Shuai X, Lin Z, et al: Association between particulate matter (PM)2.5 air pollution and clinical antibiotic resistance: a global analysis. Lancet Planet Health 7(8):e649–e659, 2023 37558346

6

Nutrition, Food and Water Insecurity, and Mental Health

Many aspects of climate change are contributing to food and water insecurity. These climate-related changes can be organized into three major categories:

1. Depletion of and damage to the soils, sources of water, oceans, and habitats that support food growth
2. Transient disruptions in the food and water supply resulting from extreme weather, drought, flooding, and so on
3. Changes in the growth patterns of food

Food security can also be impacted by human factors such as whether individuals have access to food and the stability of the food supply in relation to storage, prices, and global and local conflicts. Human emotions and behaviors around food are also affected by climate change, emerging from climate stresses and then contributing to worsened food and water management and production (Mbow et al. 2019). Climate-related food shifts have predicted nutritional effects relevant to psychiatry because of the importance of adequate food and nutrition for emotional and brain health. The aspects of climate-related changes to food and water systems with mental health implications are presented in Table 6.1.

93

Table 6.1 Climate-related food and water changes with mental health impacts

Food insecurity

Water insecurity

Decreased micronutrient and protein content

Increased risk of food toxins

As a rule of thumb, crop yield is predicted to drop about 10% for each 1.8°F increase in global temperature as warming continues. Wheat, maize, rice, and soybean production have been shown to decrease 3%–6% per 1.8°F temperature rise (Zhao et al. 2017). International development strategies that increase crop yield can help offset these impacts, but overall, climate-based losses in food production are projected to gradually and significantly outstrip improved food growth (see Fischer et al. 2005 for a detailed review). These losses will threaten the food supply of 80% of populations living in degraded environments by the end of the century, particularly those of disadvantaged and socially vulnerable groups, including women, older adults, and children (Sova et al. 2019). Loss of habitats, such as lakes and oceans for fishing or unique growing zones for fruits and vegetables, particularly threatens the sustainability of local communities and is also changing the global food economy. These global changes to food production will be associated with decreased availability of protein, iron, and zinc in particular (Beach et al. 2019; Mbow et al. 2019).

On the positive side, climate change provides an incentive to move toward a more sustainable and plant-based diet. This diet is difficult for developing nations to achieve but has the predicted benefits of reducing both land use and greenhouse gas emissions by greater than 50% and lowering cancer and all-cause mortality very significantly (Laine et al. 2021). Improved refrigeration, manure management, food transport and storage, and food-related carbon sequestration and reductions in fertilizer use, livestock dependence, and food waste will all contribute to this gain. This means that food and nutrition are an area where the negative impacts of climate change have the greatest room for positive mitigation and adaptation. Paying positive attention to food security efforts offers the additional benefit of improving nutrition-related outcomes in depression, psychosis, and disorders of early and late life described in this chapter.

Relevance of Climate-Related Food Insecurity for Psychiatry

Psychiatric Consequences of Food Insecurity

Around the world, and even in countries as wealthy as the United States, food insecurity affects about 12% of all persons and is associated with a 2%–3% negative impact on global economic productivity. In Africa, food insecurity affects more than 52% of the population, a number that is expected to rise (Trudell et al. 2021). Food insecurity is associated with numerous adverse psychiatric and medical outcomes, adding $52 billion annually—$5,527 per person—in medical costs for those on Medicare in the United States (Oronce et al. 2021).

Medically, food insecurity is not equivalent to starvation. It can be associated with both overweight and underweight habitus, as well as type 2 diabetes, hypertension, hyperlipidemia, osteoporosis, and vitamin deficiency syndromes, and, nonspecifically, a greater number of emergency department visits and inpatient hospital stays overall (Oronce et al. 2021). Psychiatrically, food insecurity is associated with several significant adverse mental health outcomes (Table 6.2). This relationship is dose-dependent and independent of physical health. It includes population-level increases in negative affective symptoms such as pain, sadness, stress, anger, and worry, which have been shown across 149 nations of all levels of affluence (Jones 2017), as well as higher rates of mental health diagnoses (Muldoon et al. 2013).

Table 6.2 Mental health impacts of food insecurity

In children	In adults
Negative affects	Negative affects
Stunting, wasting, and kwashiorkor	Sleep disorders
Depression	Anxiety disorders
Poor approach to learning, attention, and behavior	Depression
Reading, vocabulary, and math disorders	Stress and pain related to health

In children, food insecurity has adverse impacts on academic performance indicators, including reading, vocabulary, math, and approach to learning. Children with food insecurity also struggle with inattention, internalizing and externalizing behaviors, and depression (Gallegos et al. 2021; Shankar et al. 2017), often mediated in part by interactions with parental stress, the duration of food insecurity, pre-existing tendencies, and other factors (Gallegos et al. 2021). More severe inadequate food intake causing stunting or wasting (experienced by 30% of children globally) and lack of minimally acceptable diet (experienced by 84% of children globally) have similar adverse mental health consequences (Global Nutrition Report 2018). In adults, food insecurity is associated with increased positive screening for anxiety, depression, and sleep disorders in the range of 1.8- to 2.7-fold above baseline levels (Arenas et al. 2019) and with higher rates of suicide. Women are particularly vulnerable to food insecurity effects, with up to fourfold increases in related mental health diagnoses, as are HIV-positive persons and older adults (Anema et al. 2009; Trudell et al. 2021).

Regardless of socioeconomic status, and going against the intuitive expectation that gaining access to food would improve overall food consumption, food insecurity also increases the risk of disordered eating. A feast-or-famine pattern of food availability seems to increase binge-eating and also increases the compensatory behaviors for over-eating associated with restrictive eating disorders in both adolescents and adults, including vomiting, use of laxatives and diuretics, fasting, exercise, food restriction, and skipping meals. These behavioral changes are not subtle and are up to two- to tenfold more common in those with food insecurity than others: for example, more vomiting (20.4% vs. 2.6%) and laxative use (22.8% vs. 2.6%). Those with food insecurity also meet criteria for binge-eating disorder and bulimia nervosa about twice as often, and they experience higher rates of weight stigma and racial and ethnic discrimination (reviewed in Hazzard et al. 2020).

Food Insecurity, Violence, and Social Instability

Food instability is also associated with violent conflict. This association is bidirectional: violent conflict leads to food insecurity, and food insecurity leads to violent conflict. For example, the global food price crisis in 2007–2008 led to social unrest in at least 40 low- to middle-income countries. As summarized by Sova et al. (2023) for the United Nations World

Nutrition, Food and Water Insecurity, and Mental Health

Food Program USA, this causality is complex, mediated through rising food prices, lower agricultural yields, urban versus agrarian residence, and many other factors, including long-term problems for which food insecurity is the last straw of civil tolerance. Urbanization has led to 70% of food being consumed in cities. City residents are highly dependent on food imports to meet their needs, so if supplies are cut off, sudden food shortages can occur, and resultant conflicts can erupt quickly.

Highly local and temporal conditions also play a role. For example, rebel groups in sub-Saharan Africa may be more likely to attack for food in villages with high abundance if they are surrounded by areas of drought; but they may be less able to recruit from those villages, where the opportunity cost of joining the violence to gain access to food is relatively less beneficial than in villages where starving residents are wooed with food. Supporting cropland can thus have a pacifying effect (Koren and Bagozzi 2017).

Hunger, however, is not the primary driver of conflicts based on lack of food. Instead, studies demonstrate complex psychological etiologies more closely connected to perceptions, including desperation; anger at poor government action; and previous grievances related to inequality, unfairness, and ethnic group differences. Foods with cultural significance, such as the "pasta riots" in Italy and "tortilla riots" in Mexico, are more likely to gather widespread unrest because they mobilize a group identity, a sense of common distress, and a collective ability to act, findings in line with terror management theory (covered in Chapter 9, "Obstacles to Rational and Adequate Responses to Climate Change"). Climate change is a direct driver of food-related instability through its influence on extreme weather, which leads to resource losses, resource competition, and economic shocks. Since 1990, global conflict has increased by more than 60%, and civil conflict in sub-Saharan Africa may increase 30% as temperatures rise further (Jun 2017). For psychiatrists, this increased psychological and civic unrest and violence associated with food insecurity implies that more patients will present with violent trauma and that patients not directly affected may experience vicarious trauma in reality as well as in fantasy, feeling that the world is falling apart, frightening, and unpredictable, and perhaps reacting with regressive and authoritarian identifications. Helping patients navigate increased unrest while maintaining a secure and curious relationship with the outside world may increasingly require more discussion of security risks and deeper immersion in global, political, and cultural psychology.

Psychological and Cultural Factors Associated With Food Insecurity

As is evident in the data about food-based conflict in the previous section, "Food Insecurity, Violence, and Social Instability," food consumption is associated with considerable personal and cultural meaning, steeped in family, local, and national traditions. It follows that changes in food supply will shape the stories around food that patients will encounter. At a global level, narratives about the food supply system can be shaped by different concerns that can be listened for in patient sense-making of climate food issues:

- How much food is available?
- What is the quality of the available food?
- How diverse is the available food?
- Who will keep up the production of food?
- What will happen to the animals and water around us?
- How fair is our access to food?
- How stable is our access to food?
- How much agency do I have over getting and using my food?

Each of these narratives will activate various aspects of the patient's individual food psychology. For those who have been raised in poverty, those for whom food was used as punishment or reward, and those from cultures with transgenerational experiences of traumatic starvation, among others, the inability to access the types and quantities of foods to which they are accustomed will be imbued with meaning and potentially will trigger more exaggerated climate anxiety responses. Emotions of deprivation, entitlement, and greed will be active in patients' minds. Those with compulsive disorders such as obsessive-compulsive disorder and hoarding disorder, as well as those with anorexia nervosa, bulimia nervosa, binge-eating disorder, and psychotic distortions of appetite-related beliefs due to depression or schizophrenia, are likely to understand the inability to obtain particular foods or more difficulty accessing food in line with the cognitive mindsets of their psychiatric illness, with potentially maladaptive responses. The disordered eating attitudes and behaviors that might be expected to result from such psychological factors are themselves associated independently with greater depressive symptoms and suicidality and with progression to full-scale eating disorders, even in people

Nutrition, Food and Water Insecurity, and Mental Health 99

who do not fit the SWAG (skinny White affluent girl) stereotype of the anorexic patient, such as parents anxious about being able to feed their children. Food insecurity also provides psychological challenges for older adults, who often have high medical costs and may forgo needed medications in order to eat.

Each of these food narratives will also produce a different community of food concern and line of action (Béné et al. 2019) at the societal level that is associated with emotional reactions unique to each affected global culture. To take one example: Shawi men in the Amazon have described shame for their inability to bring home meat because of less animal life in the forest. They also express guilt and moral injury for actions that violate their spiritual connection to their land and animals, such as cutting trees to build roads, but feel compelled to take these actions because they bring greater wealth and access to government resources (Arotoma-Rojas et al. 2022), showing the intersectional identity issues that can arise as food sources change.

Vignette

Aliza, age 42, presented for psychotherapy, reporting work burnout at an underfunded nongovernmental organization and difficulties with her teenage daughter. The therapist learned that Aliza worked for an international food charity overstrained by climate demands and that her daughter was struggling with anorexia and complaining of both neglect and overcontrol by her mother in the limited time they had together. Aliza had been raised in relative poverty by Holocaust survivors and herself struggled with perfectionism and disordered eating, which she related to her family's worries about food adequacy and success in their new world. Her family history demonstrates climate-relevant issues of transgenerational trauma, migrant mental health, and climate-disordered eating.

Over the course of the therapy, Aliza was able to work successfully on her food issues and relationships by focusing on the local food supply and using horticulture therapy, mentoring her daughter and her friends in a community garden. The community garden inspired some of them to work in similar fields, creating new food narratives of recovery and emphasizing community building. In part through the relational experience of tending plants that then fed her, Aliza learned to recognize her interdependence with others and began interacting in a more empowering and flexible way with her coworkers, who were then able to pick up some of her load. She remained depressed, however, citing the reminders of food insecurity and traumatic stress in her work and her continual exposure to children with kwashiorkor. After consulting with a psychiatrist, she was also found to have low zinc and iron as a result of poor nutritional access in her fieldwork; repletion contributed to remission in her symptoms.

Food and Nutritional Deficiencies in Migrants and Refugees

Migrants and refugees, often forcibly displaced by natural or human-made disasters, have differing but related patterns of nutritional change. The number of climate refugees is expected to increase to as many as 400 million people by the end of this century (Hooijer and Vernimmen 2021), making an understanding of their unique status critical for successful integration into their new homes. Migrants experience numerous nutritional challenges associated with moving from one country's food environment to another, often enduring a significant period of hardship along the way. These include the following:

- The emotional losses and challenges of leaving behind native foods and acculturating to a new food environment
- The nutritional changes associated with shifting from one food culture to another
- The economic challenges of feeding oneself and one's family in a new country

The concept of the *double burden of malnutrition* refers to the common experience of migrants who begin life in circumstances of malnutrition and starvation and then become burdened in their new country by high-calorie, low-nutritional-value diets and the obesity and medical diseases associated with them. In as many as 15 countries, obesity occurs at rates of 40% or more of residents alongside the starvation measures of child wasting (15%) and stunting (30%) or high maternal thinness; the number increases to 45 countries if the obesity rate is reevaluated at 20% prevalence (Popkin et al. 2020). Rates of vitamin D deficiency can be as high as 80% in this doubly burdened group, whether overweight or underweight in their new home (Ankomah et al. 2022). This double-burden phenomenon is concentrated in the Global South and in rural and impoverished areas, and it is associated with sedentary lifestyles and nonessential food and beverage sales.

Protein-Calorie Malnutrition in the Setting of Natural Disasters

Malnutrition related to climate change is particularly important to consider in areas affected by acute and chronic natural disasters, where it concentrates particularly in infants and children and mortality rates can approach 20% (World Health Organization 2007). Malnutrition includes deficiencies of macronutrients and micronutrients such as iron, zinc, and vitamin A, which render children more susceptible to disaster-related diarrhea and pneumonia, as well as the neuropsychiatric and general health consequences of these deficiencies. These problems can begin within a few months of a natural disaster and have a high prevalence; for example, stunting and underweight were found in 50%–60% of children in drought-affected areas of India (Singh et al. 2006) and in 25% of children after an earthquake in China (Dong et al. 2014). Rates of micronutrient deficiency were also high (50%–80%) 4 months after an earthquake, and rates of anemia 25%–75% and at least 60%–65% rates of vitamin A, D, and zinc deficiencies have been found in children living in African refugee camps (reviewed in Seal et al. 2005; Yin and Dong 2015).

Various strategies for supplementing nutrition are available for use in disaster scenarios as well as global malnutrition programs. As summarized in Yin and Dong (2015) and WHO recommendations for community nutrition management (2007), these include the following:

- Complementary food supplements (ages 6 months to 3 years)—supplemented soy or cow's milk powder. Advantages include easy and safe room-temperature storage, high fat, and protein. The powder is mixed into a paste with 30 cc of boiled, cooled water and added to porridge, noodles, soup, or other food.
- Lipid-based nutrient supplements—fortified lipid-based pastes for children of all ages. No cooking or water is required, making these supplements useful when water supplies are contaminated. They are divided into ready-to-use therapeutic foods for more severe malnutrition, which contain 700 kcals and are associated with an 88% recovery rate (Gera 2010), and ready-to-use supplementary foods, which are cheaper and better for preventing widespread malnutrition in food-challenged areas.
- Micronutrient sprinkles—single-dose sachets containing micronutrients but no protein or fatty acid supplementation for

sprinkling on food in children younger than age 5. These packets are easy to transport and to mix with other foods and supplements and are shown to improve anemia (Jack et al. 2012).

The provision of these supplements requires community-based identification and referral for at-risk children. Local production of food supplements and redirection of excess foods can also shore up the local food supply.

Screening and Interventions for Food Insecurity

As food insecurity increases globally, screening for it increasingly will become the bread-and-butter of a psychiatric evaluation. A simple and accurate way to screen patients for food insecurity is by using the U.S. Food Security Scale (USFSS, www.ers.usda.gov/topics/food-nutrition-assistance/food-security-in-the-u-s/survey-tools), an 18-item assessment that can be shortened to 2 or 6 items for efficiency. Medical support staff have been shown to be more effective than clinicians in conducting this assessment. The first two questions, the so-called *hunger vital signs*, have 97% sensitivity and 83% specificity (Cutts and Cook 2017) for detecting food insecurity: Ask patients how often in the past 12 months they have

- Worried whether food would run out before they got money to buy more
- Had the food that they bought run out and did not have money to get more

If a patient reports food insecurity, numerous possible interventions can be considered. These include the following possibilities:

- Food referrals: either information about food resources or active connection to community and government food resource agencies, such as the Supplemental Nutrition Assistance Program (SNAP) or its corollary for Women, Infants, and Children (WIC)
- Fruit and vegetable vouchers
- Direct food provision: programs that provide food at a site such as a senior center or through meal delivery such as Meals on Wheels

- Community interventions to reduce food deserts and increase community gardening

Evidence suggests that home-delivered meals are most effective at improving the combined goals of food security, healthy eating, and some health-related measures. On-site food and food voucher programs work well to decrease food insecurity but may not yield healthy eating or better health. There is no strong support for other interventions, and food security in itself has not been shown to have a clear impact on health parameters such as emergency department visits, blood pressure, hemoglobin A1c levels, and BMI (De Marchis et al. 2020; Oronce et al. 2021). On-site meal provision and community gardening may be helpful for those who are more isolated because they may have the co-benefits of increasing social contact and community sustainability. Community gardens do not clearly improve food security, but they do show evidence of improving life satisfaction, social support and contact, and general physical and mental health independent of food intake in a general population (Lampert et al. 2021). Community gardens require more study to understand how to make them accessible and effective for the food-insecure group.

Water Insecurity Considerations for Mental Health

Fresh water insecurity is an additional consequence of global warming that already affects 4 billion people at least 1 month per year (Mekonnen and Hoekstra 2016). Although water insecurity is understudied in terms of its mental health implications, it is clear that water shortages increase mental distress, whether from a water crisis such as occurred in Flint, Michigan, from a drought, or from other causes. In a review of 25 studies, Kimutai et al. (2023) found a uniform association between water insecurity and mental distress, mental well-being, and common mental disorders such as depression and anxiety.

Water insecurity can exacerbate shame, anger, and gender-based violence against women, who more often are the ones to maintain the family water supply (Wutich et al. 2022). It can contribute to gender inequity when greater time obtaining water—sometimes hours in disadvantaged areas—takes away other developmental opportunities, particularly education for girls. Issues related to shared water, sanitation, financial and social capital, and justice play a significant role in this inequity and also contribute to the distress associated with inadequate drinking water service (Toivettula et al. 2023).

Water insecurity is also associated with higher rates of physical illnesses such as kidney failure and cardiac disease, poor immune function, musculoskeletal injury, low birth weight, premature aging of telomeres, and mental health effects including higher stress levels, poor concentration, and anxiety, as well as the mental and metabolic consequences of relying on alcoholic and sugared drinks as a substitute (Rosinger 2023). Those with poor mental health have more trouble collecting adequate water during shortages and feel differently about the effort, disease risk, and social reward of water-related efforts (Slekiene and Mosler 2019) and may require psychiatric support and advocacy to obtain adequate water supplies. Fluid intake and availability can be easily added to the routine monitoring of alcohol and caffeine consumption in psychiatric practice; this may contribute to greater awareness and study of the impacts of dehydration and fluid limitation on mental symptoms as more communities and individuals become affected.

Plant Toxins Increased by Climate Change and Their Health Effects

In addition to its effects on food availability, climate change is altering the makeup of soil, including its carbon and nitrogen content, soil moisture, microorganism content, and other elements that change the constituents of plant growth. Elevated atmospheric CO_2 concentrations lead crops to grow more quickly (so-called *CO_2 fertilization*). Plants that grow quickly incorporate less nitrogen into plant proteins. Additionally, both nitrates (NO_3) and nitrites (NO_2, which is more toxic) can accumulate under various meteorological circumstances linked to climate change, such as when it rains just before harvest or in a dry year. Nitrates can be toxic to animals and humans who ingest these grains, which include corn, barley, soybean, wheat, and other common crops. Rapid regrowth from irrigation or rain after a drought can also lead to the accumulation of hydrogen cyanide (prussic acid) in common food sources, including flax, maize, sorghum, and sunflower, and this can cause substantial livestock mortality. Although toxicity is rare in humans, clinical characteristics of nitrate and prussic acid poisoning in both animals and humans include the following (Stichler and Reagor 2014):

Nutrition, Food and Water Insecurity, and Mental Health

- Cellular oxygen depletion (hypoxia)
- Weakness and loss of coordination
- Tachycardia and tachypnea
- Seizures, coma, and death

As weather fluctuates more dramatically from drought to extreme rain, clinicians may be presented with cases of such poisoning syndromes.

Fungal mycotoxins are expected to increase with climate change; they currently infect 25% of the world's cereals. Additionally, drought conditions favor the production of aflatoxins by *Aspergillus* fungi (United Nations Environment Programme 2016). Aflatoxins increase in crops that are stressed by drought and insects and in warm (86°F) humid conditions. Toxicity causes nausea, vomiting, abdominal pain, and seizures, and it is associated with the following:

- Cancers connected with the *P53* gene
- Hepatitis progressing to cirrhosis and hepatic cancer
- Stunting and cognitive impairment in children
- Immunosuppression

Aflatoxin toxicity can be assessed by relevant history and the measurement of AFB1-lysine, a metabolite. No specific antidote is available, so treatment is through supportive measures (Dhakal et al. 2023; United Nations Environment Programme 2016).

The cumulative toxicity of these changes in plant growth is often referred to as the *poisoned chalice* of climate food impacts. It is likely to disproportionately affect disadvantaged groups with lesser food access, who have greater exposure to environmental chemical toxins such as pesticides, mercury, and lead (Donley et al. 2022; Jones et al. 2022). The impacts of such combined climate and environmental injustice may also be carried across generations through epigenetic changes, leaving a multidimensional *toxic legacy* of these exposures (Kryder-Reid and May 2024). These combined multigenerational effects demonstrate how climate change acts as a threat multiplier, particularly for vulnerable populations.

Vignette

Lee is a 65-year-old farmer who presents to his primary care doctor for emotional management of hypochondriasis, with chronic complaints of unexplained anorexia, fatigue, palpitations, headache, and a mild transaminitis. Aware of climate impacts, his psychiatrist tests for aflatoxin and hydrogen cyanide, and the tests return elevated levels of both. An abdominal CT scan shows an incidental early liver cancer. Lee is able to retire and relocate with remission of all his symptoms. His case prompts the collaborative care team to engage in local public health efforts to improve grain storage and groundwater testing for pesticides that may have contributed to his cancer, and to increase public health awareness of the cumulative climate and environmental toxins in their rural community. As a result, early detection of related tumors improved and rates of toxic deaths lessened.

Changes in Micronutrient and Protein Availability With Climate Change and Associated Psychiatric Outcomes

The major nutritional deficiencies expected to increase from climate change are lower food content of protein, iron, and zinc. Beach et al. (2019) have predicted climate-related decreases in the global availability of protein (19.5%), iron (14.4%), and zinc (14.6%) as early as 2050 relative to their expected increased availability from technology and improved markets at that date. Smith and Myers (2018) project that under the Representative Concentration Pathway (RCP) 8.5 emissions scenario (550 ppm CO_2), 1%–2% of the global population will be zinc- or protein-deficient, and half of the at-risk population of women and small children will be newly deficient in iron. Those with existing deficiencies will be at risk of worsening deficiency and more severe health outcomes from their deficits. Micronutrient deficiencies will be heavily concentrated in India, China, the Middle East, Africa, and South Asia (Beach et al. 2019; Smith and Myers 2018).

In planning for the health and psychiatric implications of these predicted shifts, it is important for organized psychiatric efforts to do the following:

- Consider how social, geopolitical, and economic circumstances are influencing people's ability to compensate for nutrient deficiency
- Watch for downstream effects of compensating for nutrient deficiency, such as more diagnosed cases of pica or higher rates of vitamin and other toxicity from supplements

- Account for improvements in global food supply and content due to technology and food practices
- Recognize disproportionate health consequences when micronutrient deficiencies are moderate to severe; mild deficiencies may not have significant clinical consequences, particularly in affluent societies

Psychiatric Consequences of Protein Deficiency and Treatment

The predicted dietary protein deficiency associated with climate-related food changes has implications for psychiatrists and organized mental health efforts, primarily at the beginning and end of the life cycle, as well as broad general implications for population survival. In children, malnutrition predominantly due to protein deficiency is called kwashiorkor and is found mostly in children ages 3–5 years. It is associated with abdominal distention; brittle, colorless hair; dermatitis; fatty liver; and peripheral edema. It is rare in developed countries and is predicted to remain so. Affected children are more irritable, fatigued, and vulnerable to infections and system collapse and experience stunted intellectual and physical growth. Pancreatic atrophy and cirrhosis can complicate long-term recovery. Kwashiorkor is distinguished from marasmus, in which children are deficient in protein, fat, calories, and nutrients and are small and cachectic. Both groups, however, experience similar neurodevelopmental consequences.

In late life, older adults have more difficulty consuming adequate protein because of dental disease and reduced masticatory strength as well as financial limitations. In this group, lower protein intake has been significantly associated with mild cognitive impairment, amyloid-β accumulation, and Alzheimer's disease. Supplementation with essential amino acids through therapeutic foods has been shown to improve attention, social functioning, and cognitive flexibility, and other protein supplementation improves reaction time and verbal episodic memory (Suzuki et al. 2020). Particular attention to the impacts of climate-related changes in protein consumption in both the old and young age groups is therefore warranted, and work is underway through the United Nations Global Action Plan on Child Wasting.

Psychiatric Consequences of Zinc Deficiency and Treatment

Zinc is a ubiquitous component of cellular metabolism and plays an important role in immune function, wound healing, synthesis of protein and DNA, and cell signaling, growth, and division. The National Institutes of Health (NIH) Office of Dietary Supplements and ConsumerLab provide the following summary of the role of zinc in human nutrition: Dietary zinc is primarily derived from meat and seafood (especially oysters), as well as several other foods with lesser absorption, and it is stored in skeletal muscle and bone, with body stores of 1.5 g in women and 2.5 g in men. In the United States, fortified breakfast cereals are a major zinc source. Serum levels are a poor indicator of body zinc status, but low levels suggest a need for repletion. Absorption can be reduced if zinc is taken with supplements containing more than 25 mg of iron (ConsumerLab 2024).

The recommended daily allowance for zinc varies from 3–5 mg in children to 9–13 mg in teens and older adults depending on size, with maximized recommendations for lactating persons. Supplements range from 30 mg to 50 mg and have typically been shown to contain the amount of zinc advertised. Those that can be recommended and have at least 60% absorption in adults include the following:

- Zinc picolinate
- Zinc acetate
- Zinc bisglycinate

Signs of significant zinc deficiency are predominantly immune, psychiatric, and dermatological, such as the following:

- Dermatological disorders, including alopecia, skin rashes, and breakdowns such as angular cheilitis and poor wound healing
- Increased infections, including pneumonia and malaria (important given the rise of this illness with climate change)
- Growth limitation in children
- Cognitive problems across the life span
- Depression and psychosis

High-dose (70 mg) zinc supplementation has been shown to shorten the length of colds by a third and improve outcomes in macular degeneration. Excess zinc consumption, however, can cause gastrointestinal

Nutrition, Food and Water Insecurity, and Mental Health 109

Table 6.3 Patients at high risk for zinc deficiency
People with inflammatory bowel disease
Bariatric surgery patients
Vegetarians, especially vegans
Pregnant or lactating patients
Infants exclusively breastfed beyond age 6 months
Children with sickle cell disease (due to the effects of iron chelation therapy)
People with alcohol use disorders (alcohol decreases intestinal zinc absorption and increases renal zinc excretion)

symptoms and interfere with magnesium and copper absorption and balance.

Patients at particular risk for zinc deficiency, who may be more easily tipped into deficit by climate-related factors, are listed in Table 6.3. Medications commonly taken by psychiatric patients that may also interfere with zinc absorption and transport are listed in Table 6.4.

Psychiatrically, zinc is closely associated with depression and psychosis. In the brain, zinc is found in higher levels in the amygdala, hippocampus, and cortex, where zinc inhibits glycine-mediated activation. This occurs predominantly in zinc-enriched neurons, which are glutamatergic. Zinc is also associated with increased levels of brain-derived neurotrophic factor.

Multiple human studies have demonstrated the relationship between depression and zinc. Zinc levels average 12 μg/mL lower in subjects with depression, on par with the decrease predicted from climate effects. Low zinc levels are associated with higher cortisol and C-reactive protein and with decreased neurogenesis (Wang et al. 2018). Depressive symptoms improve with zinc supplementation at doses of 30–50 mg daily, including in nondepressed people, depressed subjects, and those with treatment-resistant depression. Zinc may improve depressive symptoms in numerous ways, possibly through its complex balancing effects on neuroplasticity, its N-methyl-D-aspartate receptor inhibition, and its modulation of 5-HT_{1A} receptors (reviewed in Petrilli et al. 2017).

Zinc is also important in the development and symptomatology of psychosis, likely magnified by genetic differences in zinc transport. Patients with schizophrenia have been shown to have decreased brain

Table 6.4 Medications that interfere with zinc absorption and transport

Proton pump inhibitors and histamine H_2 antagonists

Aluminum and calcium products

Anticonvulsants (valproic acid derivatives)

Medications for diabetes

Hormones

Anti-inflammatories

Antibiotics, including quinolones, tetracyclines, penicillamines, and cephalexin

Antiretrovirals, including ritonavir, atazanavir, and integrase inhibitors

Cardiovascular medications, including amiloride

Thiazide diuretics

zinc compared with control subjects in a postmortem sample and living subjects with other cerebral diseases. Zinc levels have been shown to be particularly low in patients with schizophrenia with violent or criminal behavior, with improvements in both psychosis and aggression after supplementation of 660 mg of zinc daily. Phenothiazine antipsychotics have been shown to improve zinc uptake (reviewed in Petrilli et al. 2017).

Psychiatric Consequences of Iron Deficiency and Treatment

Iron is a mineral that has well-known roles in the function of hemoglobin and myoglobin and subsequent importance for tissue oxygenation. Most iron is stored in hemoglobin, with the remainder in ferritin and hemosiderin. Because iron-deficiency anemia occurs only with significant body iron depletion, ferritin is currently considered the most efficient and cost-effective single test for iron deficiency, with values less than 30 mcg/L considered significant.

Most residents of North America, western Europe, and Australasian nations get adequate iron from food and supplemented cereals, whereas those residing in sub-Saharan Africa and South Asia bear the greatest anemia burden (Gardner et al. 2023). Groups particularly vulnerable to

Nutrition, Food and Water Insecurity, and Mental Health 111

Table 6.5 Patients at risk of iron deficiency

Patients of childbearing age and children, particularly in Hispanic populations

Frequent blood donors

Patients with cancer

Patients with congestive heart failure

Patients with Crohn's disease, celiac disease, and ulcerative colitis

---

iron deficiency are listed in Table 6.5. For supplementation, ferrous salts containing 40–45 mg of iron taken on a daily basis are preferred over ferric or other forms. Daily iron doses of 7–11 mg are adequate for ages spanning from infants to older adults, but individuals who are in child-bearing years, lactating, or pregnant require daily doses of 15–27 mg.

Symptoms of more severe iron-deficiency anemia include weakness and fatigue, impaired concentration and cognition, and changes in immune and thermoregulatory abilities. Iron toxicity is characterized primarily by gastrointestinal effects, although large overdoses can be fatal. Excess iron intake can also interfere with the metabolism of zinc and medications, including levodopa, levothyroxine, and proton pump inhibitors (National Institutes of Health 2024).

The importance of iron chemistry in the brain is elegant, grossly underappreciated, and well worth a detailed read. Brain iron is highly stable and affects both the synthesis and signaling of dopamine, noradrenaline, adrenaline, and 5-hydroxytryptamine. Iron-dependent enzymes important for psychiatry include phenylalanine hydroxy-lase, tyrosine hydroxylase, and tryptophan hydroxylase. The brain also relies on iron for its role in mitochondrial adenosine triphosphate (ATP) generation for its high energy needs, the differentiation of oligo-dendrocytes, the synthesis of myelin components, and other functions (Hare et al. 2013).

Brain iron deficiency is associated with many developmental delays in children, including deficits in fine and gross motor skills, visual-motor integration, and verbal and total IQ. It is also associated with social and attentional problems and higher scores for anxiety and depression, although human studies have controlled poorly for related social and nutritional factors. Animal models, however, affirm these deficits. In a study of a health insurance database, Chen et al. (2013)

found high odds ratios for psychiatric disorders in children and adolescents with iron-deficiency anemia. These included unipolar depression (OR 2.34, 95% CI [1.58~3.46]), bipolar disorder (OR 5.78, 95% CI [2.23~15.05]), anxiety disorder (OR 2.17, 95% CI [1.49~3.16]), autism spectrum disorder (OR 3.08, 95% CI [1.79~5.28]), ADHD (OR 1.67, 95% CI [1.29~2.17]), tic disorder (OR 1.70, 95% CI [1.03~2.78]), developmental delay (OR 2.45, 95% CI [2.00~3.00]), and intellectual developmental disorder (OR 2.70, 95% CI [2.00~3.65]). The elevated rates of bipolar disorder and tic disorder were found only in females. In adults, iron deficiency has been associated with an adjusted hazards ratio of 1.52 (95% CI [1.45–1.59]) for anxiety and sleep disorders, depression, and psychosis (Lee et al. 2020). Other studies show both higher and lower levels of serum iron, ferritin, and chemical correlates of localized brain iron levels under conditions of stress and depression, which may reflect the role of iron in acute and chronic inflammatory changes associated with mood disorders, with further study needed (reviewed in Duarte-Silva et al. 2025). In later years, a recently discovered cell death pathway of ferroptosis and possibly excess brain iron contribute to cell loss in neurogenerative disorders, including Alzheimer's, Parkinson's, and Huntington's diseases, and brain iron deficiency may be associated with restless legs syndrome (Hare et al. 2013; Stockwell et al. 2017).

Role of Psychiatrist in Assessing and Mitigating the Nutrition and Food Impacts of Climate Change

Currently, the world produces more cereal and more meat than is needed to meet human needs (Mbow et al. 2019) but with deficits in the quantities of micronutrients and poor diversity of vegetables, fruits, and legumes. Reduced consumption of meat, which is associated with high greenhouse gas emissions, is both a health and sustainability goal. Just producing the foodstuffs needed for healthier, more diverse diets, however, does not guarantee sustainability. For example, a healthy diet of fish and fruit may result in overfishing or overharvesting or in greater greenhouse gases used in their procurement and transport, and thus can threaten the environmental sustainability of improved eating patterns. Climate-related decreases in and disruptions to food production and availability are also occurring contemporaneously with the globalization of the food market. As a result, shifts toward

Nutrition, Food and Water Insecurity, and Mental Health 113

more processed food, more colonized and sedentary ways of life, and more cultural losses are trending alongside food deficits, particularly for Indigenous groups. These combined issues raise concerns about the impact of poor quality and inadequate food on mental health.

Taken in sum, the considerations described in this chapter suggest that the average psychiatrist may be presented with a diverse set of psychological and neuropsychiatric reactions to changing and diminishing food and water supplies and efforts toward sustainable eating over the coming decades. Many other nutritional parameters have been shown to play an important role in psychiatric disorders, including B vitamins as well as vitamins C, D, and E; folate; and various fatty acids (Cornish and Mehl-Madrona 2008). Changes in food supply may equally affect the intake of these food elements. Awareness of these associations can lead to better investigation and response, including screening patients for food insecurity and food changes and understanding the accompanying psycho-emotional and psychiatric impacts. The clinician is advised to be more vigilant to the relevant symptoms and signs of worsening nutritional deficiencies overall, particularly in patients who are more vulnerable because of illness or poor baseline nutrition, and to supplement as appropriate, particularly in those with depressive, cognitive, eating, childhood, and psychotic disorders.

This role of the psychiatrist in combating the nutritional challenges of the coming climate-changed century can include individual, local, and international acts. At the individual level, an appropriate set of tasks might consist of the following:

- Asking about patients' diets and educating them about their nutritional needs
- Measuring important nutritional parameters affected by climate change, including zinc, ferritin, B_{12}, folate, and possibly essential amino acids in older adults, particularly in patients with marginal diets or food absorption
- Treating with supplements as appropriate
- Remaining vigilant to clinical signs of food insecurity, disordered eating, food toxicity, and malnutrition
- Listening for the emotional narratives that run through a patient's concerns about food and nutrition
- Referring patients to meal and meal voucher programs
- Encouraging patients to grow their own food for both emotional and nutritional benefits (Kemper 2022)

At the community level, psychiatrists can play numerous roles to ensure a healthy food and water supply for community members. These can include the following steps:

- Providing public education about how nutritional deficits and psychiatric disorders are related
- Destigmatizing food insecurity and disordered eating by raising awareness of their prevalence in the context of climate-related impacts
- Educating public officials and medical personnel about the toxins associated with climate-related food changes and their clinical effects
- Contributing to food efficiency planning, such as systems to redirect excess restaurant and grocery food to food banks, legislation to permit dumpster diving, and increasing local sourcing of difficult-to-obtain foods
- Contributing to lowering food waste and meat consumption by advocating for changes in food, food storage, and portion size at their own and other community institutions
- Advocating for community gardening programs to improve mental health

At the level of international advocacy, psychiatrists can lend their professional voice to raise empathy for those who are experiencing the greatest climate-related nutritional and food deficits. They can also lend their expertise to global nutrition programs, ensuring that populations that are more vulnerable to mental disorders due to nutritional deficits receive special attention. Because of the emotional importance of food, physician advocacy to pair climate awareness with food and water insecurity may facilitate engagement with climate change at multiple social action levels.

Key Points

- The effects of climate change on soil, food, and water systems will increasingly cause food insecurity, disordered eating, increased psychiatric disorders, and food-related impacts on violence, migration, child health, and physical illness.

Nutrition, Food and Water Insecurity, and Mental Health

- The *poisoned chalice* of aberrant food growth due to climate effects places more patients at risk of clinical toxicity from cyanide, aflatoxins, and nitrates.
- Food insecurity affects large segments of the population across countries and is associated with many difficulties, including developmental and learning disorders, disordered eating, intergroup violence, and psychological distress.
- Water insecurity clearly contributes to mental health distress but is an understudied area of psychiatric knowledge.
- Zinc, iron, and protein deficiencies are predicted to significantly increase with climate change, leading to higher rates of depression, bipolar disorder, psychosis, and cognitive disorders.
- Food systems are an area where human behavior can particularly improve outcomes, and they are laden with emotional narratives that can facilitate engagement with climate mitigation.
- Many psychiatric roles, ranging from global policy work to individual psychotherapy, can incorporate assessing for and responding to climate-related food distress.

References

Anema A, Vogenthaler N, Frongillo EA, et al: Food insecurity and HIV/AIDS: current knowledge, gaps, and research priorities. Curr HIV/AIDS Rep 6(4):224–231, 2009 19849966

Ankomah A, Byaruhanga J, Woolley E, et al: Double burden of malnutrition among migrants and refugees in developed countries: a mixed-methods systematic review. PLoS One 17(8):e0273382, 2022 35981085

Arenas DJ, Thomas A, Wang J, et al: A systematic review and meta-analysis of depression, anxiety, and sleep disorders in US adults with food insecurity. J Gen Intern Med 34(12):2874–2882, 2019 31385212

Arotoma-Rojas I, Berrang-Ford L, Zavaleta-Cortijo C, et al: Indigenous peoples' perceptions of their food system in the context of climate change: a case study of Shawi men in the Peruvian Amazon. Sustainability 14(24):16502, 2022

Beach RH, Sulser TB, Crimmins A, et al: Combining the effects of increased atmospheric carbon dioxide on protein, iron, and zinc availability and projected climate change on global diets: a modelling study. Lancet Planet Health 3(7):e307–e317, 2019 31326071

Béné C, Oosterveer P, Lamotte L, et al: When food systems meet sustainability—current narratives and implications for actions. World Dev 113:116–130, 2019

Chen M-H, Su T-P, Chen Y-S, et al: Association between psychiatric disorders and iron deficiency anemia among children and adolescents: a nationwide population-based study. BMC Psychiatry 13(1):161, 2013 23735056

ConsumerLab: Zinc supplements and lozenges review. Vernon, NJ, ConsumerLab, 2024. Available at: www.consumerlab.com/reviews/zinc-supplements-lozenges-review/zinc/?search=Zinc. Accessed November 24, 2024.

Cornish S, Mehl-Madrona L: The role of vitamins and minerals in psychiatry. Integr Med Insights 3:33–42, 2008 21614157

Cutts D, Cook J: Screening for food insecurity: short-term alleviation and long-term prevention. Am J Public Health 107(11):1699–1700, 2017 29019766

De Marchis E, Fichtenberg C, Gottlieb LM: Food Insecurity Interventions in Health Care Settings: A Review of the Evidence. San Francisco, CA, Social Interventions Research and Evaluation Network, 2020

Dhakal A, Hashmi MF, Sbar E: Aflatoxin toxicity, in StatPearls. Treasure Island, FL, StatPearls, February 19, 2023

Dong C, Ge P, Ren X, et al: The micronutrient status of children aged 24–60 months living in rural disaster areas one year after the Wenchuan Earthquake. PLoS One 9(2):e88444, 2014 24533089

Donley N, Bullard RD, Economos J, et al: Pesticides and environmental injustice in the USA: root causes, current regulatory reinforcement and a path forward. BMC Public Health 22(1):708, 2022 35436924

Duarte-Silva E, Maes M, Alves Peixoto C: Iron metabolism dysfunction in neuropsychiatric disorders: implications for therapeutic intervention. Behav Brain Res 479:115343, 2025 39557130

Fischer G, Shah M, Tubiello FN, et al: Socio-economic and climate change impacts on agriculture: an integrated assessment, 1990–2080. Philos Trans R Soc Lond B Biol Sci 360(1463):2067–2083, 2005 16433094

Gallegos D, Eivers A, Sondergeld P, et al: Food insecurity and child development: a state-of-the-art review. Int J Environ Res Public Health 18(17):8990, 2021 34501578

Gardner WM, Hagins H, Zoeckler LZ, et al: Prevalence, years lived with disability, and trends in anaemia burden by severity and cause, 1990–2021: findings from the Global Burden of Disease Study 2021. Lancet Haematol 10(9):e713–e734, 2023 37536353

Gera T: Efficacy and safety of therapeutic nutrition products for home based therapeutic nutrition for severe acute malnutrition a systematic review. Indian Pediatr 47:709–718, 2010 20972288

Global Nutrition Report: Executive summary, in 2018 Global Nutrition Report. Bristol, UK, Development Initiatives, 2018. Available at: https://globalnutritionreport.org/reports/global-nutrition-report-2018. Accessed October 23, 2023.

Nutrition, Food and Water Insecurity, and Mental Health 117

Hare D, Ayton S, Bush A, et al: A delicate balance: iron metabolism and diseases of the brain. Front Aging Neurosci 5:34, 2013 23874300

Hazzard VM, Loth KA, Hooper L, et al: Food insecurity and eating disorders: a review of emerging evidence. Curr Psychiatry Rep 22(12):74, 2020 33125614

Hooijer A, Vernimmen R: Global LiDAR land elevation data reveal greatest sea-level rise vulnerability in the tropics. Nat Commun 12(1):3592–3592, 2021 34188026

Jack SJ, Ou K, Chea M, et al: Effect of micronutrient sprinkles on reducing anemia: a cluster-randomized effectiveness trial. Arch Pediatr Adolesc Med 166:842–850, 2012 22801933

Jones AD: Food insecurity and mental health status: a global analysis of 149 countries. Am J Prev Med 53(2):264–273, 2017 28457747

Jones DH, Yu X, Guo Q, et al: Racial disparities in the heavy metal contamination of urban soil in the southeastern United States. Int J Environ Res Public Health 19(3):1105, 2022 35162130

Jun T: Temperature, maize yield, and civil conflicts in sub-Saharan Africa. Clim Change 142:183–197, 2017

Kemper KJ: Food as medicine: health professionals promoting victory gardens in light of climate crisis. Complement Ther Med 70:102869, 2022 35940342

Kimutai JJ, Lund C, Moturi WN, et al: Evidence on the links between water insecurity, inadequate sanitation and mental health: a systematic review and meta-analysis. PLoS One 18(5):e0286146, 2023 37228056

Koren O, Bagozzi BE: Living off the land: the connection between cropland, food security, and violence against civilians. J Peace Res 54(3):351–364, 2017

Kryder-Reid E, May S (eds): Toxic Heritage: Legacies, Futures, and Environmental Justice. Abingdon, UK, Routledge, 2024

Laine JE, Huybrechts I, Gunter MJ, et al: Co-benefits from sustainable dietary shifts for population and environmental health: an assessment from a large European cohort study. Lancet Planet Health 5(11):e786–e796, 2021 34688354

Lampert T, Costa J, Santos O, et al: Evidence on the contribution of community gardens to promote physical and mental health and well-being of non-institutionalized individuals: a systematic review. PLoS One 16(8):e0255621, 2021 34358279

Lee HS, Chao HH, Huang WT, et al: Psychiatric disorders risk in patients with iron deficiency anemia and association with iron supplementation medications: a nationwide database analysis. BMC Psychiatry 20(1):216, 2020 32393355

Mbow C, Rosenzweig C, Barioni LG, et al: Food security, in Climate Change and Land: An IPCC Special Report on Climate Change, Desertification, Land Degradation, Sustainable Land Management, Food Security, and

Greenhouse Gas Fluxes in Terrestrial Ecosystems. Edited by Shukla PR, Skea J, Calvo Buendia E, et al. Geneva, Switzerland, Intergovernmental Panel on Climate Change, 2019, pp 437–550

Mekonnen MM, Hoekstra AY: Four billion people facing severe water scarcity. Sci Adv 2(2):e1500323, 2016 26933676

Muldoon KA, Duff PK, Fielden S, et al: Food insufficiency is associated with psychiatric morbidity in a nationally representative study of mental illness among food insecure Canadians. Soc Psychiatry Psychiatr Epidemiol 48(5):795–803, 2013 23064395

National Institutes of Health: NIH Fact Sheet for Professionals: Iron. Bethesda, MD, National Institutes of Health, updated October 9, 2024. Available at: https://ods.od.nih.gov/factsheets/Iron-HealthProfessional/#:~:text=As%20a%20component%20of%20myoglobin,heme%20and%20nonheme%20%5B1%5D. Accessed November 24, 2024.

Oronce CIA, Miake-Lye IM, Begashaw MM, et al: Interventions to address food insecurity among adults in Canada and the US: a systematic review and meta-analysis. JAMA Health Forum 2(8):e212001, 2021 35977189

Petrilli MA, Kranz TM, Kleinhaus K, et al: The emerging role for zinc in depression and psychosis. Front Pharmacol 8:414, 2017 28713269

Popkin BM, Corvalan C, Grummer-Strawn LM: Dynamics of the double burden of malnutrition and the changing nutrition reality. Lancet 395(10217):65–74, 2020 31852602

Rosinger AY: Water needs, water insecurity, and human biology. Annu Rev Anthropol 52:92–113, 2023

Seal AJ, Creeke PI, Mirghani Z, et al: Iron and vitamin A deficiency in long-term African refugees. J Nutr 135(4):808–813, 2005 15795439

Shankar P, Chung R, Frank DA: Food insecurity with children's behavioral, emotional, and academic outcomes: a systematic review. J Dev Behav Pediatr 38(2):135–150, 2017 28134627

Singh MB, Fotedar R, Lakshminarayana J, et al: Studies on the nutritional status of children aged 0–5 years in a drought-affected desert area of western Rajasthan, India. Public Health Nutr 9(8):961–967, 2006 17125557

Slekiene J, Mosler H-J: The link between mental health and safe drinking water behaviors in a vulnerable population in rural Malawi. BMC Psychol 7(1):44, 2019 31287032

Smith MR, Myers SS: Impact of anthropogenic CO_2 emissions on global human nutrition. Nat Clim Chang 8(9):834–839, 2018

Sova C, Flowers K, Man C: Climate change and food security: a test of U.S. leadership in a fragile world. Washington, DC, Center for Strategic and International Studies, October 15, 2019. Available at: www.csis.org/analysis/climate-change-and-food-security-test-us-leadership-fragile-world. Accessed October 30, 2023.

Nutrition, Food and Water Insecurity, and Mental Health 119

Sova C, Fountain G, Zembilci E, et al: Dangerously Hungry: The Link Between Food Insecurity and Conflict. Washington, DC, World Food Program USA, 2023

Stichler C, Reagor JC: Nitrate and prussic acid poisoning. College Station, Texas Agricultural Extension Service, 2014. Available at: https://brazos.agrilife.org/files/2013/10/Nitrate-and-Prussic-Acid-Poisoning.pdf. Accessed November 28, 2024.

Stockwell BR, Friedmann A, Pedro J, et al: Ferroptosis: a regulated cell death nexus linking metabolism, redox biology, and disease. Cell 171(2):273–285, 2017 28985560

Suzuki H, Yamashiro D, Ogawa S, et al: Intake of seven essential amino acids improves cognitive function and psychological and social function in middle-aged and older adults: a double-blind, randomized, placebo-controlled trial. Front Nutr 7:586166, 2020 33324669

Toivettula A, Varis O, Vahala R, et al: Making waves: mental health impacts of inadequate drinking water services—from sidenote to research focus. Water Res 243:120335, 2023 37516073

Trudell JP, Burnet ML, Ziegler BR, et al: The impact of food insecurity on mental health in Africa: a systematic review. Soc Sci Med 278:113953, 2021 33971482

United Nations Environment Programme: UNEP Frontiers 2016 Report: Emerging Issues of Environmental Concern. Nairobi, United Nations Environment Programme, 2016

Wang J, Um P, Dickerman BA, et al: Zinc, magnesium, selenium and depression: a review of the evidence, potential mechanisms and implications. Nutrients 10(5):584, 2018 29747386

World Health Organization: Community-Based Management of Severe Acute Malnutrition. Geneva, Switzerland, World Health Organization, May 2007. Available at: https://iris.who.int/bitstream/handle/10665/44295/9789280641479_eng.pdf?sequence=1. Accessed November 24, 2024.

Wutich A, Rosinger AY, Brewis A, et al; Household Water Insecurity Experiences-Research Coordination Network: Water sharing is a distressing form of reciprocity: shame, upset, anger, and conflict over water in twenty cross-cultural sites. Am Anthropol 124(2):279–290, 2022 36108326

Yin S, Dong C: The usage of complementary food supplements for young children during natural disasters, in Handbook of Public Health in Natural Disasters. Edited by Watson RR, Tabor JA, Ehiri JE, et al. Wageningen, The Netherlands, Wageningen Academic, 2015, pp 235–250

Zhao C, Liu B, Piao S, et al: Temperature increase reduces global yields of major crops in four independent estimates. Proc Natl Acad Sci USA 114(35):9326–9331, 2017 28811375

7

Climate-Related Shifts in Infectious Diseases, Neuropsychiatric Symptoms, and Associated Issues in the Human-Microbiome Relationship

Understanding the Relationship of Climate Change to Infectious Diseases

Climate change is associated with the increasing spread of infectious diseases, including the emergence of new pathogens and the spread of existing pathogens to new areas. These diseases emerge acutely after extreme weather events, primarily through waterborne illness, and chronically from changing habitats, primarily but not exclusively through vector-borne pathogens. In response, the mental health clinician will grapple with pandemics and epidemics, as well as new neuropsychiatric disease trends and the psychological response of patients and the population to them.

Determination of which pathogens are most implicated in climate-based changes in infectious disease is more difficult than other areas of climate prediction because pathogenic organisms exist in a complex niche of habitats and hosts, all of which are undergoing their own multifactorial and interdependent shifts as temperatures warm. To say a disease will increase in frequency necessitates asking also whether the original and new habitats are hospitable now, whether they will be hospitable in the future, what original and new hosts will be present, and how all the elements of the habitat will evolve under changing conditions: moisture, temperature, the relative length of the warm season, the soil and water microbiome, foods on which the organism depends, its interaction with humanity, and many other factors. Although it is helpful to have general estimates of which diseases are most likely to proliferate in the coming decades and to prepare for this as a global medical community, it may be most helpful for the practitioner to have an understanding of these general principles and local infectious disease trends (well described in Altizer et al. 2013 and Lehmann et al. 2018).

Three examples of the interactions between host, infectious agent, habitat, and humankind illustrate the points above:

1. Diseases emerging in a new area—St. Louis encephalitis is a disease that is transmitted from common birds—dove, pigeon, robin, blue jay, and others—to mosquitoes and then to humans. Changes in precipitation and temperature are driving changes in known bird migration patterns, which sometimes span thousands of miles, as well as the duration of time birds are in the appropriate environment for transmission to mosquitoes. This may lead to outbreaks of St. Louis encephalitis in areas unfamiliar with this disease.

2. Diseases changing alongside host vulnerability—Nordic reindeer populations decreased from 4.7 million to 2.1 million in the past 20 years. The climate impacts that contributed to this decrease include new plants that have outcompeted the lichen reindeer eat; increased reindeer drowning during migrations because of less sea ice; and various new infectious diseases, including anthrax and gut nematodes that now have two breeding seasons instead of one (Russell et al. 2018). All of these factors impact reindeer health and survival, limiting the ability

of Sami and other Indigenous groups to use reindeer for food, transportation, and clothing. These local communities are faced with changes to their identities and social structures as they simultaneously confront the dangers of these new infectious diseases.

3. Diseases emerging because of new interactions between humans and their habitats—When the Zika virus broke from its geographic restriction in South America, it was not clear if it did so because of rising North American temperatures, mutations in virulence, or other factors. It is known, however, that mothers who had dengue previously have greater placental Zika infection, and mosquitoes previously infected with chikungunya are both more easily infected by Zika and better at transmitting it. Increased *Aedes aegypti* mosquito survival in warmer temperatures has tripled both chikungunya and dengue infection in South America (Taylor 2023), so that more mothers and more mosquitoes are more permissive hosts for Zika infection. As temperatures increase in North America, the *Aedes aegypti* mosquito has a greater chance of being alive in northern environments, demonstrating how intersectional increases in viral and vector hosts, reproduction, transmissibility, and range increase the total risk for fetuses and their subsequent vulnerability to microcephaly and other Zika sequelae.

Predicted Climate-Related Changes in Infectious Disease Prevalence and Type

In an effort to predict which organisms will be most impacted by climate change, McIntyre et al. (2017) modeled the sensitivity of 157 pathogens that most commonly infect both humans and animals (McIntyre et al. 2014) to 11 sets of different climate drivers. They found that two-thirds of infectious organisms were likely to be sensitive to climate change. Lyme disease, fluke, cholera, and anthrax were most sensitive to changes in these climate drivers, whereas fungi and viruses showed the least vulnerability. Other groups are modeling the temperature sensitivity of each organism across different biological environments (Alster et al. 2018). Summarizing the impacts of climate change on infectious disease, the Intergovernmental Panel on Climate Change (IPCC; Cissé et al. 2022) has said the following with high confidence:

- Climate trends favor the overall worsening of infectious diseases, despite some benefits
- Malaria has moved to higher altitudes, although the disease has decreased globally through human action
- Dengue is increasing globally
- Chikungunya virus has increased in North and Latin America, Europe, and Asia
- Lyme disease has increased in North America
- High temperatures, flooding, and heavy rainfall have increased diarrheal illnesses, including cholera

Predictive statements that can also be made with high confidence include the following:

- Malaria will increase at the edges of its distribution in Africa, Asia, and South America
- Dengue will increase broadly throughout Europe, Asia, and sub-Saharan Africa, putting 2.5 billion people at risk under Representative Concentration Pathways (RCPs) 6.0 and 8.5
- Lyme disease will continue to spread in North America
- Schistosomiasis will increase in East Africa

It can be said with medium confidence that salmonella, campylobacter, and European Lyme disease are also on the rise. Other diseases that have been increasing or are predicted to do so in the United States include tick-borne diseases (Lyme disease, Rocky Mountain spotted fever, Colorado tick fever, ehrlichiosis, anaplasmosis, Powassan encephalitis, and tick paralysis) (Bouchard et al. 2019) and mosquito-borne diseases (Zika virus; West Nile virus; St. Louis encephalitis; and Western, Eastern, and Venezuelan equine encephalitis) (summarized in Cissé et al. 2022). These changes are resulting from longer and multiple seasons of breeding and transmission, greater ranges of proliferation, and increased contact with human hosts through travel, trade, and increased population.

Flooding is another significant cause of climate-related infectious disease outbreaks. It is most associated with increases in norovirus and rotavirus gastroenteritis, hepatitis A and E, cholera, cryptosporidiosis, and typhoid fever in the Global South, as well as filariasis and disease

Climate-Related Shifts in Infectious Diseases

from fecal bacteria worldwide (Cissé et al. 2022; Wu et al. 2016). Other factors, such as temperature, stormwater management, and the availability of nonhuman reservoirs for bacteria, play a role in perpetuating these and other diarrheal illnesses. For example, chikungunya and dengue fever outbreaks occur after floods because of mosquito breeding in stagnant waters. Warmer oceans may also increasingly pose a threat: warmer ocean temperatures are associated with algal blooms that can cause illness, including neuropsychiatric illness, through shellfish contaminated by *Gambierdiscus*, *Vibrio parahaemolyticus*, *Vibrio vulnificus*, and others (Burge et al. 2014).

Drought is associated with rises in meningococcal meningitis, particularly in Africa. Although drought reduces mosquito activity and mosquito-borne diseases overall, a higher risk of malaria may occur because of temporary increases in stagnant water that can host vector-borne disease. Drought may also change human migration patterns, which leads to spread of disease or causes a paradoxical surge in infection in the home population locally when it ends because the population of nonimmune persons able to spread disease has increased through its duration (reviewed in Vajda and Webb 2017).

These summary statements do not convey the relative impacts of different infectious diseases on human mortality, which vary greatly, from 2.5 million people dying annually of respiratory infections to only 36,000 dying annually of dengue fever, despite its rapid and deadly increase. For perspective, the numbers of annual deaths from relevant infectious diseases are provided in Table 7.1.

Table 7.1 Incidence and geographical dominance of common infectious diseases

Disease	Annual deaths (2019)	Most affected region
Respiratory tract infections	2,493,200	Asia (47%)
Diarrheal illnesses	1,534,433	Asia (56%)
Malaria	643,381	Africa (92%)
Salmonella	79,046	Africa (89%)
Dengue	36,055	Asia (96%)

Source. Summarized from Cissé et al. 2022.

Infectious Disease Impacts for Practicing Psychiatrists

The needs that emerge from changes in infectious diseases invite psychiatric participation at numerous levels. Climate-related infectious diseases will present psychiatrists with the following:

- More cases of encephalitis and neuropsychiatric complications of infectious illness
- More patients challenged in their health and well-being by the physical and emotional strain and sequelae of individual disease episodes, community outbreaks, and global pandemics
- More patients with somatic fears and other adverse psychological reactions to infectious disease threats
- Great demand for psychiatrists to educate their patients and their health care systems about the neuropsychiatric manifestations of these relatively rare diseases
- Public health need for development of early warning systems and prepared community responses

Neuropsychiatric Symptoms of Climate-Related Infectious Disease

Familiarity with the psychological reactions to infectious diseases and the neuropsychiatric complications of the more common vector-borne and other climate-related infectious diseases is therefore suggested, particularly their acute manifestations in the consultation-liaison setting and the subacute and late symptoms to which the psychiatrist in outpatient practice must remain alert. These neuropsychiatric manifestations are summarized here; information on general presentation and treatment is available from the CDC, World Health Organization (WHO), and other public health sites.

Malaria is the most common mosquito-borne disease and causes at least one neurological manifestation in 60% of patients, with confusion (18%), headache (15%), and psychosis (5%) being most frequent (Singh et al. 2016). Long-term cognitive effects are common. Medications used to treat or prevent malaria, particularly quinolone treatments, can also cause aseptic meningitis, delirium, psychosis, and other neurological

Climate-Related Shifts in Infectious Diseases

complications (Nevin and Croft 2016). Dengue cases doubled from 6 to 12 million from 2023 to 2024 (Bishen 2024). Dengue causes hemorrhagic and ischemic stroke, posterior reversible encephalopathy syndrome, and autoimmune complications such as Guillain-Barré syndrome, transverse myelitis, and ocular disorders, as well as specific viral encephalitis and meningitis syndromes due to viral invasion of the central nervous system in up to 20% of patients (Guzman and Martinez 2024).

Adults with initial neurological symptoms from Zika virus can also have prolonged neuropsychiatric dysfunction, including Guillain-Barré syndrome, encephalomyelitis, peripheral neuropathy, and motor and cognitive impairment. The Zika virus has been shown to persist up to 6 months after infection. Babies with Zika virus can be born with severe microcephaly, high muscle tone or limb contracture, eye abnormalities, and hearing loss. In addition, 40% of Zika-infected babies not obviously impaired at birth go on to show developmental and motor delay later in infancy, and more than 60% develop seizures as they are followed over time (Souza et al. 2019).

West Nile virus infection has only an approximate 1% incidence of acute neuroinvasive disease, characterized most often by meningitis, encephalitis, or flaccid paralysis. However, in affected patients, symptoms persist for almost 2 years, with difficulties in learning, memory, executive and motor functions ranging from 10% to 40%, and possible contribution to dementia risk (Samaan et al. 2016; Vittor et al. 2020). Equine encephalitic diseases, although rare, cause permanent neurological impacts in 70% of infected patients and can have mortality rates up to 30% (Simon et al. 2023). How often neurological symptoms appear in chikungunya is unclear, ranging from 0.1% to 16.3%, but they occur in 60%–80% of those hospitalized with severe illness in the ICU. However, 75% of both adults and children infected by chikungunya have some CNS involvement, including encephalitis (in about 40% of this 75%), optic neuritis, sensorineural deafness, other palsies, and Guillain-Barré syndrome (Mehta et al. 2018).

Among the tick-borne diseases, Lyme disease has specific neurological manifestations in up to 40% of patients, as well as fatigue, headache, and cognitive impairment in most, thought to result from its systemic effects. Meningitis, cranial neuropathies, and radiculopathy occur most acutely, but these can also occur long after initial infection (Fallon and Nields 1994; Isaac and Larson 2014). Powassan virus, a flavivirus found in the Northeast and Midwestern United States, has increased by 671% in the past 20 years, correlated with warmer years. It causes prolonged neurological impairment in 50% of cases (Fatmi et al. 2017). Ehrlichiosis, caused by a family of gram-negative bacteria endemic to the Central and Eastern United States, has increased eight-fold in the past two decades and is associated with neuropsychiatric symptoms in 20% of patients (Ismail et al. 2010).

> *Vignette*
>
> Susan is a 63-year-old woman with a history of rheumatoid arthritis treated with methotrexate who presented with a first seizure and pos-tictal psychosis. Taking a social history, the consultant psychiatrist learned that Susan had not felt well since a recent family reunion at a North Carolina beach, during which she had played hide-and-seek with her grandchildren in the scrub vegetation around the house. Testing revealed ehrlichiosis, a disease found predominantly in mid-Southeastern states that can be severe if untreated, particularly in immunosuppressed individuals. Susan responded well to treatment with doxycycline and was able to discontinue all neuropsychiatric medicines over several ensuing months.

Among the waterborne diseases, *Vibrio parahaemolyticus*, *Vibrio vulnificus*, norovirus, rotavirus, and hepatitis only rarely cause neurological disease, although cases have been reported, and they may cause seizures in children (Deb et al. 2023). Cholera is also less likely to cause neurological difficulties but may affect infants, and the prognosis when it does is poor (McEntire et al. 2021). *Naegleria fowleri* is an amoeba that thrives in very warm surface waters—between 86°F and 114°F—and it can cause an amoebic meningoencephalitis that is 97% fatal (Ahmad Zamzuri et al. 2023). *Gambierdiscus* microalgae species, found in the livers of fish that graze on coral reefs, produce ciguatoxins (potent neurotoxins) that activate voltage-gated sodium channels and potentially inhibit potassium channels. This leads to neuronal excitability, with clinical symptoms marked by painful paresthesias, including urogenital pain, cold dysesthesia, numbness, pruritus, electric shocks, and bradycardia, with relapses to symptoms such as polymyositis and ataxia possible months after exposure. Fatality is less than 1% but can be 50% in children (L'Herondelle et al. 2020).

Treatment Considerations

The descriptions in the previous sections give some idea of the range of acute and long-term neuropsychiatric symptoms that may emerge with climate-related infectious diseases and may require workup, referral, and treatment. Many of these diseases can be rapidly fatal. Testing for them is algorithmic; depends significantly on the stage of illness and the location of exposure; and uses a combination of polymerase chain reaction (PCR), antibody, histological, and cell-culture techniques (Rodino et al. 2020), so that treatment often proceeds empirically at first. To respond to these diseases, psychiatric practitioners need to be more cognizant of infectious disease updates. This is particularly important for practitioners who provide consultation-liaison services and may be the first to see emergent illness patterns representing a new epidemic. The general psychiatrist can be helpful to patients by educating them about the diseases and treatments and about how to avoid illness through good hygiene and vigilance during travel. They can also help patients with anxiety disorders calm catastrophic reactions that impede taking reality-based action when threats do occur.

Community Interventions to Decrease Infectious Disease Outbreaks

In addition to taking the measures needed to care for their patients, psychiatrists can help community efforts to combat new infectious diseases by reporting unusual symptom clusters to local authorities, taking leadership roles in patient education within their institutions and communities when new diseases emerge, and educating others about effective strategies for working with hard-to-reach groups that may otherwise become superspreaders of disease, including people with chronic mental illness; unhoused people; and people with intellectual limitations, substance dependence, or paranoid disorders.

Community and national responses to new emerging diseases currently focus on disease containment, although efforts to rebalance ecosystems are increasingly gaining traction. This containment includes systems for the following:

- Surveillance for new emerging illnesses
- Planning for early warning and education systems to control population spread
- Vector and host wildlife management
- Vaccine development and distribution
- Improved stormwater management

- Improved access to potable water, including backup systems for disasters
- Information delivery to the public

These systems are part of larger national resilience efforts for climate adaptation and mitigation, covered further in Chapter 13, "Coordinating the Climate Psychiatry Response," and Chapter 14, "Community Psychiatry and Its Role in Climate Mitigation and Adaptation."

Psychological Responses to Infectious Disease Relevant to Climate Effects

Beyond their role as physicians treating infectious diseases that have neuropsychiatric manifestations, psychiatrists must also respond to the psychological aspects of infectious diseases, including both the individual and social enactments that comprise human emotional reactions to microbiological disease. Infectious diseases increase illness anxiety and pathological coping for both individuals and groups. The fact that they cannot be seen or otherwise perceived makes them frightening, leading to a state of high uncertainty and high alert to the risks of illness, death, and potential deprivations of food and income for individuals and their families. Media sensationalism, disinformation, and misinformation contribute to higher anxiety. When it is unclear whether care will be available, or if seeking medical attention will lead to even worse sickness, help-seeking behavior deteriorates. Being unable to control how others behave—those who deny they are sick and become superspreaders or those who will not wash or vaccinate—adds to perceived vulnerability and triggers paranoia, avoidant coping, and social isolation.

Historically, infectious disease epidemics have also been associated with stigmatization, xenophobia, and irrational labeling of out-groups, from the labeling of the *scellerati* (evil ones) during the Black Death to the QAnon conspiracy fears of the "Illuminati" that occurred during the coronavirus disease 2019 (COVID-19) pandemic. These paranoid fears contaminate trust in authority, leading to a situation in which health information is irrationally rejected and self-professed expertise, rumors, and other unscientific sources are overvalued. This occurs in parallel with fear and paranoid distrust on one hand and overtrust of false prophets on the other. Some individuals may experience dispro-portionate fear alternating with magical thinking about easy, risk-free rescues. People who rely more on observational learning (observing the reactions of others to assess information, a form of mimicry) and those who are narcissistic, suspicious, gullible, interested in the para-normal, less educated, and low in media literacy and analytic thinking are more at risk of such paranoid and irrational reactions (Taylor 2019).

Germ Panic: Associations and Dangers

Excess health anxiety associated with illness anxiety disorder, somati-zation disorder, and other somatoform syndromes affects about 6% of the population, and these individuals experience higher distress dur-ing illness outbreaks. Some also have a specific germ phobia, or myso-phobia, often in association with obsessive-compulsive disorder. Illness anxiety is associated with high distress, repetitive checking, obsessive-compulsive behaviors, and reassurance seeking. Those with high neu-roticism, high body vigilance, and higher trait anxiety, particularly its subelements of overestimation of threat and intolerance of uncertainty, are likely to be particularly anxiously preoccupied. Infectious disease anxiety also activates the behavioral immune system, a conscious and unconscious system of social awareness and aversion that alerts us to illness and includes disgust sensitivity and visual cueing in response to those who are ill (Taylor 2019).

Such anxiety about infectious diseases can lead patients to several maladaptive and dangerous behaviors that are clinically significant, including the following:

- Excessive decontamination practices leading to skin burns, chem-ical fires, use of unverified treatments, and other consequences
- Social withdrawal so severe it leads to failure to thrive
- Doctor-shopping, leading to confusion from contradictory health information and iatrogenic illness
- Misinterpretation of or failure to respond to real illness symptoms
- Use of quack cures and folk remedies, such as drinking hydro-gen peroxide
- Mistreatment or killing of people and animals perceived to be infected

- Fear contagion and other forms of mass hysteria
- Panic buying, rioting, and other impulsive and antisocial behaviors

All of these reactions can be the purview of the psychiatrist as both clinician and consultant in an era when pandemics and other infectious scourges will arise unpredictably.

Infectious Disease in the Context of the Planetary and Individual Microbiotic Health

Human-Planetary Microbiome Relationship

The "germ panic" just described focuses on reacting emotionally and practically to eliminate a pathogenic organism hostile to individual survival. A different way of promoting patient health vis-à-vis climate-changed infectious diseases embeds this conversation in the larger context of the human and planetary microbiome. By implication, it asks the psychiatrist to spend more time vividly imagining their patient not only as surrounded by a web of human relationships, imbued with a network of neurobiological processes and as a product of outside environmental influences, but also as a "bag of bugs" embedded in a microscopic web of life as well. Although this point of view may seem initially far out, it is in line with several important matters:

1. The actuality of the relationship between human and microbiological life-forms (Sender et al. 2016)
2. Evolving science about the role of the microbiome in human health, including neurological and mental disease (Hou et al. 2022)
3. Gaia theory (Lovelock 2009), which posits human and planetary health as a cohesive, interdependent, self-regulating, and evolving conscious system, the awareness of which is necessary for the transition from the Anthropocene to the Symbiocene

Function of Microorganisms

In raw numbers of cells, a human being is 50% microbial, and 90% of ocean life-forms are microbiological organisms. These microorganisms are the life-support system of the biosphere and for human life. They perform essential functions in humans that include development of the immune system, digestion, synthesis of vitamins and hormones, and provision of cellular nutrients and defense, and in nature they harvest solar energy, fix carbon and nitrogen, clear toxins, and perform thousands of other processes critical for life (Timmis et al. 2019).

The Hygiene Hypothesis and Its Medical and Psychiatric Consequences

Industrialization, sanitation, availability of potable water, and scientific advances in treating infectious diseases have been associated with hygienic measures such as sterilization of surfaces; use of antibiotics; preterm and cesarean birth; decreased breastfeeding; decreased contact with animals, plants, and soil; and having a home environment that is dirty enough to trigger adequate microbial exposure. Contact with helminths and parasites has particularly decreased. The *hygiene hypothesis* (reviewed in Pfefferle et al. 2021) states that we have gone too far with such sterilizing approaches, leading to increased illness and worsening antibiotic resistance. Far fewer than 1% of microbes are human pathogens. Exposure to these benign microorganisms is critical for health, training the immune system with proinflammatory but nonthreatening stimuli.

As summarized by Arleevskaya et al. (2019), inadequate microbial exposure is thought to cause an imbalance in helper T cells that predisposes a person to allergic and autoimmune diseases including asthma and inflammatory bowel disease. In particular, type 1 helper T cell responses to harmless antigens in the skin, mouth, and gut downregulate the type 2 helper T cell response, training the immune system not to attack its host or harmless molecules in the air or intestine. Specific understanding now exists of how the immune development of the infant is triggered by exposure to the more than 200 organisms acquired through breast milk and the birth canal, how antigen responses to helminth exposure reduce symptoms of multiple sclerosis, and other examples of critical microorganism synergy for human wellness (Rook et al. 2003, 2014).

Overly hygienic attitudes of the past century are also thought to have contributed to the disproportionate rise in depression in industrialized countries over the same period by altering the types of cytokines produced under stress (Raison et al. 2010). Antidepressants, alcohol, and benzodiazepines, among many other medication and lifestyle factors, change gut microbiota (Falony et al. 2016; Rukavishnikov et al. 2023). In animal models, gut microbiota have influences on social behaviors, anxiety systems, and neuromotor function (Hou et al. 2022). Understanding of the relationship between gut dysbiosis and depression is progressing rapidly, with studies showing a depletion of *Coprococcus*, *Faecalibacterium*, and *Blautia* genera and greater numbers of proinflammatory species. Treatments based on microbiome improvement are underway (Liu et al. 2023), although they are not standardized or considered in light of climate-based changes in microbial life.

Restoring Health to the Human and Global Microbiome

Global warming is changing the global microbiome in many ways that affect the overall carbon balance (Cavicchioli et al. 2019). In response to this and the cumulative health consequences of decreased and adverse human microbiome interactions, leading groups have called for greater microbial literacy for all people and more cultivation of relationships with beneficial microorganisms in human bodies and nature (Timmis et al. 2019).

Time in nature may facilitate such positive microbial contact while also decreasing a person's stress response and supporting immune function. Although it is difficult to study links of specific microbial species to specific immune markers after time in nature (Tischer et al. 2022), forest bathing has been associated with clear and positive immune effects, including increased natural killer cell function and numbers lasting for up to 30 days (Li 2010), and farm exposure has been associated with lesser allergic disease (Ober et al. 2017). This microbio-psychosocio-environmental approach also has potential psychological co-benefits, including greater knowledge of lesser-known microbe groups (Robinson et al. 2021) and decreased fears of "creepy crawlies" (Hosaka et al. 2017). By participating in such microbial literacy and conceptualizing the infectious disease challenges of climate change as a need for greater support for microbial diversity and promotion of individual immune health through microbial contact, the psychiatrist may achieve substantial benefits for a patient:

Climate-Related Shifts in Infectious Diseases

- Better mental health
- Better physical health
- Improved immune function
- Deeper understanding of the symbiotic relationships supporting microbial survival
- Fewer maladaptive and anxious responses when infectious outbreaks do occur

Key Points

- Climate change is altering the epidemiology of infectious diseases through complex effects on microbial habitats and the environmental niches occupied by their hosts.
- Familiarity with the neuropsychiatric effects of increasingly prevalent pathogens such as malaria, dengue, Lyme disease, and other vector-borne illnesses is part of climate-informed psychiatric practice.
- Psychiatrists can contribute to public health identification and containment of epidemics and pandemics from emerging infectious diseases with neuropsychiatric symptoms.
- Psychiatrists have a unique role to play in clarifying and mitigating anxiety and irrational individual and societal health behaviors in response to microbial illness.
- Contributions from Gaia theory, climate ethics, the hygiene hypothesis, and human microbiome health data suggest that a microbio-psychosocio-environmental conceptualization of the patient can support mental health.

References

Ahmad Zamzuri MI, Abd Majid FN, Mihat M, et al: Systematic review of brain-eating amoeba: a decade update. Int J Environ Res Public Health 20(4):3021, 2023 36833715

Alster CJ, Weller ZD, von Fischer JC: A meta-analysis of temperature sensitivity as a microbial trait. Glob Change Biol 24(9):4211–4224, 2018 29888841

Altizer S, Ostfeld RS, Johnson PTJ, et al: Climate change and infectious diseases: from evidence to a predictive framework. Science 341(6145):514–519, 2013 23908230

Arleevskaya MI, Aminov R, Brooks WH, et al: Editorial: shaping of human immune system and metabolic processes by viruses and microorganisms. Front Microbiol 10:816, 2019 31057521

Bishen S: The world is in the grip of a record dengue fever outbreak: what's causing it and how can it be stopped? Cologny, Switzerland, World Economic Forum, 2024. Available at: www.weforum.org/stories/2024/11/dengue-fever-outbreak-climate-change. Accessed December 29, 2024.

Bouchard C, Dibernardo A, Koffi J, et al: N increased risk of tick-borne diseases with climate and environmental changes. Can Commun Dis Rep 45(4):83–89, 2019 31285697

Burge CA, Eakin CM, Friedman CS, et al: Climate change influences on marine infectious diseases: implications for management and society. Annu Rev Mar Sci 6(1):249–277, 2014 23808894

Cavicchioli R, Ripple WJ, Timmis KN, et al: Scientists' warning to humanity: microorganisms and climate change. Nat Rev Microbiol 17(9):569–586, 2019 31213707

Cissé G, McLeman R, Adams H, et al: Health, wellbeing, and the changing structure of communities, in Climate Change 2022: Impacts, Adaptation and Vulnerability. Contribution of Working Group II to the Sixth Assessment Report of the Intergovernmental Panel on Climate Change. Edited by Pörtner H-O, Roberts DC, Tignor M, et al. Cambridge, UK, Cambridge University Press, 2022, pp 1041–1170

Deb S, Mondal R, Lahiri D, et al: Norovirus-associated neurological manifestations: summarizing the evidence. J Neurovirol 29(4):492–506, 2023 37477790

Fallon BA, Nields JA: Lyme disease: a neuropsychiatric illness. Am J Psychiatry 151(11):1571–1583, 1994 7943444

Falony G, Joossens M, Vieira-Silva S, et al: Population-level analysis of gut microbiome variation. Science 352(6285):560–564, 2016 27126039

Fatmi SS, Zehra R, Carpenter DO: Powassan virus—a new reemerging tick-borne disease. Front Public Health 5:342, 2017 29312918

Guzman MG, Martinez E: Central and peripheral nervous system manifestations associated with dengue illness. Viruses 16(9):1367, 2024 39339843

Hosaka T, Sugimoto K, Numata S: Childhood experience of nature influences the willingness to coexist with biodiversity in cities. Palgrave Commun 3:17071, 2017

Hou K, Wu Z-X, Chen X-Y, et al: Microbiota in health and diseases. Signal Transduct Target Ther 7(1):135, 2022 35461318

Isaac ML, Larson EB: Medical conditions with neuropsychiatric manifestations. Med Clin North Am 98(5):1193–1208, 2014 25134879

Ismail N, Bloch KC, McBride JW: Human ehrlichiosis and anaplasmosis. Clin Lab Med 30(1):261–292, 2010 20513551

Lehmann P, Ammunet T, Barton M, et al: Complex responses of global insect pests to climate change. bioRxiv, 2018. Available at: https://doi.org/10.1101/425488. Accessed December 12, 2024.

L'Herondelle K, Talagas M, Mignen O, et al: Neurological disturbances of ciguatera poisoning: clinical features and pathophysiological basis. Cells 9(10):2291, 2020 33066435

Li Q: Effect of forest bathing trips on human immune function. Environ Health Prev Med 15(1):9–17, 2010 19568839

Liu L, Wang H, Chen X, et al: Gut microbiota and its metabolites in depression: from pathogenesis to treatment. EBioMedicine 90:104527, 2023 36963238

Lovelock J: The Vanishing Face of Gaia: A Final Warning. London, Allen Lane, 2009

McEntire CRS, Song K-W, McInnis RP, et al: Neurologic manifestations of the World Health Organization's list of pandemic and epidemic diseases. Front Neurol 12:634827, 2021 33692745

McIntyre KM, Setzkorn C, Hepworth PJ, et al: A quantitative prioritisation of human and domestic animal pathogens in Europe. PLoS One 9(8):3103529, 2014 25136810

McIntyre KM, Setzkorn C, Hepworth PJ, et al: Systematic assessment of the climate sensitivity of important human and domestic animals pathogens in Europe. Sci Rep 7(1):7134, 2017 28769039

Mehta R, Gerardin P, de Brito CAA, et al: The neurological complications of chikungunya virus: a systematic review. Rev Med Virol 28(3):e1978, 2018 29671914

Nevin RL, Croft AM: Psychiatric effects of malaria and anti-malarial drugs: historical and modern perspectives. Malar J 15:332, 2016 27335053

Ober C, Sperling AI, von Mutius E, et al: Immune development and environment: lessons from Amish and Hutterite children. Curr Opin Immunol 48:51–60, 2017 28843541

Pfefferle PI, Keber CU, Cohen RM, et al: The hygiene hypothesis—learning from but not living in the past. Front Immunol 12:635935, 2021 33796103

Raison CL, Lowry CA, Rook GA: Inflammation, sanitation, and consternation: loss of contact with coevolved, tolerogenic microorganisms and the pathophysiology and treatment of major depression. Arch Gen Psychiatry 67(12):1211–1224, 2010 21135322

Robinson JM, Cameron R, Jorgensen A: Germaphobia! Does our relationship with and knowledge of biodiversity affect our attitudes toward microbes? Front Psychol 12:678752, 2021 34276497

Rodino KG, Theel ES, Pritt BS: Tick-borne diseases in the United States. Clin Chem 66(4):537–548, 2020 32232463

Rook GAW, Martinelli R, Brunet LR: Innate immune responses to mycobacteria and the downregulation of atopic responses. Curr Opin Allergy Clin Immunol 3(5):337–342, 2003 14501431

Rook GAW, Raison CL, Lowry CA: Microbial 'old friends', immunoregulation and socioeconomic status. Clin Exp Immunol 177(1):1–12, 2014 24401109

Rukavishnikov G, Leonova L, Kasyanov E, et al: Antimicrobial activity of antidepressants on normal gut microbiota: results of the in vitro study. Front Behav Neurosci 17:1132127, 2023 37035624

Russell DE, Gunn A, Kutz S: Migratory tundra caribou and wild reindeer, in Arctic Report Card 2018. Edited by Osborne E, Richter-Menge J, Jeffries M. Silver Spring, MD, National Oceanic and Atmospheric Administration, 2018. Available at: https://arctic.noaa.gov/Report-Card. Accessed December 12, 2024.

Samaan Z, McDermid Vaz S, Bawor M, et al: Neuropsychological impact of West Nile virus infection: an extensive neuropsychiatric assessment of 49 cases in Canada. PloS One 11(6):e0158364, 2016 27352145

Sender R, Fuchs S, Milo R: Revised estimates for the number of human and bacteria cells in the body. PLoS Biol 14(8):e1002533, 2016 27541692

Simon LV, Coffey R, Fischer MA: Western Equine Encephalitis. Treasure Island, FL, StatPearls Publishing, 2023

Singh VB, Kumar H, Meena BL, et al: Neuropsychiatric profile in malaria: an overview. J Clin Diagn Res 10(7):OC24–OC28, 2016 27630883

Souza INO, Barros-Aragão FGQ, Frost PS, et al: Late neurological consequences of Zika virus infection: risk factors and pharmaceutical approaches. Pharmaceuticals (Basel) 12(2):60, 2019 30999590

Taylor L: Dengue and chikungunya cases surge as climate change spreads arboviral diseases to new regions. BMJ 380:717, 2023 36972905

Taylor S: The Psychology of Pandemics: Preparing for the Next Global Outbreak of Infectious Disease. Newcastle Upon Tyne, UK, Cambridge Scholars, 2019

Timmis K, Cavicchioli R, Garcia JL, et al: The urgent need for microbiology literacy in society. Environ Microbiol 21(5):1513–1528, 2019 30912268

Tischer C, Kirjavainen P, Matterne U, et al: Interplay between natural environment, human microbiota and immune system: a scoping review of interventions and future perspectives towards allergy prevention. Sci Total Environ 821:153422, 2022 35090907

Vajda ÉA, Webb CE: Assessing the risk factors associated with malaria in the highlands of Ethiopia: what do we need to know? Trop Med Infect Dis 2(1):4, 2017 30270863

Vittor AY, Long M, Chakrabarty P, et al: West Nile virus-induced neurologic sequelae-relationship to neurodegenerative cascades and dementias. Curr Trop Med Rep 7(1):25–36, 2020 32775145

Wu X, Lu Y, Zhou S, et al: Impact of climate change on human infectious diseases: empirical evidence and human adaptation. Environ Int 86:14–23, 2016 26479830

8

Climate Change, Extreme Weather, Natural Disasters, and Human Displacement

Disaster psychiatry is a large and growing subfield of psychiatry, the scope of which is well beyond this book. At the same time, extreme weather and natural disasters are the more commonly experienced and identifiable impacts of climate change for most people. This chapter, therefore, is geared toward providing enough clinical material for psychiatrists working with people affected by disasters to be a useful reference, while also highlighting larger conceptual and systemic matters related to the relationship between climate change and disaster psychiatry.

Climate Change Is Increasing Natural Disasters and Their Damage

Climate change is increasing the frequency and intensity of natural disasters (Cissé et al. 2022), contributing to unfamiliar types of extreme weather such as bomb cyclones and atmospheric rivers, and

139

intensifying flooding, fire, and drought and their associated damage. For example, Hurricane Maria in the United States (2017) delivered up to 37 inches of rain, damaged or destroyed 300,000 homes, killed between 3,000 and 5,000 people, and incurred costs of $93.6 billion.

Between 1970 and 2019, there have been approximately 11,000 disasters, 90% of which have affected developing countries, with a five- to tenfold increase in frequency since 2010 compared with the 1970s and earlier (Institute for Economics and Peace 2022; World Meteorological Organization 2021; see also EM-DAT public data at www.emdat.be). The number of billion-dollar disasters annually correlates strongly with increases in atmospheric carbon. The costs of these natural disasters are skyrocketing, reaching more than $2 trillion from 1980 to 2021 in the United States alone, not adjusted for inflation or the value of lost natural capital and life. These numbers, representing more than $5,500 per United States resident during these four decades, are thus significant underestimates, whereas the benefits of climate mitigation are 4:1 for every dollar spent (reviewed in Bhola et al. 2023).

The disasters that have caused the greatest loss of life during these decades include droughts (approximately 800,000 people in Africa) and storms (300,000 from Cyclones Gorky and Nargis), followed by heat waves and floods (World Meteorological Organization 2021). The Asia-Pacific region, followed by sub-Saharan Africa, Central America, and the Caribbean, have been and are predicted to be the areas most affected in the twenty-first century (Institute for Economics and Peace 2022). Extreme heat events, currently not considered as natural disasters, may be given this status in the future, adding to this load.

Defining Natural Disasters and Emerging Climate Disaster Patterns

A disaster is defined as an event that causes widespread human, material, environmental, or economic losses and harm, leading to personal and social disruption. Many definitions also stipulate that the suffering caused by the event exceeds the capacity of the affected community to respond (United Nations Office for Disaster Risk Reduction 2024). This latter element is conceptually important for psychiatry and carries relational, psychological, psychiatric, public health, and ethical implications.

Disasters can arise from all types of hazards and can be natural or technological and acute or chronic in nature. Climate-related disasters contain all of these types. Disasters created by human action or error have been considered to be more likely to cause conflict, and climate change falls partly into this category. The increasing frequency and intensity of disasters with the progression of climate change also means that communities may often experience multiple disasters at the same time, or one disaster on the back of another before having adequate time for recovery. For example, in summer 2022, Florida was simultaneously affected by particularly heavy Saharan dust, heat waves with heat indexes close to 110°F, and a disproportionately high rate of coronavirus disease 2019 (COVID-19) infection. A concurrence of disaster events of this type is termed a *compound disaster*. When disasters happen one after another without adequate recovery in between, they are termed *consecutive* or *cascading disasters*, the latter implying that the earlier disaster sets off the latter. The 2011 Tohoku earthquake in Japan was a cascading disaster because the earthquake triggered a tsunami, which then caused a nuclear disaster. Disasters are considered *recurrent* when the same type of disaster occurs more than once within 1 year but without overlap (Leppold et al. 2022). Disadvantaged groups can also experience *neglected disasters*, as can older adults (Ayalon et al. 2023), particularly if smaller disasters do not receive media recognition or fall in the shadow of a larger event. These terms (Table 8.1) are just beginning to be formalized, and the broader concepts of the *polycrisis, metacrisis*, and *permacrisis* (Table 8.2) often associated with climate disaster are not yet part of the disaster psychiatry lexicon.

Conceptual Issues in Disaster Psychiatry and Climate Change

Issues Related to Disaster Intensification and Repetition

Understanding the differences in mental health effects of these intensifying multiple concurrent climate-related disasters compared with the effects of a single disaster is an important area just opening to research. In their review of all studies of public health and multiple disasters up to 2021, Leppold et al. (2022) found 150 articles, only a few of which compared their findings with those of a single disaster exposure.

Table 8.1 Types of natural disaster

Type of disaster	Description
Recurrent disasters	More than one separate disaster in a single location within 1 year
Consecutive disasters	Two or more disasters in succession, occurring before recovery from the previous event is completed
Compound disasters	The combination of two or more extreme events, simultaneously or almost simultaneously
Cascading disasters	Extreme events that overlap and in which the earlier event sets off or contributes to the destructiveness of the subsequent event
Neglected disasters	Disasters receiving inadequate support because of size, timing, or social prejudice

Importantly, mental health was the largest impact theme, identified in 35% of these studies. Most studies found that recurrent disaster exposure increased ongoing mental health symptoms or triggered a relapse of the mental health symptoms of prior disaster exposure. Recurrent disaster exposure also led to more poor physical health, often mediated by factors related to mental illness or stress. In terms of mental health, studies also showed the following:

- Individuals, communities, and governments were generally slow to change behaviors or policies even with repeated disaster occurrence
- Responders and response systems were severely strained by recurrent disasters
- Too few studies and efforts have been dedicated to mitigating these damages by improving resilience and well-being for future events
- Impoverished and disadvantaged groups experienced more distress
- Trends in terms of public complacency were inconclusive; most people did not change behaviors in response to recurring events, but a very severe event such as evacuation or relocation was likely to precipitate behavioral change

Extreme Weather, Natural Disasters, and Human Displacement   143

Table 8.2 Emerging crisis vocabulary

Type of crisis	Description
Polycrisis	Multiple simultaneous crises, such as when many natural systems decline
Permacrisis	A state of unremitting crisis, such as during a prolonged pandemic or climate change
Metacrisis	A larger crisis, such as climate change or crises in human psychology and behavior, that underlies and contributes to emerging crises

The developmental, genetic, toxic, and transgenerational impacts of these multiple stressors form another important set of concerns related to climate change and compounding disasters. In utero and immediately postnatal exposure to natural disasters predisposes children to more cognitive problems, negative affect, and emotional dysregulation, likely through maternal stress biology, which also correlates with suicide, autism, and anxiety in later life (Buthmann et al. 2019). Children experience nonlinear increases in trauma in areas of repeat disaster, such as the recurrent fires in Sonoma County, California, in part arising from the compounding impacts of repeat disasters on violence, substance use, poverty, and other social determinants of health (Diamond 2022), and adolescent mental distress can be up to 25% higher in the several years following disaster exposure (Auchincloss et al. 2024).

Compound and recurrent disasters also increase the broader neuropsychiatric toll of these events. For example, for those who experience wildfires, not only does haze from the smoke increase negative emotions across the population, but wildfire smoke contains both particulate matter and toxins that are associated with more respiratory events; changes in cerebral hemodynamics (Eisenman and Galway 2022); and predicted risk of stroke, myocardial infarction, cancer, and dementia. Toxins in fire exposure include benzenes, butadienes, formaldehyde, dioxins, asbestos, arsenic, and other compounds associated with various cancer risks (Soteriades et al. 2019). Of these, a significant portion is related to perfluoroalkyl and polyfluoroalkyl substances in firefighter personal protective equipment (Wolffe et al. 2023). These impacts add to the multiple acute and chronic traumas of the initial event. As reviewed in Gonzalez et al. (2024), firefighters suffer high rates of sudden cardiac events from metabolic, thermoregulatory, and cardiovascular exertional strain and oxidative damage as well as rates of occupational cancers 9% higher than those of the average population. Additionally, they carry burdens of depression and PTSD that are similar to those of other first responders and have high rates of suicide (72% greater than that of the average population).

Multiple disasters raise other risks for responders as well. Although they generally benefit from high trust, loyalty, cohesion, and skills in their work groups, responders are at higher risk of depression, anxiety, and posttraumatic stress disorder (PTSD) if they have preexisting physical or mental disorders, concurrent losses or stresses, overwork, or sleep disruption. They are exposed to the stress of dead bodies, catastrophic injuries, and challenging conditions in their work. The culture of responders also demands they privately shoulder emotional burdens by virtue of its rigid work values, work conditions that can isolate them from family and friends, distrust and high concern for confidentiality in divulging symptoms, avoidant coping, and a tendency to deflect the concern of others, all of which must be considered when offering them support (Kronenberg et al. 2008).

In multiple disasters, these risks multiply concurrently with the demand that responders stretch their work capacities even further. Bernstein (2021) reported that in the Paradise Fire of 2018, 300 of 2,200 county staff in Butte County, California, lost their homes, while at the same time, demand for case management services increased 700% and call volume to a distress line increased 400%. This county then endured two events, the Dixie Fire and Oroville Dam collapse, in the subsequent 4 years, further straining these responder systems. Another study (Mash et al. 2022) had surveyed 681 Florida county workers between the 2004 and 2005 hurricane seasons. This proved to be serendipitous because in 2005, there were 14 named hurricanes, including three Category 5 storms (National Centers for Environmental Information 2006), allowing the impacts of the second year on these workers to be studied. Trouble recovering from the 2005 disasters was associated with longer 2004 recovery time (OR 5.22, 95% CI [3.01–9.08]), personal injury or damage (OR 3.08, 95% CI [1.70–5.58]), less support, lower pre-disaster work productivity (OR 1.98, 95% CI [1.08–3.61]), and higher initial 2005 emotional distress. Understanding such factors can help in planning for enhanced support for individuals and parts of the system more vulnerable to overlapping disaster stress.

These observations on the psychology and psychiatry of these events suggest a great need for public education and research around multiple disasters and more efforts to augment support and maximize resilience

Extreme Weather, Natural Disasters, and Human Displacement

for individuals and community systems. One model proposed for identifying such multiple disaster-related needs (Machlis et al. 2022) uses topographical mathematics to map the spatial overlap, duration, periodicity, and expansion rates of disaster impacts as well as interdisaster infrastructure repair. This model can be used for sequential disasters to identify *legacy conditions* such as saturated ground, deforestation, and areas of weakened civic systems and public trust that predispose to greater future disaster vulnerability. For example, areas of drought that are more susceptible to fire lose their surface cover and become more vulnerable to mudslides, greater stormwater, and flooding during wet weather events, and housing damaged during earthquakes is more vulnerable to the impacts of hurricanes. Identifying where these concentrated areas of risk are is helpful for community planning. Similar modeling could be used for mental health claims or visits to show where populations are stressed, or particular populations known to have mental health conditions or risk could be surveyed topographically for their geographic overlap with areas of climate disaster risk, to begin to plan multiple disaster services and infrastructure.

Another model (https://marccd.info), developed by a coalition of Vibrant Emotional Health, the Group for the Advancement of Psychiatry, and Decision Point Systems, organizes multiple disaster responses by a diathesis-stress model, highlighting the characteristics of four phases of disaster response (anticipation, impact, adaptation, and recovery) and the ways to mitigate stress for survivors, community leaders, and responders at three defined phases (foundationally, acutely, and chronically) to keep the total impacts of recurrent disasters within the thresholds of the human ability to regulate stress in healthy ways.

Vignette

Supported by a mayor who had lost a grandson in a flood and had experienced post-traumatic growth, Dr. M was asked to fill a public health role by providing a disaster recovery plan for a community that had experienced the compound disasters of flooding and landslides after a long drought. The request came as they prepared for the spring melt from a record snowfall (extreme weather). As part of disaster planning, Dr. M met with town leaders to explain the Vibrant model for complex cyclical disasters and the different risks and needs of first responders and other groups. As the leaders came to understand the need to keep citizens and employees within nonpathogenic stress levels per this diathesis-stress model, they allowed Dr. M to screen all civil workers for anticipatory eco-anxiety and pretraumatic stress disorder and to set up mental health support for those at risk of PTSD from the coming stress.

In preparation for the next disaster, local occupational toxins were identified and stored properly. After an asset mapping of the town, community-wide delivery of mental health preparation was established. Lay groups were enlisted to pair adults with local teens for mentoring in emergency skills, set up a phone check system, and disseminate public health materials. The materials included information on how to prepare a go kit; education about normalcy bias and brain function during emergencies, with loud graphics that said "Do something! Do anything!"; videos of deep breathing and other stress-reduction techniques for grounding and presencing; a list of shelters and other resources; and mental health referrals. The graphics became a running gag with local kids, who later in life credited them with preventing several opioid deaths. Residents who had lost more in the first floods (neglected disasters) were identified, and they received personal outreach and anticipatory funds to prepare better. This act of environmental justice helped with a just transition for the community and decreased the potential for conflict. After being educated about the tendency to underestimate risk (common planning errors), the town practiced climate adaptation by using money from the Inflation Reduction Act to dig 10-foot-deep reservoirs three times larger than planned. These reservoirs were ultimately protective against the breakage of a local dam and contributed to local green space in the summers, providing time in nature for residents.

Psychologically, the more frequent and intense disasters of the climate crisis disrupt patterns of thought that contribute to a sense of personal stability, safety, and hope. The frequently encountered cycle in disaster recovery models (impact stress, heroic effort, stress impacts, reassessment, and resilient recovery) in response to challenges is disrupted when a second event befalls a still-vulnerable psyche. The overall stability of the natural world around us is also a core aspect of both reality testing and individual consciousness, processed unconsciously and in language. A typical person uses metaphors to describe themselves multiple times per minute (Steen et al. 2010), many of them based on natural phenomena (e.g., cooling off, going downhill). In this way, natural imagery contributes preconsciously to the processing of events, and the radical disruption of natural patterns and imagery by disasters can derail structures of thought and language that support identity, which often are already destabilized in patients with mental illnesses. The seasons and patterns of nature and landscapes that contribute to an individual mindset of cyclical repair, self-continuity, and familiarity are also more radically interrupted by repeated natural disasters and extreme weather events. One descriptive study of an area hit by successive tornadoes found high levels of disorientation to place, "like a bomb going off," as if "shit and goo" had coated all aspects of the self, leaving them feeling that they were "living but not living" (McKinzie 2018). Nature metaphors may be grounding for patients with postdisaster anxiety in this regard (Nguyen and Brymer 2018) and may also help them process and appreciate the dangers of impending disasters more realistically (Hauser and Fleming 2021).

Issues Related to Displacement and Migration

Natural disasters often lead acutely to forced displacement from home and land, and chronic disasters can lead to human migration. Migration is also occurring as low-lying sea islands go underwater and areas of drought become uninhabitable. Many social and economic factors determine climate-related migration, including livelihood, financial capital, food security, resource security, environmental degradation, political stability, health, social capital, and aid programs (Nabong et al. 2023). Although often described as international, such migration tends to be temporary, and the migrants tend to stay within their country of origin, moving from rural to urban areas. The Intergovernmental Panel on Climate Change (IPCC) projects that 31–143 million people per year will be displaced by climate conditions by 2050, including acute displacement from floods and storms and chronic displacement by drought and heat, and the IPCC states with high confidence that such movement contributes to violent conflict (Cissé et al. 2022). Displacement from home, whether permanent or temporary, has been associated with worse postdisaster outcomes, including multiple aspects of place attachment, such as notions of what is historical, stable, normal, and safe.

It is helpful in thinking about how patients may understand and react to climate displacement and migration to delineate the conceptual biases that have underlain its study. Initially, climate-induced migration was represented as a pathology to be prevented; next, it was understood as a matter of refugee rights. The media use metaphors such as floods and waves to describe migrants as an overwhelming influx of uncontrolled masses, sensationalizing what is already a field with complicated environmental justice, human rights, and jurisdictional issues.

The assumption of mass international climate migration has also been used for political purposes by governments to strengthen and protect national, regional, and international borders. The fearmongering about hordes of climate refugees has not borne out yet in reality, but it is shaping an increase in "othering" and fear of migrants.

All of this has happened in the absence of firm evidence that it will occur. Research in fact shows the opposite: that many factors, climate being only one, push a population to move from its ancestral homelands, and often this movement will be only temporary and local until conditions improve. From this perspective, mass climate migration is merely one resilient action, and it can be prevented by mitigation. However, even this positive research information was immediately co-opted by some to say that climate-related migration is the free choice of responsible individuals, "facilitating the movement of labor." This stance is then exploited to further the myth that there is a docile, cared-for population supported by the liberal order (Methmann and Oels 2015) and to neglect migration traumas and conflict. Understanding the overlay of such ideologically and emotionally charged societal narratives may help psychiatrists clarify patient fears and difficulties, whether migrant or host citizen.

Climate migration research is difficult because it must account for the numerous hazards and psychologies that could contribute to the end process and the many types of population movement—internal, external, circular, temporary—in calculations. Overcontrolling for factors such as economic status or conflict can lead researchers to minimize the way climate may have exacerbated these factors in tandem with increased migration. It is difficult to use preexisting knowledge to account for how migration will be impacted by new phenomena such as the melting of the Andes glaciers. Migration decisions represent a host of interpersonal and personal change factors: they can be made by households or by individuals, delayed by strategic waiting or because of wealth or a transient climate-related liquidity of it in a wealthy individual, and myriad other influences (Hoffmann et al. 2021).

Boas et al. (2019) argue that the securitization of climate migration studies is preventing more nuanced and relevant understandings of human movement in response to weather that would undergird decisions about where to invest in measures such as building codes and infrastructure that might allow people to remain in their home territory. Hirsch (2023) notes that alarmist international securitization of climate migration is also paradoxically and sadistically used to forcibly contain and immobilize populations, particularly encasing those that are Indigenous or nomadic, undergirded by historical and unconscious "settler logics of elimination." The psychology of immobilization and entrapment vis-à-vis climate change, such as might be experienced by people stuck on nonarable land, has not received adequate attention, but several studies show that prolonged detention in refugee camps for those who have tried to flee adverse conditions leads to a steady increase in suicide, acute health problems, and mental health problems by an OR of 1.03 per 10% increase in length of stay (CI not disclosed), correlating to 40 mental health presentations per night in a population of 100,000 (van de Wiel et al. 2021).

In fact, movement-based ways of living have always allowed Indigenous and nomadic peoples to respond more successfully to changing weather and to maximize access to abundant resources. These groups conceptualize home in different terms. The Fijians do not consider one's "dwelling as a motionless empty container of security that is placeless and interchangeable"; instead, they have the concept of *banua*, which considers home to be "meaningful relations with land, ocean, and place" (Hirsch 2023). Native Americans describe a web of relationships between kin, animals, land, spirits, the Earth, territories, and ancestors that is not bound to a physical structure (Bowra and Mashford-Pringle 2021). These psychologies of entrapment versus flow in relationship to place may also be more generally applicable for working with patient fears about entrapment on the declining Earth and an inability to adapt. For the working psychiatrist, the psychological narrative of movement needs to be considered in light of all of these factors and others that pertain to the psychological and psychiatric experience of the immigrant forced to leave or the victim trapped in dangerous climate conditions.

Issues Related to Climate-Related Resilience and Posttraumatic Growth After Disasters

Resilience has been defined in many ways, but is generally an ability to recover from adversity over time that has been defined as a fundamental characteristic of normal coping, a particular individual ability, an imperviousness to feeling stress, greater resistance to the impact of negative stress, or bouncing back from states of stress more quickly than most. Definitions also differ as to whether positive coping, which is the ability to use traumatic circumstances to fuel growth and improve baseline adaptation, should be included in the concept of resilience (Sisto et al. 2019). *Resilience* here refers to recovery from climate-intensified natural disasters and extreme weather, and adaptation to evolving weather conditions, such as changed shorelines, less predictable growing seasons, and other weather effects, both for individuals and for communities. Resilience that leads to adaptive change is sometimes called transformational resilience (Asadzadeh et al. 2022), but this concept should be distinguished from the practice of Transformational Resilience discussed in Chapter 12, "Psychotherapy Considerations and Approaches for Climate-Related Distress."

Resilience after natural disasters can be eroded by financial stress and loss of previous supports. Particularly for those of lower educational attainment or financial means, disasters can start a downward spiral related to property losses, a delayed return to employment, inadequate insurance, costs of displacement and rebuilding, lesser skills and knowledge for accessing resources, and other longer-term strains that follow the acute disaster event. Decisions by insurance companies to pull out of whole areas chronically affected by disaster further destabilize housing, property values, and tax-based services for whole areas, thus starting a spiral of social decline (Flavelle et al. 2024). Across diverse types of disasters and individuals, poverty, being in a marginalized ethnic group, younger age, neuroticism, and female gender work further against resilience (Saeed and Gargano 2022). These vulnerabilities are of particular concern when the next disaster strikes.

In their original work on posttraumatic growth, Calhoun and Tedeschi (2014) insisted that posttraumatic growth required events "seismic" enough to force individuals to reassess their representation of themselves and others, their world, and the future. They felt there had to be something extreme enough to break through the hypnotic trance of normalcy, and the individual and the group had to struggle with the meaning of it as well. As noted by Leppold et al. (2022), more severe and frequent climate-related disasters meet these criteria: they demand that we learn and change so that we can survive going forward. Calhoun and Tedeschi called such moments of awareness cognitive engagement, linked to two questions:

1. Why did this happen?
2. What implications does this have for my life?

Assessment of resilience is covered further in Chapter 11, "Assessment of the Patient." Such moments often occur several years after the inciting event, which can be unfortunate in relation to natural disasters because rebuilding efforts must start earlier. Whether more frequent or overlapping disasters will have this growth effect remains to be seen, perhaps delivering a final blow too far down an injured road, or perhaps the rock bottom that initiates recovery, as happens when experiencing addiction. Religious, spiritual, meaning-making, and acceptance coping can contribute to more growth, as can positive reframing, openness, hope about events, and experiences of high belongingness (Henson et al. 2021). These processes may be engaged to facilitate earlier and increased transformative recovery from disasters.

Transformative capacity in the wake of disasters is not the work of individuals, however, but rather of collectives of individuals acting in a deliberate, conscious way to enact shared goals in an uncertain and changing environment. In studies of adaptive responses, it has been shown to be more effective to do this in ways that include diverse voices and disciplines, empower vulnerable populations, implement trauma-informed care in schools and health care settings, provide education and infrastructure for housing and money pre- and postdisaster, and create dialogue specifically about accepting and understanding climate change (Everett et al. 2020). Central to such efforts is empowering agency within all participants to overcome avoidant, maladaptive coping patterns such as fatalism, denial, and wishful thinking. In complex socioecological systems requiring postdisaster reorganization of this type, adaptive capacities require the following:

- Creative work with social and ecological memory
- Disruptive, experiential, and experimental types of learning
- Allowing for process-oriented, self-organizing, and chaotically evolving governance structures

At the same time, those involved also follow best practices at the level of objective resources and external structures that allow such adaptation to proceed (Brown and Westaway 2011). Community adaptation planning for climate impacts is discussed further in Chapter 14, "Community Psychiatry and Its Role in Climate Mitigation and Adaptation."

Ethical Problems Associated With Promoting Climate-Related Resilience

The promotion of resilience to climate change is highly problematic ethically. It shifts responsibility for responding to conditions that can be prevented through the rapid reduction of fossil fuels to communities and individuals, and away from those who continue to impose hardship and adversity on others through fossil fuel industry and use, in the manner of a parent who tells a child whom they are abusing not to be so weak. Disaster psychiatry is inherently a responsive field, intervening after events and often led by militarily trained psychiatrists with strong loyalty to established structures. Although disasters are the current face of climate change because of the attention-grabbing nature of disaster events, disaster psychiatry is, as such, not optimal as a leader of a needed paradigm shift to a public health focus on prevention. It falls to the leaders of disaster psychiatry, then, to reject their traditionally prescribed identities and to envision new models for disaster recovery that address the human contributions to what have until now been seen as acts of God.

Providing Care for the Physical and Mental Health Impacts of Disasters

Psychiatric Risks of Acute Disasters

Disasters activate the stress response through injury, fear, and uncertainty, leading to both acute and chronic effects. The acute stress response after a disaster most commonly does not trigger a psychiatric illness; the most common symptoms are listed in Table 8.3.

Disaster-related stress, however, can trigger an exacerbation of an existing psychiatric condition or cause a trauma- or stressor-related disorder, as shown in Table 8.4.

The incidence of the most common disorders after disasters varies widely across studies, from 2.2% to 84% for anxiety, 3.23% to 52.70% for depression, and 2.6% to 52% for PTSD (Keya et al. 2023), although wider ranges have been reported. Studies vary by whether they are cross-sectional or longitudinal, the time frame after the disaster, whether methods are geared to pick up as much symptomatology as possible or only that which is more rigorously defined, and how they delineate acute from ensuing and more chronic impacts on outcomes (Chen et al. 2020). Higher rates of psychiatric sequelae are correlated with the intensity of the acute exposure, the perceived threat to oneself or one's family, loss, death, property loss, relocation, displacement, and physical

Table 8.3 Acute psychological disturbances associated with natural disasters

Sleep disturbance

Changes to eating behavior

Irritability and difficulties with concentration

Increased substance use, particularly alcohol and tobacco

Over-dedication or avoidance

Intergroup conflict

Increased domestic violence and child and elder abuse

pain and illness (reviewed in Saeed and Gargano 2022). The relationship between natural disasters and the sequela of eco-anxiety has not been formally studied, although it is clear from eco-anxiety surveys that the experience of a natural disaster triggers greater awareness and fear of climate change for some.

Risk factors for mental disorders after natural disasters span many domains of psychiatric health. Individuals with poor social support, prior stress, preexisting mental illness, substance abuse, neuroticism, avoidance coping, and difficulty finding spiritual or other meaning do particularly poorly, whereas a positive relationship with God is protective for mental health. Over the longer term, economic and property losses are increasingly important. Children exposed to disasters accrue

Table 8.4 Psychiatric disorders associated with natural disasters

Generalized anxiety disorder

Panic disorder

Major depressive disorder

Adjustment disorder

Substance use disorder

Acute stress disorder

Posttraumatic stress disorder

Brief psychotic disorder

long-term psychiatric risks, including higher rates of anxiety, mood, and substance use disorders as adults (Maclean et al. 2016). Neurobiologically, genes involved in contextual fear learning and fear extinction systems may play a role in outcomes. For example, variants in tropomyosin-related tyrosine kinase B (TrkB), a brain-derived neurotrophic factor receptor, distinguished children who had recovered from PTSD 3 years after an earthquake from children who had not (Li et al. 2020).

Physical Risks of Acute Disaster Exposure

The acute phase of a disaster is marked by destruction of property and surroundings. Beyond mortality, the most common associated acute physical risks to patients are injuries from blunt trauma and human-made hazards and from stress-related events such as myocardial infarctions. The profile of disaster-associated physical illness depends somewhat on the disaster, but within a few days, the greatest source of new morbidity and mortality shifts toward wound infections, communicable respiratory and gastrointestinal diseases, and vector-borne illnesses. Exacerbations of chronic illnesses such as diabetes and hypertension are also common. The physical risks of natural disasters are shown in Table 8.5.

Disasters also release toxins into the environment. Table 8.6 shows toxic hazards associated with major extreme weather events.

With this information in mind, a general conversation to reduce the physical risks of natural disasters can be useful and might include practical education and advice, such as that found in Table 8.7.

Improving Mental Function and Outcome in an Acute Disaster Through Rehearsal and Preparation

During an acute disaster, high or low temperatures, wind, water, smoke, and other environmental factors often decrease the accuracy of sensory perception. In addition, the stress response impairs thought processes and increases dissociation (Ripley 2008). Above a heart rate of 145, hearing is muffled, vision tunnels, and the perception of time is slowed (Ripley 2008). The typical human response goes through phases of denial and deliberation before the individual takes action to escape a threat, and cognitive biases such as the normalcy bias (downplaying information about threats such as gunshots) and social proof (looking

Table 8.5 Physical risks associated with natural disasters

Injuries (broken limbs, lacerations, and wounds)

Electric shock and other injuries from human-made hazards

Stress-related physiological events such as myocardial infarctions and strokes

Wound infections from *Staphylococcus*, *Streptococcus*, and tetanus

Waterborne illnesses, including cholera, E. coli, hepatitis A and B, leptospirosis, and dengue

Diseases of crowding (acute upper respiratory infections, measles, and meningitis)

Vector-borne illnesses (malaria, leishmaniasis, and rabies)

Source. Summarized from Burns et al. 2023; Jafari et al. 2011.

Table 8.6 Toxic hazards from major hydrometeorological events

Toxic gases

Combustible gases

Carbon monoxide

Sulfur dioxide

Hydrogen sulfide

Cyanide

Hydrocarbons

Aliphatic compounds (methane, butane, butadiene, propane)

Aromatic compounds (benzene, toluene, xylene)

Heavy metals

Lead (Pb)

Arsenic (As)

Mercury (Hg)

Cadmium (Cd)

Polychlorinated chemicals

Polychlorinated dibenzo-*p*-dioxins (dioxins)

Polychlorinated biphenyls (PCBs)

Table 8.6 Toxic hazards from major hydrometeorological events (*continued*)

Pentachlorophenol (PCP)

Fertilizers

Ammonium phosphates

Nitrates

Pesticides

Insecticides (organophosphates, carbamates, pyrethroids)

Herbicides (glyphosates)

Rodenticides (zinc and aluminum phosphides, brodifacoum)

Caustic agents

Acids (sulfuric acid, hydrochloric acid, hydrofluoric acid)

Alkalis (sodium hydroxide, potassium hydroxide)

Pulmonary carcinogens

Asbestos

Natural venoms

Hymenoptera (bees, wasps, ants)

Source. Used with permission from Erickson et al. 2019.

for what others are doing) impede a rapid response. It is most important to do something, anything, rather than allow precious minutes to pass.

Practicing for such experiences can help patients avoid the freezing response, which may cost them their lives, by creating automatic procedural memories for what to do. Techniques that have been shown to improve outcomes in high-risk situations include the following:

- Rehearsal—Fire, earthquake, tornado, active shooter, and similar drills help the body move effectively when cognitive processes are hampered by the fear response.
- Scripting—Similar to rehearsal, this is a practice of deliberating on what one would do if a threat emerged, such as on an airplane or in a movie theater. Patients might count the number of rows to the nearest exit, visualize themselves running in a haphazard way toward a door, look for fabrics or a fire extinguisher that could be used to douse a fire, and so on.

Extreme Weather, Natural Disasters, and Human Displacement   **157**

Table 8.7 Education and advice for all patients related to extreme weather and disasters

Obtain up-to-date vaccinations for measles, meningitis, tetanus, and hepatitis B; people traveling to endemic areas should also obtain cholera vaccination and prescriptions for antimalarial medication and a broad-spectrum antibiotic

Use good hand hygiene and low-concentration chlorine solutions against fungal spores, viruses, and bacteria

Use insect repellent and protective clothing

Be aware of the risks of carbon monoxide poisoning from charcoal, gas, and propane heaters; pressure washers; cars; generators; and other warming devices

Be aware of other safety issues, including dangers of standing water and electric power lines and equipment, contact with wild animals, improper use of power saws, gas leaks, and drowning and fall risks

- Combat breathing—Inhale through the nose, hold, exhale through the mouth, hold.
- Calm and shift—This is a cognitive sequencing for when one has decided on a plan of action: repeat the phrase "calm and shift" to oneself, slow breathing, engage in positive self-talk, focus on the moment and its needs, and then shift to visualizing and executing the steps to a positive outcome.

Patients with anxiety and anxiety disorders, as well as those with prior trauma and dissociation, have trouble working through such threat scenarios. They can nonetheless gain mastery through anticipatory practice and be supported to diminish the use of worry as avoidance. All patients should additionally have a go kit. Table 8.8 lists recommended and useful items. Go kits are most successful, however, when they are tailored to the needs of the particular patient and their family.

Psychiatric Support in the Acute Aftermath of a Disaster

Well-intentioned psychiatrists may often wish to provide psychological support in affected areas in the immediate aftermath of a disaster. Unfortunately, such helpers can do more harm than good, becoming

Table 8.8 Building a go kit for disasters

Water (1 gallon per person per day)

Canned food (3-day supply) and can opener

Prescription medications

Battery-powered or hand-crank radio

NOAA weather radio

Flashlight

Extra batteries in a sealed container

Matches and fire-starter in a sealed container

First aid kit with bandages and nonprescription medication

Whistle

Dust mask

Wrench or pliers

Sleeping bags

Soap and hand sanitizer

Infant formula and supplies

Pet food and water and medications

Cash

Candy, books, and games for children

Feminine hygiene products

Change of clothes

Paper towels and camping mess kits

Copies of family documents (birth and marriage certificates, social security cards, passports, insurance records)

High rubber boots or waders

Life jackets

Cell phone chargers

Fire extinguisher

Note. NOAA=National Oceanic and Atmospheric Administration.

Extreme Weather, Natural Disasters, and Human Displacement 159

another mouth to feed or another medical casualty of the situation. Practical help rather than psychotherapeutic support is often more immediately needed, and a psychiatrist may be more useful working on public messaging, fundraising, or other off-site tasks. Such outside help can assist inside helpers such as teachers and local emergency personnel, who are more familiar with the culture and norms of the community (Saeed and Gargano 2022).

If a psychiatrist does choose to participate, it is important to be affiliated with a disaster response organization and trained in appropriate techniques for emotional support in advance of participation, although "just-in-time training" may be available (Kantor and Beckert 2011, p. 12). Understanding the hierarchy of command and having a clear understanding of the various organizational roles and limits of one's own capacities are critical. Numerous governmental agencies are engaged in disaster responsiveness, as detailed in Table 8.9. The American Psychiatric Association Committee on Psychiatric Dimensions of Disaster (www.psychiatry.org/psychiatrists/practice/professional-interests/disaster-and-trauma) and the Center for the Study of Traumatic Stress (www.cstsonline.org/fact-sheet-menu/disasters) provide many useful materials for supporting disaster engagement.

For clinicians participating in providing direct psychological support in the acute setting, Psychological First Aid (PFA) has evolved to be the most widely recognized and deployed psychological intervention strategy for the acute postdisaster setting, despite questions about its cross-cultural usefulness. The goals of PFA are as follows (Fox et al. 2012):

- To make contact and provide empathic, unintrusive emotional support
- To enhance safety and physical comfort
- To calm those who are distraught and engage the positive coping of each individual
- To gather information, help articulate needs, and provide resources and practical assistance in response
- To connect victims with family and social supports, now and in the future
- To provide information about the psychological impacts of disasters and promote active recovery

Providing PFA can be a meaningful contribution for any volunteer or professional responding to a disaster. Empathic listening skills, however, may require more than the usual one-day training and should

Table 8.9 Disaster response systems in the United States

Agency	Description
National Incident Management System (NIMS)	A system focused on interagency and interjurisdictional cooperation during a disaster
National Response Framework (NRF)	A group for coordinating intergovernmental agency responses established by G.W. Bush, with an emphasis on preplanning
Incident Command System (ICS)	The basic emergency response structure of FEMA
Federal Emergency Management Agency (FEMA)	Lead disaster response agency under the Department of Homeland Security
National Disaster Medical System (NDMS)	Mobile medical teams under the Department of Health and Human Services (HHS) authorized for medical care and evacuations
Disaster Medical Assistance Teams (DMATs)	Fully functional mobile medical teams operating under NDMS
American Red Cross (ARC)	The ARC provides shelters, family assistance, social support, health screening, and basic mental health care
Community Emergency Response Teams (CERTs)	A federal citizen corps program, under FEMA, which can be an area of engagement for psychiatrists
Medical Reserve Corps (MRCs)	Often also called the Civilian Volunteer Medical Reserve Corps, MRCs aim to augment the disaster response of communities; they are under HHS, often offer mental health support, and can be an entry point for psychiatrists wishing to serve

include modeling, practice, feedback, and future supervision, including for mental health professionals (Movahed et al. 2022). When done correctly, PFA is associated with reduced anxiety, distress, depression, and PTSD, as well as better safety, connectedness, and sense of control (Hermosilla et al. 2023). Other treatments that may reduce development of PTSD after trauma have not been adequately validated but may include prophylactic glucocorticoids and brief cognitive-behavioral therapy (Howlett and Stein 2016).

Office-Based Assessment and Treatment of Psychiatric Disorders After Disasters

The first task for a psychiatrist assessing a patient presenting after a disaster is to differentiate normal from pathological responses to disaster and to recognize any neuropsychiatric conditions that may require urgent referral, such as toxic or infectious encephalitis. Attention can then be directed to the treatment of the presenting symptoms, including grief and loss, depression, anxiety, stress disorders, substance abuse, and interpersonal violence. Assessment should attend to vulnerabilities due to social determinants of health; the intersectionality of the patient in terms of race, culture, individual traits, and roles; and particularly to disruptions to identity that may have come from the loss of historical places or objects or displacement to an alien culture.

Standard medication treatments can be used, with the exception of benzodiazepines for anxiety, which may worsen long-term trauma-based outcomes. Although only paroxetine and sertraline have FDA approval for the treatment of PTSD, fluoxetine and venlafaxine have also been shown to be effective. Many clinicians find prazosin to be helpful for nightmares and risperidone to help with anger and hyperarousal, although studies are smaller and more mixed (Stein et al. 2006). Psychotherapy, however, is often the optimal treatment for PTSD and can include cognitive-behavioral therapy, cognitive processing therapy, prolonged exposure therapy, and mindfulness training, all of which have a strong evidence base. These therapies are described in Table 8.10. Virtual reality, ketamine, and 3,4-methylenedioxymethamphetamine (MDMA) are new treatments for PTSD that have not yet been researched in the disaster setting (Boydstun et al. 2021).

Table 8.10 Psychotherapy for PTSD after natural disasters

Therapy	Description
Cognitive-behavioral therapy	Cognitive-behavioral therapy is a structured treatment with homework focused on identifying automatic thoughts that contain distortions such as overgeneralization or arbitrary inference and challenging these with new thoughts and beliefs.
Cognitive processing therapy	Cognitive processing therapy is a 12-session manualized treatment shown to be effective in many populations, including combat veterans, sexual assault victims, and refugees. Sessions include patient education about PTSD symptoms, how treatment can help, articulating the thoughts and feelings to be focused on, teaching how to question these thoughts and feelings, and working to recognize how traumatic events have shaped the patient's identity and belief system and imagine new ways of being and believing. Sometimes the patient provides a written account of the trauma and reads it to decrease avoidance.
Prolonged exposure	In prolonged exposure (which is based in emotional processing theory), PTSD-related fearful reactions are viewed as units containing representations of the trauma, fear responses, and meanings given to it that are distorted by avoidance, overreaction, and incorporating safe elements as threatening. After psychoeducation and training in relaxation techniques, patients go through imaginal and in vivo exposure to feared situations, with reprocessing of the reaction. Prolonged exposure is highly effective (45%–90% response) regardless of type of trauma or time since exposure.

Table 8.10 Psychotherapy for PTSD after natural disasters (*continued*)

Therapy	Description
Mindfulness training	Mindfulness takes a nonjudgmental, "decentered" (i.e., observational) approach to thoughts and feelings while returning the focus of attention to the present when the mind strays. Practices include meditation, breathwork, relaxation, mindful execution of a task, and exercises that focus attention on a small element of the body or environment.

Source. Boyd et al. 2018; Watkins et al. 2018.

Key Points

- Climate change is increasing the frequency and severity of disasters, particularly natural disasters, around the world, leading to new multidisaster effects.
- Disasters take an enormous toll on the social and financial health, infrastructure, mental and physical health, and resilience of communities and individuals.
- Psychiatrists can participate in climate disaster psychiatry by researching the emerging phenomena of multiple and overlapping disasters and climate migration and by cultivating skills for disaster preparation, transformational resilience, and posttraumatic growth for individuals and communities.
- The traditional reactive approach of disaster psychiatry to single events can better mitigate climate disaster mental health impacts by shifting their orientation toward their preventable cause and interdisaster proactive adaptation efforts.

References

Asadzadeh A, Khavarian-Garmsir AR, Sharifi A, et al: Transformative resilience: an overview of its structure, evolution, and trends. Sustainability 14(22):15267, 2022

Auchincloss AH, Ruggiero DA, Donnelly MT, et al: Adolescent mental distress in the wake of climate disasters. Prev Med Rep 39:102651, 2024 38405174

Ayalon L, de Mendonça Lima CA, Banerjee D, et al: Older persons in climate change-induced hazards and building forward better: International Psychogeriatric Association, World Psychiatric Association—Section of Old Age Psychiatry, and NGO Committee on Ageing in Geneva position statement. Int Psychogeriatr 35(11):589–591, 2023 37655740

Bernstein D: Unpublished data, December 2021

Bhola V, Hertelendy A, Hart A, et al: Escalating costs of billion-dollar disasters in the US: climate change necessitates disaster risk reduction. J Clim Change Health 10:100201, 2023

Boas I, Farbotko C, Adams H, et al: Climate migration myths. Nat Clim Chang 9:901–903, 2019

Bowra A, Mashford-Pringle A: More than a structure: exploring the relationship between Indigenous homemaking practices and wholistic wellbeing. Wellbeing Space Soc 2:100007, 2021

Boyd JE, Lanius RA, McKinnon MC: Mindfulness-based treatments for posttraumatic stress disorder: a review of the treatment literature and neurobiological evidence. J Psychiatry Neurosci 43(1):7–25, 2018 29252162

Boydstun CD, Pandita S, Finkelstein-Fox L, et al: Harnessing virtual reality for disaster mental health: a systematic review. Transl Issues Psychol Sci 7(3):315–331, 2021

Brown K, Westaway E: Agency, capacity, and resilience to environmental change: lessons from human development, well-being, and disasters. Annu Rev Environ Resour 36:321–342, 2011

Burns P, Myers C, Yzermans J, et al: Physical health impacts of disasters, in Disaster Health Management: A Primer for Students and Practitioners, 2nd edition. Edited by FitzGerald GH. Abingdon, UK Routledge, 2023, pp 149–160

Buthmann J, Ham J, Davey K, et al: Infant temperament: repercussions of Superstorm Sandy-related maternal stress. Child Psychiatry Hum Dev 50(1):150–162, 2019 30030653

Calhoun LG, Tedeschi RG (eds): Handbook of Posttraumatic Growth: Research and Practice. New York, Psychology Press, 2014

Chen S, Bagrodia R, Pfeffer CC, et al: Anxiety and resilience in the face of natural disasters associated with climate change: a review and methodological critique. J Anxiety Disord 76:102297, 2020 32957002

Cissé G, McLeman R, Adams H, et al: Health, wellbeing, and the changing structure of communities, in Climate Change 2022: Impacts, Adaptation and Vulnerability. Contribution of Working Group II to the Sixth Assessment Report of the Intergovernmental Panel on Climate Change. Edited by Pörtner H-O, Roberts DC, Tignor M, et al. Cambridge, UK, Cambridge University Press, 2022, pp 1041–1170

Diamond E: Unpublished data, 2022

Eisenman DP, Galway LP: The mental health and well-being effects of wildfire smoke: a scoping review. BMC Public Health 22(1):2274, 2022 36471306

Erickson TB, Brooks J, Nilles EJ, et al: Environmental health effects attributed to toxic and infectious agents following hurricanes, cyclones, flash floods and major hydrometeorological events. J Toxicol Environ Health B Crit Rev 22(5–6):157–171, 2019 31437111

Everett A, Sugarman O, Wennerstrom A, et al: Community-informed strategies to address trauma and enhance resilience in climate-affected communities. Traumatology 26(3):285–297, 2020

Flavelle C, Rojanasakul M, Ratje P: Insurers are deserting homeowners as climate shocks worsen. New York Times, December 18, 2024. Available at: www.nytimes.com/interactive/2024/12/18/climate/insurance-non-renewal-climate-crisis.html. Accessed December 27, 2024.

Fox JH, Burkle FM, Bass J, et al: The effectiveness of psychological first aid as a disaster intervention tool: research analysis of peer-reviewed literature from 1990–2010. Disaster Medicine and Public Health Preparedness, 6(3):247–252, 2012 23077267

Gonzalez DE, Lanham SN, Martin SE, et al: Firefighter health: a narrative review of occupational threats and countermeasures. Healthcare (Basel) 12(4):440, 2024 38391814

Hauser DJ, Fleming ME: Mother Nature's fury: antagonist metaphors for natural disasters increase forecasts of their severity and encourage evacuation. Sci Commun 43(5):570–596, 2021 34489614

Henson C, Truchot D, Canevello A: What promotes post traumatic growth? A systematic review. Eur J Trauma Dissociation 5(4):100195, 2021

Hermosilla S, Forthal S, Sadowska K, et al: We need to build the evidence: a systematic review of Psychological First Aid on mental health and well-being. J Trauma Stress 36(1):5–16, 2023 36300605

Hirsch E: Forced emplacement: flood exposure and contested confinements, from the colony to climate migration. Environ Soc 14(1):4–22, 2023

Hoffmann R, Šedová B, Vinke K: Improving the evidence base: a methodological review of the quantitative climate migration literature. Glob Environ Change 71:102367, 2021

Howlett JR, Stein MB: Prevention of trauma and stressor-related disorders: a review. Neuropsychopharmacology 41(1), 357–369, 2016 26315508

Institute for Economics and Peace: Ecological Threat Report 2022. Sydney, Australia, Institute for Economics and Peace, October 2022. Available at: www.visionofhumanity.org/wp-content/uploads/2022/10/ETR-2022-Web-V1.pdf. Accessed December 11, 2024.

Jafari N, Shahsanai A, Memarzadeh M, et al: Prevention of communicable diseases after disaster: a review. J Res Med Sci 16(7):956–962, 2011 22279466

Kantor EM, Beckert DR: Preparation and systems issues: integrating into a disaster response, in Disaster Psychiatry: Readiness, Evaluation, and Treatment. Edited by Stoddard FJ, Pandya A, Katz CL. Washington, DC, American Psychiatric Publishing, 2011, pp 3–17

Keya TA, Leela A, Habib N, et al: Mental health disorders due to disaster exposure: a systematic review and meta-analysis. Cureus 15(4):e37031, 2023 37143625

Kronenberg M, Osofsky HJ, Osofsky JD, et al: First responder culture: implications for mental health professionals providing services following a natural disaster. Psychiatr Ann 38(2):114–118, 2008

Leppold C, Gibbs L, Block K, et al: Public health implications of multiple disaster exposures. Lancet Public Health 7(3):e274–e286, 2022 35065004

Li Y, Lv Q, Li B, et al: The role of trauma experiences, personality traits, and genotype in maintaining posttraumatic stress disorder symptoms among child survivors of the Wenchuan earthquake. BMC Psychiatry 20(1):439, 2020 32894097

Machlis GE, Román MO, Pickett STA: A framework for research on recurrent acute disasters. Sci Adv 8(10):eabk2458, 2022 35263123

Maclean JC, Popovici I, French MT: Are natural disasters in early childhood associated with mental health and substance use disorders as an adult? Soc Sci Med 151:78–91, 2016 26789078

Mash HBH, Fullerton CS, Morganstein JC, et al: Responding to repeated disasters: time to recovery in public health workers. Disaster Med Public Health Prep 17:e172, 2022 35770776

McKinzie AE: In their own words: disaster and emotion, suffering, and mental health. Int J Qual Stud Health Well-being 13(1):1440108–1440111, 2018 29493424

Methmann C, Oels A: From "fearing" to "empowering" climate refugees: governing climate-induced migration in the name of resilience. Secur Dialogue 46(1):51–68, 2015

Movahed M, Khaleghi-Nekou M, Alvani E, et al: The impact of Psychological First Aid training on the providers: a systematic review. Disaster Med Public Health Prep 17:e120, 2022 35332859

Nabong EC, Hocking L, Opdyke A, et al: Decision-making factor interactions influencing climate migration: a systems-based systematic review. WIREs Climate Change 14(4):e828, 2023

National Centers for Environmental Information: Annual 2005 Tropical Cyclones Report, Atlantic Basin. Asheville, NC, National Centers for Environmental Information, 2006. Available at: www.ncei.noaa.gov/access/monitoring/monthly-report/tropical-cyclones/200513#:~:text=14%20hurricanes%20formed%20during%20the,are%20over%20$100%20billion%20dollars.&text=Five%20named%20storms%20formed%20(Cindy,is%20the%20most%20on%20record. Accessed December 10, 2024.

Nguyen J, Brymer E: Nature-based guided imagery as an intervention for state anxiety. Front Psychol 9:1858, 2018 30333777

Ripley A: The Unthinkable: Who Survives When Disaster Strikes—and Why. New York, Three Rivers Press, 2008

Saeed SA, Gargano SP: Natural disasters and mental health. Int Rev Psychiatry 34(1):16–25, 2022 35584023

Sisto A, Vicinanza F, Campanozzi LL, et al: Towards a transversal definition of psychological resilience: a literature review. Medicina (Kaunas). 55(11):745, 2019 31744109

Soteriades ES, Kim J, Christophi CA, et al: Cancer incidence and mortality in firefighters: a state-of-the-art review and meta-analysis. Asian Pac J Cancer Prev 20(11):3221–3231, 2019 31759344

Steen GJ, Dorst AG, Herrmann JB, et al: Metaphor in usage. Cogn Linguist 21(4):765–796, 2010

Stein DJ, Ipser JC, Seedat S: Pharmacotherapy for post traumatic stress disorder (PTSD). Cochrane Database Syst Rev 2006(1):CD002795, 2006 16437445

United Nations Office for Disaster Risk Reduction: Definition: Disaster. Geneva, Switzerland, United Nations Office for Disaster Risk Reduction. Available at: www.undrr.org/terminology/disaster#:~:text=A%20serious %20disruption%20of%20the,and%20environmental%20losses%20and %20impacts. Accessed December 10, 2024.

van de Wiel W, Castillo-Laborde C, Francisco Urzúa I, et al: Mental health consequences of long-term stays in refugee camps: preliminary evidence from Moria. BMC Public Health 21(1):1290, 2021 34215237

Watkins LE, Sprang KR, Rothbaum BO: Treating PTSD: a review of evidence-based psychotherapy interventions. Front Behav Neurosci 12:258, 2018 30450043

Wolffe TAM, Robinson A, Dickens K, et al: Cancer incidence amongst UK firefighters. Sci Rep 12(1):22072, 2023 36627291

World Meteorological Organization: Atlas of Mortality and Economic Losses From Weather, Climate and Water Extremes (1970–2019). WMO-No 1267. Geneva, Switzerland, World Meteorological Organization, 2021

PART III

Psychological Responses to Climate Change, Assessment, and Psychotherapeutic Response

9

Obstacles to Rational and Adequate Responses to Climate Change

History of Climate Change and the Failed Human Response

Over the 150 years since global warming was first predicted and the 50 years that humankind has been aware that urgent action is needed, we have continued to pursue a destructive climate course against our own interests, threatening our own extinction. Scientists have been surprised by human climate irrationality. Their original prediction, known as the Gateway Belief Model, was that people would develop environmental concern and adjust their behavior as soon as they became aware of the scientific consensus on global warming. Instead, human unconscious reactions, defenses, emotional resistances, cognitive biases, and personality styles; the conceptual, spiritual, and philosophical complexities of grasping climate change; and the miscommunications, deliberate and inadvertent misinformation, shortsightedness, and failures of our cultural, political, and economic systems have contributed to perverse and destructive actions. In this chapter, I cover these problems: the history, denialism, and societal forces that have led to our

172   Handbook of Climate Psychiatry and Psychotherapy

current existential emergency, and the obstacles within human consciousness and in the nature of climate change itself that impede a sane and sustainable response.

Global warming was first formally predicted in 1861 by John Tyndall, who hypothesized that burning coal would increase global temperatures because CO_2 absorbs heat (Tyndall 1861). The greenhouse effect, however, had been noted by scientists such as Joseph Fourier and Claude Pouillet as early as 1824 and soon after by the undercredited American scientist and feminist Eunice Newton Foote, who in 1856 formally published the hypothesis that higher CO_2 would change the climate (Foote 1856). Swiss chemist Svante Arrhenius subsequently made the specific prediction that the Arctic would warm 15°F if CO_2 levels (295 ppm) at that time increased two- to threefold (Arrhenius and Holden 1897). In 1938, the first actual evidence of global warming was collected by Guy Callendar, who used weather station data to calculate that global temperature had risen 0.54°F over the previous 50 years (Callendar 1938). These predictions were formally codified in the work of Charles Keeling, who from 1958 onward conducted critical experiments to measure actual CO_2 concentrations in the air for the first time at the Mauna Loa Observatory in Hawaii, proving that CO_2 concentrations in the atmosphere were rising and were derived from fossil fuels. These measurements and their extrapolation to further elevations in CO_2 became the Keeling Curve (Keeling et al. 1976), which continues to correlate closely with changes in Earth's temperature.

Over the next three decades, the Nimbus satellites allowed scientists to gather data on the concentration of greenhouse gases in the atmosphere, the ozone layer, sea ice thickness, and Earth temperatures, increasing certainty about global warming. Antarctic ice cores obtained in 2004, reaching 3 km and recording nearly 800,000 years of ice, allowed scientists to measure the concentrations of greenhouse gases trapped in bubbles in the ice in relationship to ice layer thickness, a measure of temperature. These measurements showed that global temperatures, despite periods of fluctuation, have maintained a predominantly stable climate for essentially the past million years, rising this dramatically only in the nineteenth century and in direct correlation to greenhouse gas emissions. The science of global warming has continued to explode in recent decades, allowing high certainty now that the collapse of the Arctic ice sheets is inevitable, along with worsening weather and species and habitat loss.

These main points of debate about the mechanism and legitimacy of climate change were settled by 1979. Within that decade, led by the

Obstacles to Rational and Adequate Responses 173

efforts of dozens of leaders in the United States and abroad, human-kind endorsed a binding framework to reduce emissions. In the United States, many Republican administrations were on board to solve the problem. Fossil fuel industries were acknowledging the need to change energy strategies and were investing in solar and nuclear energy. But throughout the subsequent two decades, climate policy blew ineffectively in the political wind, abetted by the dismantling of environmental legislation that was particularly fierce and destructive during the Reagan administrations of 1981–1989, and further worsened during the Trump administration of 2017–2021, despite the extraordinary efforts of many committed and bipartisan government officials. The second Trump administration, at the time of this writing, was anticipated to dramatically eliminate climate protections.

The public opinion that permitted this unraveling resulted from a concerted campaign of denialism funded by a grant from Exxon that began in the late 1990s when more than 30 conservative groups bonded together as the Cooler Heads Coalition to form an echo chamber of climate denialism that has reverberated through United States climate policy since. Between 2000 and 2016, the fossil fuel industries spent $2 billion to defeat climate change legislation. This story—who said what, which reports received support and which were buried—evolved because of the psychological vicissitudes of alarm and moderation, delay and urgency expressed by reasonable people with various character styles whose spectrum of responses ultimately resulted in inaction. Its history is available in fine detail in *Losing Earth: A Recent History* by Nathaniel Rich (2019). It is a fundamentally psychological story, one from which organized psychiatry and psychiatrists have been alarmingly absent. As a result, the United States now ranks fifty-seventh among major nations in climate change performance, is one of nine nations responsible for producing 90% of global coal (Burck et al. 2024), and dominates per capita emissions.

In contrast to this discouraging history, a record number of Americans, and people in other countries around the world, show strong interest in climate realities and favor aggressive action to mitigate them. In the United States in 2023, 46% of people felt that they and others in America were being harmed by global warming, and 56% felt that global warming should be a high governmental priority, rising up to 85% when asked about particular policies rather than global warming as a phenomenon. Yet 65% of Americans rarely talk about climate change, and only 20% hear something about it more than once a month (Leiserowitz et al. 2023a, 2023b).

How can we understand this history of advancement and retrenchment, knowledge and inaction? Answers abound, most of them political and economic. But politics and economics are just the end product—the result of the obstacles, paradoxes, limits, and irrationalities of human thought and the feelings and actions that divert us from what would be best to do: factors that are the province of psychotherapy and psychiatry. In the remainder of this chapter, I will explore these obstacles to an adequate climate change response.

Factors That Interfere With People Understanding Climate Change

Climate change is a difficult thing for the human mind to grasp in its entirety. Problems with mentalizing climate change as a phenomenon, summarized in Table 9.1, make it more challenging to work on its emotional impacts and more difficult to take meaning-based action. These difficulties can be divided into four categories: epistemic (science- or knowledge-based), socioecological (the total environment), psychological or emotional, and ontological (related to the nature of a thing itself). Ontologically, climate change is difficult to mentalize because of its scope, complexity, and uncertainty. Ways of organizing one's thinking about these inherent traits in its nature include thinking of climate change as:

- A hyperobject
- An emergent system
- A wicked problem

Climate Change as a Hyperobject

Hyperobjects are hard to mentalize. They are defined as such: something so vast and diffuse that its totality is unknowable from any one point of reference (Morton 2013). With hyperobjects, the relationship between cause and effect is so remote and dispersed that causal connections cannot be easily made. Without causal connection, it becomes difficult to connect the dots between one's personal actions and what happens to the planet or to argue with certainty against other points of view for why climate effects are happening. It is equally difficult to connect any specific individual policy of governments or product

Obstacles to Rational and Adequate Responses 175

Table 9.1 Factors that impede the human climate response

The hyperobject nature of the climate problem

The wicked problems of climate change

The emergent properties of climate change

The uncertainty and ambiguity of climate outcomes

Epistemological challenges in knowing enough about climate change

Denialism

Disavowal

Cognitive biases

Emotional reactions

Reactions to existential and mortality threats

American values

Capitalism

Self-interest and the tragedy of the commons

Cultural and social factors

Perversity and irrationality in climate thought

---

of an industry directly to global climate-related increases in natural phenomena such as hurricanes. At some point, in trying to think about how to respond to all the systems of life interacting together to affect one's future, the mind exceeds its capacity and gives up.

Clinically, this may be reflected in feelings of fatalism, lack of agency, or irrelevance: "I just can't figure out how all of this will affect me," "What I should do?" or "There's nothing I can do—it's too big and too far away." Like the proverbial elephant examined by a blind man, such a problem is best approached from multiple points of view: both one's own over time, learning different angles of approach, and approaching the problem together with others, using their knowledge, to avoid defeatist outcomes. The dialectical behavioral therapy technique of chaining may also be useful to help patients keep cause and effect connected between small actions they might take and their remote benefits for the climate problem as a whole.

Psychiatrists, as well as patients, may struggle to keep the climate hyperobject in the focus of clinical care because it may feel both imminently and maximally important as well as dispersed and remote from the everyday well-being that is the concern of most visits. Psychiatrists may feel an ethical pressure to keep the focus on the patient's presenting problems and an equal pressure not to let the importance of climate impacts, like any other significant threat, become a neglected aspect of care due to countertransference minimization. Clinicians must keep an active focus on climate the same way they would for anything patients tend to push aside that is critical to their well-being. Keeping attention on such neglected matters can help cultivate long-term trust, increasing the patient's faith that the clinician can be counted on to take care of and remember the patient's safety needs and notice when the patient is evading an important area of function.

Climate Change as a Complex and Emergent System

In addition to being so large as to defy an encompassing view, climate change is also difficult to grasp because the planetary systems that determine its outcome are complex and emergent. In a straightforward but complicated system, such as a watch, each piece acts precisely and separately in a way that does not change over time and is easily monitored. In complex systems, however, components can interact. When these interactions have the potential to lead to new and evolving forms of organization and behavior, the system is defined as emergent. The properties of emergent systems are listed in Table 9.2.

The downsides of emergent systems—their chaotic, complex, and unpredictable natures—can lead to psychic tuning-out or overwhelm. But these characteristics are also what give them transcendent possibility. Emergent systems produce butterfly effects—possibilities that a small action will lead to an exponential response, moving a system along quickly to a higher level of function. They thus offer theoretical support for hope that an individual or collective action that tries something new or takes a step into uncertainty could change the world. Because human consciousness is also an emergent system, psychiatrists may be well attuned to appreciate and support these possibilities.

Climate Change as a Wicked Problem

Climate change is also difficult to grasp because it falls into the category of what decision science calls a wicked problem. The term *wicked*

Obstacles to Rational and Adequate Responses 177

Table 9.2 Characteristics of emergent systems

The system is rich and layered, as are its many subsystems

The elements of the system interact dynamically

Individual elements cannot know the full behaviors of the system in which they are embedded

Through the actions of individual elements, the system can evolve to new behaviors

There are diverse behaviors in the elements of the systems

The system is not in equilibrium

Feedback loops contribute to self-organization

The system is open and operates in nonlinear and chaotic ways

The system's chaotic, unbalanced, new organizations lead to evolution

problem was developed by Rittel and Webber (1973) to describe problems that cannot be easily or completely solved. Wicked problems do not have binary, clear answers, nor are their solutions binary in a moral or ethical sense. Problems can be solved in ways that are better or worse, more or less accurate, but not in ways that are good or bad, true or false: wicked problems never come fully clear. With wicked problems such as climate change, solutions to one part of the problem often create a new problem to solve, or require revision of the previously arrived-at solutions to another part of the problem. This further complicates a person's ability to feel they have a handle on the issues or can find answers to cope with them. The transition to clean energy is such an example: it raises a host of new questions about reemployment for people in fossil fuel industries and the environmental impacts of the new energy technologies.

Wicked problems are also characterized by the inability to fully test solutions in advance of implementing them. Psychiatrists are positioned to respond to this challenge in climate comprehension because of their long experience with supporting patients to find the best possible compromise formations. Through compromise formations, patients resolve multifaceted conscious and unconscious feelings and internal and interpersonal conflicts, reiteratively revising each best compromise over time, in a very similar process. The teaching "not to make

178 Handbook of Climate Psychiatry and Psychotherapy

perfect the enemy of the good" in psychological progress can also be brought to bear in the climate response.

Vignette

Jodi, age 42, had worked for years with her local conservation group to promote solar power legislation in her state. When it finally came through, the state authorized new lithium mining. Jodi found herself at odds with her former activist friends, who opposed all actions that might endanger local habitats. She was confused by the multitude of perspectives and conflicting facts presented by the two sides (hyperobject). Her therapist helped Jodi realize it would help to bring together a larger coalition to clarify the facts, find the least invasive sites to minimize mining damages, and broker the various problems that arose out of this negotiation (wicked problems). Later, to everyone's surprise, the redirection of water associated with the mine brought in some new organisms that led to a flourishing of local species that had been on the verge of extinction (emergent properties).

Epistemic Challenges of Climate Change

Climate Change Contains Several Types of Knowing

In addition to the challenge in absorbing the scale and emergent nature of climate change as a phenomenon, climate information is complicated to digest. To fully understand what is happening requires an understanding of magnetic radiation, chemistry, physical systems, feedback effects, chaos theory, and numerous other scientifically and mathematically complex topics. Evaluating the quality of scientific information requires an understanding of statistics and the scientific method, the relationship between high-probability events and certainty, and the relationship between the truly extraordinary accuracy of scientific climate predictions and the tremendous nonmeasurable risks and uncertainty of interacting natural systems.

Many levels of knowledge may be required to adequately mentalize climate change. These include the following (Gifford 2011):

- Knowing enough about the problem
- Knowing how to assess the relevance of the problem for you and others

Obstacles to Rational and Adequate Responses

- Knowing enough about its solutions
- Knowing enough to assess the relative benefits of these solutions, such as whether a solar panel system or an electric car is a better financial investment

These ontological barriers can be formidable enough to de-skill even motivated environmentalists, who have been shown to cite as their primary reasons for climate inaction that they are not skilled enough, are not as good as others for the task, do not know how to get involved, and need further training and encouragement (Latkin et al. 2023). However, a shared knowledge base is essential to unite the public cohesively around a climate action plan. Making accurate information and recommendations available in culturally accessible, simple terms is an important part of the sustainable transition. Even with simplified messaging, people require administrative support to sort through government climate program benefits. Studies have shown that talking about health, local issues, family benefits, and solutions is most effective in engaging people in climate information and action (ecoAmerica et al. 2015).

Uncertainty Introduces Ambiguity to Climate Understanding

Uncertainty about climate change introduces further difficulty in sorting through information to decide what to do. Climate uncertainty includes both uncertainties about what we know and uncertainties in factors that contribute to personal and social change. How uncertainty is discussed can play a significant role in climate outcomes (Kause et al. 2021).

Uncertainty about what we know can be helpfully divided into five categories:

- Uncertainties in static factual knowledge about the current climate system and the past
- Uncertainties about dynamic processes, whether current, future, or past (e.g., future emissions)
- Uncertainties that arise from contradictions within the system
- Uncertainties linked to the strategies of current actors (how humans will respond)
- Uncertainties linked to emerging elements and advances in what we know

These categories can be further refined in terms of the following (Fertel and Waaub 2013):

- Uncertainties due to breaks from the past, continuities, and discontinuities (e.g., leapfrogging effects in solar adaptation, changes in the political status of actors)
- Uncertainties related to reversibility and irreversibility (e.g., tipping points)
- Uncertainties related to scientific and technological innovation
- Uncertainties related to the eruption and evolution of contradictory forces in societies and people
- Uncertainties related to the evolution of thoughts, values, and behavior across generations
- Uncertainties related to the speed of processes and other time-related factors

Psychologically, the uncertainties of climate change introduce ambiguity, which can present both difficulty and opportunity in the clinical situation. The clinician can identify, label, and validate the type of uncertainty a patient is feeling and also normalize the experience of uncertainty as a starting point for interesting creative work. The patient may, however, require support to avoid polarizing their reaction to evolving climate information as "totally unclear" or "absolutely certain" and may become either phobic or counterphobic in taking action within uncertain outcomes.

A recently introduced concept of volatility may be useful. *Volatility*, as defined by Krause and Eriksen (2023), includes an acknowledgment of the greater flux and uncertainty in the emerging crisis but highlights the benefits of a volatile life, such as greater flexibility, self-mastery, attentionality, and improvisational and creative adaptation. Embracing volatility means adapting—without trying to control, acquire, or bounce back, and with greater freedom from colonizer norms. A skill of interactive reassessment may facilitate this kind of flow in uncertain or unstable times, given that things will change, and then they will change again. Further techniques for containing the anxiety of climate uncertainty are discussed in Chapter 12, "Psychotherapy Considerations and Approaches for Climate-Related Distress."

Obstacles to Rational and Adequate Responses **181**

Denialism Corrupts Knowledge-Gathering About Climate Change

Uncertainty also leaves people more vulnerable to climate disinformation. Denialism can then step into the gap and corrupt the intellectual clarity and unity necessary to motivate a social response to climate change. Denialism is not the systematic practice of the psychological defense of denial; rather, it is a systematic discrediting of truth to promote the agenda of a particular person or group—a socioecological undermining of knowledge-gathering. Denialism uses various tactics and techniques to undermine knowledge, including the following:

- Creating confusion and ambiguity

  - Saying there is no consensus about the facts
  - Saying that the evidence is contradictory or inadequate
  - Cherry-picking facts and evidence
  - Pushing oversimplified, hastily generalized, or circular arguments
  - Introducing logical fallacies and spurious arguments

- Pitting people against each other to create hate and division

  - Presenting minority views as having equal validity
  - Presenting fake experts to support marginal views
  - Linking interpretations of the facts and evidence to polarized political views and emotions
  - Launching ad hominem attacks on a person's character rather than the validity of their view
  - Introducing a conspiracy theory

- Delaying and stalling the resolution of conflict

  - Moving the goalposts of the debate so that a past acceptable standard is surpassed or overlooked
  - Creating delay by adding another reason climate action should be reexamined or postponed
  - Diverting attention to other issues

Patients may not have formal education in identifying logical fallacies and noting the distortions in how information is presented, although

Table 9.3 Therapeutic highlighting of denialism

"It sounds like they were almost *trying* to make you feel confused when you got it just fine."

"They seem to think picking on that one little thing will keep you from seeing the whole picture."

"It seems pretty manipulative to say that if you have a different view you can't be on their team."

"It's like they expect you to believe that one opinion as much as the opinions of people who have been working on this for years."

"It's like even though they know you're right, they want to kick the can down the road."

"It doesn't necessarily follow that A leads to B leads to C, but they talk like it does."

"A lot of other things would have to happen for that one thing to do all that."

"It really seems like they just wanted to divert your attention from the real issue."

"I don't know how you sort out the facts with all those emotional appeals and insults."

gut instincts are likely to tell them something is amiss. Labeling these denialist techniques when they occur, whether in a family argument or when reviewing climate issues in a session, may be helpful. Table 9.3 shows some simple comments a clinician might make to call attention to denialism in climate information.

Numbing Leads to Neglect of Climate Information

Information about climate change is also affected by environmental information numbing, defined by Gifford (2011) as habituation to repeated climate messaging or selective neglect of information that does not affect our immediate environment, such as conditions in the Global South. Varying the groups with which one communicates, engaging with groups with differing points of view, and taking time for self-care and leisure can keep approaches to climate information fresh.

Human Optimism Reduces Awareness of Threats

In contradistinction to environmental numbing, human optimism can also keep us from appreciating climate threats. Overall, optimism is adaptive, but it has also been shown that people significantly underestimate their personal vulnerability in general (Weinstein and Klein 1996) and their vulnerability to environmental hazards in particular (Pahl et al. 2005). Gently querying what climate adversity is like for a patient or modeling that the therapist expects problems to arise for themselves may be helpful; reviewing insurance actuarial tables may also provide a tolerable reality check of the likelihood of events (e.g., flood or fire damage probabilities).

Cognitive Biases Distort Logic

Cognitive biases are an additional and powerful reason that people struggle to process climate-related information logically. These biases operate both to distort information processing and to provide emotional motivation for how information is heard and used, so they fall between psychological and epistemological resistances to climate awareness and action. Our mental apparatus is poorly adapted for the climate crisis in particular because it has evolved to survive in the immediate present for the following reasons:

- To take care of ourselves and our small group
- To respond to immediate dangers
- To hoard useful resources

It has not evolved for the tasks that face individual people now:

- To preserve the larger group of all humanity and nonhuman beings
- To preserve larger natural resource systems over our own needs
- To deal with dangers that are, mostly, at least in the moment, far away and nonthreatening

Cognitive biases act also to shape attitudes that more readily preserve preexisting views, including those of one's identity and valued group. They also steer us away from uncertainty and from engaging in unnecessary or risky change. The backfire effect, self-serving bias, and conservation bias are cognitive biases that act to preserve existing views and affiliations rather than adopt new information. Examples of cognitive biases that work against psychological adaptation to climate change are presented in Table 9.4. Pointing out such habits of thought when noted may allow patients to make safer choices.

Environmental Amnesia Changes Our Ability to Know

Environmental amnesia is another way we can "not know" about climate change. Environmental amnesia refers to forgetting past natural realities over generations. Those who have never seen snow are unlikely to mourn its loss. Just as we do not routinely mourn the absence of dinosaurs in daily existence, future generations may not mourn lost species.

Social Barriers to Climate Responsiveness

Societal pressures also stall a rapid adaptive response. Social structures, organized around beliefs, practices, and existing norms and rules, can cause climate responses to languish through various attitudinal, financial, and political means that can be assessed for both individuals and institutions (Eisenack et al. 2014). Social barriers include the following:

- Lack of technical and economic means to change
- Lack of societal knowledge on how to adapt
- Institutional pressures (on companies as well as individuals) to remain the same
- Pressures to avoid unnecessary financial and structural destabilization and risk by waiting until action is unavoidable
- Cultural and normative pressures that favor preexisting behaviors
- Inadequate or biased top-down or bottom-up leadership
- Conflicting goals or timescales
- Institutional crowding or institutional voids that weaken individual actors

Examples of cultural pressures impeding climate responsiveness include cultural beliefs in having large families, behavioral norms in

Obstacles to Rational and Adequate Responses **185**

Table 9.4 Cognitive biases with relevance for climate change

Cognitive bias	Influence on thought process	Optimal thought process for climate responsiveness
Anchoring (e.g., common source bias, conservatism bias)	Overusing familiar information: overuse of the same source, failure to revise with new evidence	Openness to new information; adopting new points of view as conditions change
Ambiguity effect	Avoiding uncertainty, even if the outcome is worse	Confronting and experimenting with uncertainty
Availability heuristics (future discounting)	Overestimating the future likelihood or importance of things fresh in memory	Imagining changing frequencies of events on the basis of data rather than those we have seen
Bystander effect	Waiting to act until others do, even in emergencies	Innovating and being early adopters; allowing oneself to stand out
Confirmation biases (e.g., backfire effect, selective perception, Semmelweis reflex)	Reacting to disconfirming evidence by digging into old beliefs, seeing what you expect to see, rejecting evidence that contradicts a familiar paradigm	Appreciation for shifts in conditions as representing actual change; cognitive and emotional flexibility of trying on new ways of thinking and being
Egocentric biases (e.g., illusory superiority, unnoticed bias, illusory validity, naïve realism, false consensus effect)	Believing one is less biased, more valid in judgment, superior, and more able to see reality accurately, and that others all agree	Ability to question one's point of view when futures are unknown, to try on alternative descriptions of what is happening or ideas about what to do; ability to respond to disagreement or dissent

186   Handbook of Climate Psychiatry and Psychotherapy

Table 9.4 Cognitive biases with relevance for climate change (*continued*)

Cognitive bias	Influence on thought process	Optimal thought process for climate responsiveness
Endowment effect	Valuing what one already has, including a way of life, as greater than its actual worth	Understanding the equal or greater possibilities and values associated with giving up old ways and modes of production
Hyperbolic discounting (future discounting)	Preferring immediate payoffs; minimizing future costs	Making decisions that are better for long-term sustainability
Logical fallacies (e.g., sunk cost fallacy, plan continuation bias, zero-sum bias)	Continuing to invest in old strategies even if evidence suggests change; failure to recognize the need to change; seeing the possibilities as zero-sum so changing is losing	Investment in new strategies and lifestyles; ability to see the degree of threat; appreciating the positives of change that is unfamiliar
Ostrich effect	Sticking one's head in the sand to avoid anxiety about things that are critical for one's survival	Courageously confronting difficult truths and taking in their personal relevance emotionally; living in a fact-based world
Prospect theory: ambiguity effect, dread aversion, loss aversion, status quo bias/system justification	Preferring knowns to unknowns; overvaluing or savoring what one has because of dread of change; keeping the status quo even when unwise	Gritty, courageous forays into uncertain new technologies and ways of life; ability to evaluate the negatives of the status quo

Obstacles to Rational and Adequate Responses   **187**

Table 9.4 Cognitive biases with relevance for climate change (*continued*)

Cognitive bias	Influence on thought process	Optimal thought process for climate responsiveness
Truth judgment: illusory truth effect, subjective validation	Believing something to be true because it is easier to process or because one's beliefs demand it be true	Ability to comprehend complex systems and realities and question one's beliefs and assumptions about how to live

some cultures that prevent women from acquiring needed skills such as the ability to swim to escape a flood, beliefs in the fertility powers of consuming endangered species, or pressures in the fashion industry or elite groups to dress or travel a particular way. These social barriers can be systematically reviewed with patients and in civic structures and workplaces interested in improving their sustainability. Futures thinking can then be applied to help them overcome inertia and plan creative and effective responses. Bringing in data from the mental health literature on what contributes to individual and social happiness and well-being is an additional role for the clinician.

American Character Armor

For most Americans, one of the most difficult social barriers in responding to climate change arises from our national ethos. Founded on values of individualism and expansion, our national character is poorly suited to a cooperative, self-limiting global response that supports interdependence and group welfare. The following are some of the values that disadvantage the climate responsiveness of Americans compared with other cultures (Kohls 1984):

- Individualism—neglects the role that group and planetary welfare play in individual well-being
- Competition—rewards individual victories more than victories that result from group cooperation
- Materialism—espouses a more-is-better mentality that hinders the capacity to recognize what is enough, to feel the kind of

lightened happiness associated with having less, and to not seek happiness from the acquisition of material goods

- Action and work—reduce attention to the value and pleasures of just being and work against care for and appreciation of the vitality and value of elements of the natural world that just are, such as rocks and trees
- Change—works directly against preservation-oriented mind-sets that value history and continuity of resources and systems
- Speed—places a utilitarian emphasis on productivity, which opposes the gains of thoughtful, slow interactions that enhance attachment to and concern for other humans and other beings
- Control—de-emphasizes the role of fate and forces beyond one's control in outcomes and makes it more psychologically challenging to see the roles that larger forces, such as climate effects, have in one's personal circumstance and future

In contrast, European and Asian cultures tend to value group cooperation, group welfare, sacrifice, and conceptions of the self that place it in larger historical, spiritual, and universal contexts. Dedicating oneself to sustainability is more consonant with that ethos, in part explaining why it may come more naturally to countries in these areas.

Capitalism

In addition to the values held by many Americans, the U.S. capitalist economic system makes climate adaptation more difficult to mentalize and to make behavioral changes toward. Climate demands challenge the capitalist way of life Americans have been raised to aspire to and their most treasured institutions. As an economic structure currently dependent on accumulation and on the extraction of fossil fuels and other resources to obtain perpetual growth, capitalism is associated with negative societal effects that include climate change, pollution, wasting of resources, commodification of human and nonhuman beings, inequality, and unemployment (Schot and Kanger 2018).

As articulated by writer David Wallace-Wells (2019), psychological attitudes toward capitalism vary dramatically, from growth-oriented conservatives to anti-capitalist liberals. Climate-related beliefs about capitalism also vary to extremes, from those who feel it must be replaced by a postcapitalist fully circular nonhierarchical economy to those who see it as critical to any sustainable transition (reviewed in Baer 2023).

Obstacles to Rational and Adequate Responses 189

Human thought around climate and capitalism easily becomes distorted, with difficulties such as the following:

- Exaggeration of capitalism as the most viable economic system, when co-ops, family networks, local exchanges, and social solidarity can be equally effective
- Irrational consideration of scale and benefit (e.g., thinking that changing capitalism is more difficult than changing its environmental costs, despite financial evidence)
- Reliance on devaluation and splitting to feel positive about its benefits (e.g., deliberately suppressing awareness that workers in Saudi Arabia are dying from the global warming effects of the oil they have produced)

These views lead to meta-narratives about the value of capitalism that can be explored in psychotherapy. An approach to the reform of capitalism that is psychologically intuitive is Deep Transition theory. This model defines a deep transition as "a series of connected and sustained fundamental transformations of a wide range of socio-technical systems in a similar direction" and is built on two socioeconomic models: the techno-economic paradigm and the multi-level perspective. It considers human techno-industrial progress in terms of multiple overlapping waves. Everything so far is part of the first deep wave, and the green energy and informational conditions created by artificial intelligence, high-speed Wi-Fi, and global sharing of information are part of the just-beginning second wave (Schot and Kanger 2018). This way of thinking takes into account the emergent nature of complex systems and provides hope that such complex techno-economic systems can progress without minimizing the way that capitalism and other economic structures permeate and support our social landscape and must be integral to sustainable living.

Vignette

Sharon, age 20, presented to session infuriated at her "stupidity" during a conversation with her conservative uncle, who told her wind farms were a nonviable energy source and attacked the ignorance of her favorite professor. Her therapist pointed out that her emotions and self-evaluation were more a response to the ad hominem attacks and cherry-picked information than the data (denialism) and gently helped her to confront the cognitive biases (anchoring) about wind farms that made her so certain of her righteousness. Talking about the relationship increased Sharon's empathy for her uncle's experience as an older American (American character armor). This work helped Sharon to confront her own certainty about building wind farms (defensive optimism) and explore her underlying fear about climate uncertainty (uncertainty). After doing more detailed research, she was able to engage her uncle in a productive conversation about the current and future benefits of alternative energy sources that shifted his pattern of political and charity donations.

Tragedy of the Commons

Tragedy of the commons is a term used to describe the downside of high levels of individual consumption, which can be a social barrier to climate responsiveness. Exploiting free resources that are common to all is beneficial for short-term personal gain, but over time it leads to the depletion or destruction of the resource for both the individual and the group (Hardin 2009). Until that point, however, it is beneficial for the person to take as much as possible. Such phenomena as people rushing to buy a rare hardwood or taste the declining roe of a sturgeon before it is "gone" are examples of such irrational behavior, in which straining the resource further hastens its collapse. Rather, by prioritizing the benefits to the commons of shared sustainable action, the resource as well as the community interested in it can be supported and even enhanced.

Disavowal as a Defense Against Awareness of Climate Change

Unlike the defenses that block climate awareness, disavowal is defined as a defense in which we are aware of a problem or conflict but act as if we are not. Disavowal is one of the defenses identified by Sigmund Freud, along with denial and dissociation, that requires a splitting of reality (Blass 2015). It is distinguished from repression, in which the problem is wholly pushed out of consciousness temporarily but can be brought back by various triggers; from suppression, in which we push only our anxiety out of awareness but remain in full awareness of the problem; and from denial, in which the problem is forced completely into the unconscious and we are literally unable to acknowledge or feel it. Disavowal is typically considered a lower-level defense associated with high anxiety because the split-off reality we ignore is still close to awareness and pressing to break through. It brings preconscious guilt

Obstacles to Rational and Adequate Responses **191**

from pretending that one's actions are all right when one knows better. Disavowal is a common climate defense to reconcile our social and climate realities, which often include social norms that pressure us to live as if we are not aware of the implications of this lifestyle. The costs, however, include threats to authenticity and superego integrity, which manifest as free-floating guilt and anxiety.

Perverse Defenses and Irrationality in the Climate Response

Perverse Thinking

Perverse defenses also play a role in climate inaction, often arising from disavowal. The essence of the perverse thought or defense is pretending that something does not have the meaning or function that it does—metaphorically turning a sow's ear into a silk purse, followed by lavish fawning over how wonderful the silk is. Perverse thinking is stubborn, and persistent in seeing something that is patently untrue as true, as, for example, when a subway frotteur insists that rubbing his penis against someone disgusted by it is a private pleasurable experience. Perversion thrives on ambiguity, illusion, and collusion: the child I am molesting likes it; the odd specialness that others witness between us represents love. Through silencing and devaluing opposition, the perverse fantasy and its false ideology are forced on what is actually happening. Perversion is a more severe form of psychic retreat from a psychodynamic perspective: it is disconnected from the feelings, needs, and realities of the other.

Many aspects of the human response to climate change are perverse. Colloquially, we say something is "perverse" when it is wrongheaded, unreasonable, corrupt, improper, and incorrect (*Merriam-Webster,* accessed July 30, 2023). Examples of perverse thinking associated with climate change include the following:

- The technological solution fantasy—that mechanical inventions can compensate fully for our bio-physiological dependence on nature
- The scientific solution fantasy—that science, which has supplied the nitrogen fixation and fossil fuel extraction that have led to a population explosion on a hot planet, is inherently and purely prone toward doing good

- The capitalist fantasy—that an unmodified expansionist economic model dependent on the use of resources can continue and provide solutions to the problem of diminishing resources
- The secret weapon fantasy—that, deprived of the communal support of his allies by a destructive enemy, a sole male individual will come up with an invention that will restore peace and fertility to a conflict-ridden, depleted global family (Sontag 1961)
- The suprahuman power fantasy—that even though humankind created the climate problem, something suprahuman (Mother Nature, God) will reverse it
- The recycling fantasy—that recycling is a sufficient personal action to mitigate a global energy problem

Paul Hoggett (2013) identified the way perversion is created and maintained in "gaps," which create a space between the thing and the way it is seen. In modern society, the complexities of shipped products; products that are easily replaced in a throwaway culture; products that are digital; and digital communication that allows us to distance the appearance, voice, and every other aspect of the essence of a thing have moved us further and further into perverse modes. So also has profit-based capitalism, which continually exploits the gap between the value of a thing and its cost to others.

Chasseguet-Smirgel (1984), Steiner (1994), and others have looked at perversion as a way of not coming to terms with conscious and unconscious feelings of loss, deprivation, and neglect, such as we might experience if we appreciated the damage done to nature by its exploitation, or the damage done to another by sexually perverse acts experienced as unwanted assaults. For the pervert, frotteur, voyeur, pedophile, and exhibitionist, access is never denied on the basis of its unwantedness, because they are imagined away through fantasies that deny the experience of the other. It is in a similar pretending way—that things will be OK, that we will not have to change, give some things up, or be in danger—that perverse thinking prevents effective climate action. Through this perverse enactment, valued aspects of the self are protected, but at high cost.

Terror Management Theory

Another way of understanding individual and social resistance to rapid climate adaptation similarly linked to the preservation of identity over adaptation is terror management theory. This theory states that terror

Obstacles to Rational and Adequate Responses **193**

arises at both conscious and unconscious levels because of the tension between self-preservative instincts and our adaptive awareness of death, which shows us that we cannot survive regardless of our efforts. Because we are aware we cannot live, we instead act to preserve our identity by improving self-esteem and creating symbolic meaning for our lives in ways that will transcend mortality: through alliances with larger national, communal, and cosmic identities and through belief in religion, the afterlife, and our superiority over animals (Solomon et al. 2015). This way of thinking posits that people faced with existential fears will act to preserve their identity as well as their life, using two main propositions:

- Proposition 1—People will respond to threats of death with health behaviors
- Proposition 2—People will respond to unconscious awareness of death with efforts to maintain meaning and self-esteem through affiliation with something larger, valuable, and enduring

Mortality Salience Theory

Mortality salience theory is linked to terror management theory. Proponents of this theory hypothesize that increased attention to or awareness of death will lead to an increase in behaviors that restore a sense of identity or invulnerability. Anti-vaccination attitudes are an example of a behavior linking oneself to one's larger political group, consistent with terror management and mortality salience theories. Mortality salience theory offers an explanation for how humans have responded to waves of increased climate awareness with an entrenchment in their existing ways of acting and thinking, including at the cost of preserving or prolonging life—for example, choosing smoking or visits to tanning salons to preserve one's style (Cox et al. 2009; Jessop et al. 2008). Studies (Glad 2022; Vess and Arndt 2008) have demonstrated decreased environmental concern after increasing mortality stress. This behavior, however, was mediated by preexisting beliefs—both people accustomed to contemplating death and those with preexisting pro-environmental beliefs increased their self-esteem and endorsement of pro-environmental views after contemplation of a death threat, whereas those not immersed in these issues retrenched to a less pro-environmental stance (Glad 2022). It follows, also, that creating sustainability narratives that link desired new behaviors to both existing

Emotional and Unconscious Reactions to Climate Change

In addition to the difficulties of processing climate change cognitively, our reactions are shaped by many uncomfortable emotions that can interfere with our rational and adequate response to it. These emotions include the following:

- Sadism—We are the ones destroying the planet and its creatures for our pleasures
- Guilt—We continue to do things that worsen climate conditions when we know better
- Betrayal—Those who had responsibility for stewarding the planet have placed us in jeopardy
- Rage—We feel betrayal and climate injustice and feel powerless to bring those responsible to justice and to force change
- Envy—Others who are blissfully unaware and unconcerned do not carry this burden
- Dependency—We are dependent on Nature to keep us alive and on others to respond to the climate crisis
- Fear—We will be annihilated or will experience starvation, disease, and injury from worsening conditions
- Grief—We grieve for what is being destroyed and what will be destroyed for future generations
- Emptiness—We feel numb from an identification with the death and losses we see around us
- Disgust—We are disgusted at carboniferous excess consumption
- Narcissistic injury—We feel the loss of imagined legacies in children and grandchildren, and pain from our inability to address the problem
- Uncertainty—We face the destabilization of our identities, social structures, and futures

These emotions, many of which are covered in Chapter 10, "Emotional Reactions and Syndromes Associated With Climate Change," are uncomfortable to bear and can lead to avoidance. By exploring and

Obstacles to Rational and Adequate Responses

articulating them, the values that lead to these feelings can be identified, and meaningful forms of participation can be found.

Key Points

- Human failure to respond to global warming is based on psychology and behavior, in which psychiatric and other mental health practitioners must play a critical role.
- Climate change is difficult to respond to because of its hyperobject, emergent, and wicked nature.
- Adequate and accurate knowledge about climate change is limited by complexity and uncertainty, denialism, and cognitive biases.
- Social norms and cultural forces also impede climate responsiveness, leading to disavowal and perverse thinking in the face of evolving threats.
- Mortality terror and emotional responses to climate change can lead to avoidance of facing climate realities.

References

Arrhenius S, Holden ES: On the influence of carbonic acid in the air upon the temperature of the Earth. Publ Astron Soc Pac 9(54):14–24, 1897

Baer HA: Climate change and capitalism, climate dystopia, and radical climate futures. J Aust Polit Econ 91:107–127, 2023

Blass RB: Conceptualizing splitting: on the different meanings of splitting and their implications for the understanding of the person and the analytic process. Int J Psychoanal 96(1):123–139, 2015 25684617

Burck J, Uhlich T, Bals C, et al: Results: Climate Change Performance Index: Monitoring Climate Mitigation Efforts of 63 Countries Plus the EU— Covering More Than 90% of the Global Greenhouse Gas Emissions. Bonn, Germany, Germanwatch, 2024. Available at: https://ccpi.org/wp-content/uploads/CCPI-2024-Results.pdf. Accessed February 2, 2025.

Callendar GS: The artificial production of carbon dioxide and its influence on temperature. Q J R Meteorol Soc 64(275):223–240, 1938

Chasseguet-Smirgel J: Narcissism and perversion, in Creativity and Perversion. New York, WW Norton, 1984, pp 24–34

Cox CR, Cooper DP, Vess M, et al: Bronze is beautiful but pale can be pretty: the effects of appearance standards and mortality salience on suntanning outcomes. Health Psychol 28(6):746–752, 2009 19916643 ecoAmerica, Lake Research Partners; Krygsman K, Speiser M, et al: Let's Talk Climate: Messages to Motivate Americans. Washington, DC, ecoAmerica, 2015

Eisenack K, Moser SC, Hoffmann E, et al: Explaining and overcoming barriers to climate change adaptation. Nat Clim Chang 4:867–872, 2014

Fertel C, Waaub J-P: Climate change, uncertainty and ethical perspectives: the role of decision-making tools. Int Soc Sci J 64(211–212):39–54, 2013

Foote E: Circumstances affecting the heat of the Sun's rays: read before the American Association, August 23, 1856. American Journal of Science and Arts 22(66):382, 1856

Gifford R: The dragons of inaction: psychological barriers that limit climate change mitigation and adaptation. Am Psychol 66(4):290–302, 2011 21553954

Glad J: A strength model of mortality salience: can practicing thinking about death encourage environmental concern? PhD Thesis. Ann Arbor, MI, ProQuest, 2022

Hoggett P: Climate change in a perverse culture, in Engaging With Climate Change: Psychoanalytic and Interdisciplinary Perspectives. Edited by Weintrobe S. Hove, UK, Routledge, 2013, pp 56–71

Hardin G: The tragedy of the commons. J Nat Resour Policy Res 1(3):243–253, 2009

Jessop DC, Albery IP, Rutter J, et al: Understanding the impact of mortality-related health-risk information: a terror management theory perspective. Pers Soc Psychol Bull 34(7):951–964, 2008 18453389

Kause A, Bruine de Bruin W, Domingos S, et al: Communications about uncertainty in scientific climate-related findings: a qualitative systematic review. Environ Res Lett 16(5):53005, 2021

Keeling CD, Bacastow RB, Bainbridge AE, et al: Atmospheric carbon dioxide variations at Mauna Loa Observatory, Hawaii. Tellus 28(6):538–551, 1976

Kohls LR: The Values Americans Live By. Washington, DC, Meridian House International, 1984

Krause F, Eriksen TH: Inhabiting volatile worlds. Soc Anthropol 31(4):1–13, 2023

Latkin C, Dayton L, Bonneau H, et al: Perceived barriers to climate change activism behaviors in the United States among individuals highly concerned about climate change. J Prev 44(4):389–407, 2023 36264403

Leiserowitz A, Maibach E, Rosenthal S, et al: Climate Change in the American Mind: Beliefs and Attitudes, Fall 2023. New Haven, CT, Yale Program on Climate Change Communication, 2023a

Leiserowitz A, Maibach E, Rosenthal S, et al: Climate Change in the American Mind: Politics and Policy, Fall 2023. New Haven, CT, Yale Program on Climate Change Communication, 2023b

Morton T: Hyperobjects: Philosophy and Ecology After the End of the World. Minneapolis, University of Minnesota Press, 2013

Obstacles to Rational and Adequate Responses

Pahl S, Harris PR, Todd HA, et al: Comparative optimism for environmental risks. J Environ Psychol 25(1):1–11, 2005

Rich N: Losing Earth: A Recent History. New York, MCD/Farrar, Straus and Giroux, 2019

Rittel HWJ, Webber MM: Dilemmas in a general theory of planning. Policy Sci 4(2):155–169, 1973

Schot J, Kanger L: Deep transitions: emergence, acceleration, stabilization and directionality. Res Policy 47(6):1045–1059, 2018

Solomon S, Greenberg J, Pyszczynski T: The Worm at the Core: On the Role of Death in Life. New York, Random House, 2015

Sontag S: The imagination of disaster, in Against Interpretation and Other Essays. New York, Picador, 1961, pp 209–225

Steiner J: A theory of psychic retreats, in Psychic Retreats: Pathological Organisations in Psychotic, Neurotic, and Borderline Patients. London, Routledge, 1994, pp 1–13

Tyndall J: The Bakerian Lecture: On the absorption and radiation of heat by gases and vapours, and on the physical connexion of radiation, absorption, and conduction. Philos Trans R Soc London 151: 1–36, 1861

Vess M, Arndt J: The nature of death and the death of nature: the impact of mortality salience on environmental concern. J Res Pers 42:1376–1380, 2008

Wallace-Wells D: The Uninhabitable Earth: A Story of the Future. New York, Penguin, 2019

Weinstein ND, Klein WM: Unrealistic optimism: present and future. J Soc Clin Psychol 15(1):1–8, 1996

10

Emotional Reactions and Syndromes Associated With Climate Change

Symptoms and Prevalence of Climate Distress

Distress about climate change can express itself in many ways. It is natural to feel anxious, overwhelmed, terrified, betrayed, angry, sad, heartbroken, helpless, fatalistic, guilty, isolated, numb, uncaring, paralyzed, nostalgic, or any other feeling when facing climate threats to one's life, the lives of others, and other living beings. It is expected that people will have strong reactions when they are powerless to change those who are perpetuating damage to the things they care about (Albrecht 2019; Pihkala 2020). In this chapter, I explore these emotions and the emotional syndromes (Table 10.1) that may accompany climate distress.

Although empirical study of the emotions and syndromes of climate distress is just beginning, the widespread prevalence of distress about climate change has been validated through many large surveys. In an annual international study conducted by the Yale Program on Climate Change Communication, about 90% of respondents expressed worry

Table 10.1 Emotional syndromes associated with climate change

Eco-anxiety

Pretraumatic stress disorder

Existential or global dread

Eco-grief

Solastalgia

Eco-paralysis

Cassandra syndrome/moral injury

Ostrich syndrome/climate denial

Eco-rage/terrafuria/ecotage

Biophobia/ecophobia/topoaversion

Nature-deficit disorder

Ecocide/tierracide/eco-necrophilia

about climate change in seven countries, and a majority expressed worry in most of the other 192 countries and territories surveyed (e.g., Leiserowitz et al. 2022). Climate distress is particularly intense among young people: in a 2021 international survey of 10,000 young people, more than half said they were "very" or "extremely" worried about climate change, while also expressing high rates of other emotions such as anger and betrayal (Hickman et al. 2021). An annual poll by the American Psychiatric Association found in 2024 that 53% of Americans believe climate change is affecting their mental health currently (American Psychiatic Association 2024) and in 2022 found that more Americans were worried about the impact of climate change on the planet (51%) than were worried about their own mental health (39%) (American Psychiatric Association 2022). This high prevalence implies that psychiatrists and other mental health clinicians should be asking all patients about climate distress.

Eco-anxiety

Eco-anxiety has been the most common term used for climate distress and has been defined in several ways, including as

Emotional Reactions and Syndromes

- A chronic fear of environmental doom
- A sense that the ecological foundations of existence are collapsing

The term *eco-anxiety* can be considered both synonymous with and a subcategory of ecological distress, or eco-distress, and it can also be used synonymously with the term *climate anxiety*. Eco-anxiety may contain elements of worry, angst, habitual anxiety, anticipatory anxiety, existential anxiety, or raw panic, or it may be "practical," meaning adaptive and solution-oriented; the equivalent term across languages can contain different elements of these near-synonyms (Pihkala 2020). Eco-anxiety may encompass clinically significant symptoms related to specific anxiety disorders and their physiological manifestations (Clayton and Crandon 2024; Pihkala 2020). The term eco-anxiety can also broadly refer to distress about many different concerns, including extreme weather, habitat and species loss, and unmitigated carbon emissions. Additional manifestations of eco-anxiety that have been reported in the literature or described in the lay press include carborexia, a phobic or avoidant fear response to consuming too much carbon (Kaufman 2008); obsessive-compulsive symptoms (Jones et al. 2012); counterphobic risk-taking driven by a sense of hopelessness (Bodnar 2008); and reports of delusions (Wolf and Salo 2008) and suicides (Conroy 2019) directly linked to climate fear.

Eco-anxiety can be conceptualized in terms of biological fear response systems and trauma-based models of anxiety. The evaluation of complex threats and their risks takes place in the ventral prefrontal cortex and orbitofrontal cortex and activates the amygdala and other aspects of the behavioral inhibition system (Fitzgerald et al. 2021; Mobbs et al. 2015). Among trauma models, the continuous traumatic stress model (Herman 1992) can be suggested as the best fit for climate stress, because people with climate distress share with chronically abused children the experience of powerlessness, entrapment, and ongoing psychic immersion in multiple traumatic realities (Woodbury 2019). Somatic symptoms, depression, vigilance to risk, future preoccupation, mental exhaustion, dissociation, and changes in identity are some of the effects that have been found with such chronic stress exposure (reviewed in Goral et al. 2021; Itzhaky et al. 2017). Eco-anxiety can also be conceptualized in terms of insecure attachment resulting from ongoing fossil fuel industry and sociopolitical interference in the ability to preserve a secure relationship to nature, or in terms of complicated bereavement in the sense of a distressed state of continuous psychic separation and grief resulting from losses accruing in the natural world.

Existential or Global Dread

The terms *existential dread* and *global dread* are sometimes used to describe a particularly severe kind of eco-anxiety. These terms can be taken in two ways:

- Dread or terror about catastrophic climate outcomes
- Existential concerns such as control, dignity, continuity, finitude, aloneness, responsibility, meaning, death, and suffering related to climate change, usually in terms of more catastrophic outcomes

Global warming that exceeds 5.4°F will lead to catastrophic change; change greater than 9°F is beyond scientific predictive ability—unknowable, and potentially beyond language to describe. Without dramatic emissions reductions, the predicted impacts will include 74% of people subjected to deadly heat (and potentially 4 billion people dying), 90% of species at risk of extinction, and untold suffering for hundreds of millions of refugees, children, and others along the road to their deaths (Xu and Ramanathan 2017). Rumination on such possibilities can become obsessive and disabling, leading to overwhelm, disorganization, despair, numbing, and even suicide.

Empirical Evidence for Clinical-Level Climate Anxiety

One of the first questions the psychiatrist will confront in a patient with climate anxiety or other climate emotional distress is whether a psychiatric disorder is also present. Conceptually, this asks us to consider whether people with strong climate emotions have the same epidemiological and characterological patterns of mental health as others. That is to say, do those most engaged with the climate crisis have less, equal, or more psychiatric burden, or are they unique in their psychiatric profile in some way, compared with population norms? The current database of studies addressing this question includes work in the United States, Europe, India, and Asia (Tam et al. 2023) using the Climate Change Anxiety Scale (CCAS) developed by Clayton and Karazsia (2020). To date, this work supports the idea that climate anxiety overlaps with clinical psychiatric symptoms that cause functional impairment at a rate approximately equivalent to the rates of these disorders in the general population. These studies (Schwartz et al. 2022; Wullenkord et al.

Emotional Reactions and Syndromes   203

2021) have shown 3%–10% rates of frequently experienced depression and anxiety and 20%–25% rates of intermittent depression and anxiety, correlating with scores on the nine-item Patient Health Questionnaire (PHQ-9) and seven-item Generalized Anxiety Disorder (GAD-7) scale. In the United States, Schwartz et al. (2022) found significant associations between climate anxiety and generalized anxiety disorder, and functional impairment from climate anxiety was associated with major depression. More recently, Uppalapati et al. (2023) used the GAD-2 and PHQ-2 to form a four-item measure that was scaled on five degrees of severity and found that 3% of Americans (including 10% of Hispanics and 4%–5% of young people from Gen X, Gen Z, and Millennial groups) may be experiencing serious levels of both climate-related anxiety and climate-related depression.

Other Syndromes and States Associated With Climate Distress

Pretraumatic Stress Disorder

The term *pretraumatic stress disorder* has been used to refer to anticipatory anxiety about future climate changes. Originally satirized in *The Onion* and then developed as a conceptual response to dystopian climate and sci-fi futures by E. Ann Kaplan (2015), the term was picked up by Berntsen and Rubin (2015), who devised a pretraumatic stress disorder checklist of responses to possible future stressful events (PFSE) based on PTSD scales and demonstrated evidence of validity in Danish soldiers awaiting deployment. The scale includes the following items:

- Repeated, disturbing, unwanted images of PFSE
- Repeated disturbing dreams of PFSE
- Suddenly acting as if a PFSE is already happening
- Feeling very upset or having strong physical reactions when reminded of PFSE
- Avoiding reminders of PFSE
- Trouble imagining PFSE
- Blaming oneself or others for PFSE

Berntsen and Rubin emphasized that intrusive thoughts of the past and future are common, occurring about 20 times per day, and that these kinds of thoughts develop in unique windows in childhood, have associations with affective disorders, and are predictive of combat-related PTSD, thus making them an important neurocognitive process. Their work supports the idea that pretraumatic stress disorder and PTSD share common neurological processes, sometimes called the *remembering-imagining system* (Conway et al. 2016), that could be leveraged to intervene in excessive anticipatory climate distress, PTSD prevention, and other adaptive and mitigative climate emotion responses.

Eco-grief

The term *ecological grief,* or *eco-grief,* is often used to describe sadness over losses in and degradation of the natural world. As treasured species go extinct and coral and other habitats die, people for whom these are beloved mourn. Eco-grief is linked to solastalgia (described in the subsection "Solastalgia") in that both emerge from attachment, but eco-grief is a broader term encompassing climate losses other than place-based losses and has been less studied and defined at an empirical level (Comtesse et al. 2021). Numerous qualitative studies have addressed the intangible losses to ways of life and personal identity for Indigenous and rural peoples experiencing climate-related losses to habitat and livelihood (Cunsolo and Ellis 2018). This is politically and legally relevant in reference to the potential effects of eco-grief on the other stressors and risks to mental health that Indigenous and rural people face and the scope of reparations that need to be made.

Although few data are available to outline the qualities of eco-grief, it can be expected to include sadness, yearning, bitterness, anger, and more severe emotional collapse when losses are multiple, violent, unexpected, or intimate. Additional elements may frequently occur regarding climate change and complicate the grieving process:

- Anticipated grief from known future losses
- Maturational forms of grief from losses of legacy and longtime companionship from nature
- Catastrophic grief when the loss is unbearably large, such as the mass death of animal or human life
- Chronic unrelenting sadness, repeatedly triggered by declining habitats and species loss
- Ambiguous forms of loss—unanswered questions such as whether the loss of snowy winters will be permanent or whether a decision not to have children will have been wise—similar to losses that lack closure, such as divorce

Emotional Reactions and Syndromes

- Disenfranchised grief due to a lack of social recognition of the importance of climate-based losses and accompanied by alienation, envy, and even distrust
- Grief from intangible losses, such as the loss of identity, culture, connection to others, social status, world order, sovereignty, meaning, faith, or hope, when efforts and energies have been spent on failed climate efforts
- Vicarious grief witnessing unjust suffering in disadvantaged countries and groups

Pihkala (2024) and others focus on how ecological grief is disenfranchised because it is often only a partial loss of an environment or is not noticed by others, leaving the individual alone in ambiguous and incomplete loss, alienated from a culture that is ego-dystonic to them. Ecological losses also disrupt transmission of knowledge about the things that are gone, which carries consequences for precious aspects of transgenerational and cultural identity. Climate apathy has been linked to ecological grief as an arrested mourning resulting from intolerance of the loss and our own ambivalent destructiveness in creating it (Lertzman 2013). Pihkala (2024) has suggested organizing the losses of climate change as shown in Table 10.2.

Because of the complexity of eco-grief, and because of the inherently aversive and intense emotions of the grief process itself, acknowledging and staying with feelings of loss are considered important for effective processing of climate distress. In relation to the natural world, we are still attached, even if it is a painful attachment. Resistant mourning is a nonpathological and triumphant concept that describes this process of remaining in melancholia as a demonstration of connection and commitment to the natural world, challenging the usual regulation and

Table 10.2 Climate change losses

Categories of ecological grief	Eco-specific types of grief
Tangible vs. intangible losses	Transitional loss and grief
Ambiguous losses	Lifeworld loss
Incomplete or nonfinite losses	Loss from shattered dreams
Loss from shattering of basic assumptions	

censorship of prolonged grief responses and promoting more sustained consciousness of the deterioration of the natural environment.

Eco-paralysis

Eco-paralysis is a term used for a state of limbo in which there is no ability to take meaningful climate action. The term has not been studied, but it has been used by writers including Glenn Albrecht and Renée Lertzman (Albrecht 2011; Lertzman 2013) to refer to a climate-related emotional state of numbness and inability to act. Eco-paralysis may occur temporarily or long-term, and it is likely to reflect other emotions such as fear, sadness, burnout, defeat, or anger. It may be used to reflect societal states or practical problems, such as the inability to afford an electric car.

Solastalgia

Solastalgia is a climate-related syndrome of nostalgia for landscapes that have undergone irrevocable unwanted change as a result of human activity or climate-related degradation, both acute and chronic. Originally introduced by writer and philosopher Glenn Albrecht (Albrecht et al. 2007), it has been defined by Galway et al. (2019, p. 2,662) as "the distress caused by the unwelcome transformation of cherished landscapes resulting in cumulative mental, emotional, and spiritual health impacts." The feelings of sadness and longing encapsulated by this term are related to ecological grief and anxiety but are more narrowly focused on place-based attachment. Solastalgia is thus also a marker of a secure connection to home and nature, which Galway and colleagues have called *landscape identity*.

Solastalgia has been described through more than 50 qualitative studies, mostly using the Environmental Distress Scale (EDS). The EDS is an 81-item survey that looks at the frequency of environmental hazard events; the observations people make about them; the perceived threats to self, family, health, emotions, economics, and community; the feelings related to solastalgia; and the performance of environmental actions (Higginbotham et al. 2006). The following feelings included in the EDS are relevant to place-based attachment and can be queried in patients:

- Feelings of sadness when looking at changed landscapes
- Feeling that what makes the place unique or valuable is being lost forever

Emotional Reactions and Syndromes 207

- Missing the peace, quiet, and unique aspects of nature
- A loss of the sense of belonging to the place
- Feelings of shame at the way the place looks
- Feeling one's way of life and family home threatened by the loss of good land and water
- Feeling powerless to stop unwanted changes

Solastalgia has been documented in a wide range of communities, including those affected by mountaintop removal to mine coal, those living on the Great Lakes, Inuit and Aboriginal peoples, and people in places such as Palestine, Indonesia, Norway, and the Australian wheat belt. Further refinement is needed in the ways people-place relationships are defined; how the ability to control one's local outcomes affects the potency of solastalgia; and how solastalgia varies with gender, locale, and culture and across generations (Galway et al. 2019).

Cassandra Syndrome

In Greek mythology, Apollo fell in love with Cassandra and granted her the gift of prophecy in exchange for a promise of favors. When she reneged on her promise, he doomed her never to be believed. Originally conceptualized by Richard Grigg (1992) at the University of Hawaii, Cassandra syndrome was used to describe the difficulties of raising concerns about coral reef death. Vis-à-vis climate change, it has been used to describe the distress experienced by climate scientists, activists, and younger generations when they try to raise climate awareness and are met with toxic disbelief. Outside the climate literature, the term Cassandra syndrome is used to describe the deprivation of sense-making and the emotional invalidation experienced by people in relationships with abusive, narcissistic, and neurodivergent partners. Although little studied, the Cassandra syndrome experience is similarly one of traumatic invalidation and moral injury, about which there are ample data. Traumatic invalidation (Linehan 1993) is the delegitimization or punishment of reasonable information and feelings, such as in the following:

- The denial of abuse, gender preferences, racist treatment, or medical symptoms
- Discouragement of negative affect
- Minimizing of problems
- Blaming of distress on personal flaws

Cassandra syndrome includes these experiences, as well as the decades of challenges that many climate scientists and youth climate activists have encountered:

- Disbelief
- Apathy
- Denialism
- Legal and political challenges
- Mockery, character assassination, and career assassination
- Other denigration and aggression toward their work

Leading climate scientist Jim Hansen was arrested six times, was shunned by colleagues, and almost lost his career for his Earth-changing work, and Nobel Prize–winning climate activist Greta Thunberg has been subject to widespread attack, mockery, and even death threats.

Traumatic invalidation has been associated with the development of borderline personality disorder, self-harm, and future suicide in children, and with negative affect, anxiety, higher physiological arousal, lesser capacity for self-expression, PTSD, and depression in adults (reviewed in Lee et al. 2022). Invalidation also activates the shame system, reducing the orientation toward and capacity for self-compassion that is needed for self-soothing (Naismith et al. 2019). Decreasing tolerance for self-pity may create a vicious cycle in this way, encouraging the over-dedication that leads to even more burnout by exaggerating the perceived need for self-improvement. These findings support the clinical experience of Cassandra syndrome, which is characterized by high levels of the following:

- Self-criticism and shame
- Rumination, depression, and anxiety
- Somatic hyperarousal and fatigue
- Burnout and disillusionment
- Moral injury
- Hopelessness and, in some cases, fatalism, destructive behaviors, or suicidality

Moral injury has been described as the experience of being forced to participate in or bear witness to something that violates one's core beliefs, or the conflictual need to betray a trusted authority or other important relationship in order to express one's core beliefs in action. Examples of moral injury include soldiers killing innocent civilians in combat;

Emotional Reactions and Syndromes 209

doctors being forced to provide or deny abortion care; first responders failing to save an accident victim; and doctors being attacked, sued, or disbelieved by patients they are trying to treat. It might also include someone being undermined in their goals (e.g., by inadequate military or medical leadership).

Like PTSD, moral injury (reviewed in Griffin et al. 2019) can be conceptualized as a response to a traumatic event, but its outcomes and symptoms are distinct and include guilt, shame, anhedonia, social cynicism, perceived rejection, loss of trust, hopelessness, and loss of meaning. Moral injury can be divided into betrayal-based and perpetrator-based types, characterized by anger at those who have undermined the ability to conduct right action or by guilt or shame for failing to live up to one's moral standards, respectively. Moral injury carries numerous significant psychophysiological risks, including social exclusion, spiritual conflict, pain sensitivity, depression, and suicidal thoughts and actions. Familiarity with moral injury may assist in understanding patients presenting with Cassandra syndrome. Psychotherapy techniques targeting moral repair may be helpful and might include practicing self-compassion and forgiveness, contextualization of what happened, restoring connections to family and community, and applying acceptance and commitment therapy principles of meaning-based action.

Ostrich Effect and Climate Denial

Individuals immersed in climate data who experience moral injury or Cassandra syndrome butt up against those who show its near opposite: information avoidance or, more colloquially, the ostrich effect. The *ostrich effect* can be used to describe the increasingly incomprehensible and delusional psychology of ignoring the intensifying threats of climate change, despite the dangers of doing so for an individual's near-term decision-making, health, survival, and genetic legacy. The science of information avoidance is linked to this effect and includes irrational human tendencies to believe in false prophecies and paranoid conspiracies (e.g., Y2K) more than valid information about dangers and to seek and prefer apparently useless information when better is available (e.g., public interest in ivermectin over vetted antiviral treatments for coronavirus disease 2019 [COVID-19]). The science of information avoidance tells us that people ignore information that could help them make better decisions for many reasons, such as the following:

- Avoiding negative affect
- Inattention
- Selfishness
- Maintaining "moral wiggle room"
- Confirmation biases (e.g., anchoring bias)
- In-group biases

These or similar factors may contribute to better mental health by reducing immediate distress (Golman et al. 2017), but at the cost of damage from denied risks. Terror management theory and mortality salience theory are additional concepts for conceptualizing the psychological motivations for the ostrich effect response (see Chapter 9, "Obstacles to Rational and Adequate Responses to Climate Change") and can be useful when considering why individuals and groups choose to defend business as usual when climate information carries mortality and identity threats.

Eco-rage, Terrafuria, and Ecotage

Eco-rage and *terrafuria* (Albrecht 2019) are terms used for anger about the destruction of the natural world. Although eco-rage (and more minor eco-frustration) has not been extensively studied, data indicate that it is a unique climate emotion that is experienced at least as often as, if not more often than, eco-anxiety or eco-depression. Stanley et al. (2021) found that eco-rage was moderately correlated with lower anxiety, depression, and stress and strongly correlated with both individual and collective climate action. These findings are in line with the longstanding sociological observation that anger motivates collective action, particularly in deprived groups with a strong sense of identity (van Zomeren et al. 2008). *Ecotage*, also called eco-sabotage or ecoterrorism, is a form of eco-rage in which protesters act to stop fossil fuel expansion and call attention to the climate crisis through destructive action or illegal forms of protest (Izak 2022). Eco-saboteurs, and increasingly lawyers and other climate activists around the world (Hans 2023), believe their actions are justified by the lethality and destructiveness of the fossil fuel industry and by the failure and slowness of policy and government action. Exploring courage, triumph, hopelessness, and self-destruction may be clinically helpful when working with eco-saboteur patients.

Emotional Reactions and Syndromes   211

Vignette

Hanna, age 30, is a geophysicist expressing homicidal ideation (eco-rage) toward local authorities after she was given the choice of betraying her friends (moral injury) or facing arrest with tribal members who had damaged an oil pipeline disrupting the water supply (ecotage) on their Native American reservation. She talks about how her dissertation on local oil shale has been completely neglected by pipeline environmental assessments (Cassandra syndrome), and then breaks down crying about a local child who died from an environmental toxin (eco-grief). A review of her history shows she has not been able to find a tenured position because of her eco-activism (climate developmental phase problem) and has decided to forego children because of the climate crisis.

States of Aversion, Avoidance, and Destructiveness Toward the Natural World

In contrast to the conditions emerging from love of the natural world in the previous sections, numerous emotional states have been described as ways of relating to the natural world that turn away from it, including aversion, avoidance, or even active destruction. This biophobia and related animal phobias may have a genetic component. The urbanization-disgust hypothesis posits that biophobia and nature avoidance may be increasing with global development and less time in nature due to competing contact with technology. This may result in a vicious cycle of further decreased contact with the natural world and increased nature ignorance, fear, and avoidance. These emotional states can be enhanced by frightening experiences in nature, parental nature fears, and media exposure to natural dangers. People with nature phobias and nature avoidance have less pro-biodiversity attitudes, undervalue the benefits organisms provide society, and are more likely to kill species they fear or eliminate aspects of their natural environments. It is therefore important to make these aversions a focus for climate-related psychotherapy (reviewed in Soga et al. 2023) for successful preservation of these resources.

Psychologist Richard Louv used the now-popularized term *nature-deficit disorder* to describe the physical and emotional effects of alienation from nature on contemporary children, including myopia, obesity, and risks of physical illness. In his book *Last Child in the Woods* (Louv 2005), he reviewed the beneficial effects of time in nature on vision, physical activity, weight, ADHD, and school performance, as well as its contributions to creativity, wonder, resilience, healing from trauma, and nature-based knowledge. These findings are generally supported by the literature (Bell et al. 2008; Lingham et al. 2021; Zamora et al. 2021).

As we grow up, we naturally become more caught up in the preoccupations of our adult human activities, consumed by the familial, social, occupational, and bureaucratic concerns that can take us away from a mindful appreciation of the precious places and things within the natural world that are typically a source of delight in childhood. Originally proposed officially by Liam Heneghan (2013) but also mourned in writings from Plato through Wordsworth and Thoreau (Griffith 2017), the term *toponesia* has been used to describe this amnestic turning away from the paradisial delights of nature that are readily appreciated by children. At its opposite end is *endemophilia*, described by Albrecht (2019) as being truly at home within one's place and culture. Many ecotherapy techniques, from mindfulness to other exercises based on deep immersion in and practiced appreciation for nature, seek to restore this endemophilic sense of delight and connection.

As alienation from nature progresses across the generations and nature wisdom is lost, environmental generational amnesia further turns us away from the natural world. Younger generations take whatever impoverished environmental conditions they are raised with as normal experiences. Those who have not forgotten, however, can become averse to seeing the worsening landscapes they have loved and may avoid contact with them. This has been called topoaversion by Albrecht and others.

At the extreme of turning away from nature is the state of *eco-necrophilia*. Derived from the definition of necrophilia used by Erich Fromm in *The Heart of Man*, necrophilia is not the perversion of erotic arousal by corpses but a love of all that is mechanical and does not grow, a desire to "transform the organic into the inorganic" and to "possess [it].... He loves control, and in the act of controlling he kills life" (Fromm 1964, p. 2). Eco-necrophilia is the opposite of biophilia and, when extended into ecological terms, refers to delight in the objectification and control of nature and the ability to own or kill it without empathy for what is destroyed. Examples of eco-necrophilia include trophy hunting, excessive taming of wild and wilderness spaces, indifference to violence and

Emotional Reactions and Syndromes 213

death due to climate change, and neoliberal capitalist processes that turn nature and its inhabitants into commodities, described by Sally Weintrobe as a "culture of uncare" emerging from entitlement and narcissism (Weintrobe 2021). Its consequences are ecocide, the killing of ecosystems (reviewed in de Pompignan 2007), and tierracide (Albrecht 2019), the killing of planet Earth.

Overlap of Climate Emotional Syndromes With Other Psychological Concerns

In young people, as well as older adults, the climate distress syndromes described in this chapter are often connected to more general developmental and existential issues, including the following:

- Developmental issues across the life span
- Universal existential struggles about life, death, meaning, and purpose
- Valued aspects of the self, such as capabilities, career development, love of nature and animals, moral or spiritual strivings, or dreams for the future
- Desired roles of parent, grandparent, leader in society, caregiver, and others

It is important that climate distress not be invalidated as "really about" these other life issues; that is, a defensive displacement of other psychological problems onto climate distress. Nonetheless, their overlap is important to consider. These other psychological issues may exist in numerous different relationships to climate distress. They may

- Contain parallel concerns or co-occur with climate distress
- Overlap directly with climate issues
- Magnify climate distress
- Serve as a container for or displacement of climate anxieties
- Be minimized in their developmental and life importance through containment by or displacement onto climate anxieties

A few hypothetical examples of these relationship overlaps are presented in Table 10.3.

Table 10.3 Possible relationships between climate distress and general psychological challenges of the human condition

Climate experience	Psychological challenge	Relationship
Lack of safety; an unstable world	Loss of a relationship	Magnifying, parallel concerns
Fear of future climate breakdown	History of trauma	Magnifying
Death of beloved nature and animals	Death of close other	Parallel concerns, magnifying
Conflict with unconcerned others	Familial, social, or occupational invalidation	Magnifying, overlapping
Loss of future	Adult milestones, legacy	Overlapping, displacement
Helplessness and powerlessness	Autonomy, independence	Overlapping, containing
Institutional or civic betrayal	Adult role maturation	Overlapping, impeding
Damage to future generations	Parenting, grandparenting	Overlapping, magnifying
Existential threats	Death	Parallel concerns, magnifying

Overlap of Climate Emotions With Psychiatric Syndromes

In addition to considering the psychological and developmental issues that may accompany climate syndromes, clinicians must also consider whether a climate syndrome is a manifestation of a co-occurring psychiatric disorder, while also taking care not to prejudice interpretation of appropriate distress in this direction. Examples of psychiatric disorders associated with similar climate concerns include the following:

- Ecological grief with bereavement
- Ecological grief with major depressive disorder and persistent depressive disorder

Emotional Reactions and Syndromes

- Eco-anxiety with generalized anxiety disorder
- Eco-anxiety with posttraumatic stress disorder
- Eco-paralysis with major depressive disorder
- Climate-related phobias with specific phobia and separation anxiety disorder

Because anxiety and depressive disorders are the two categories of psychiatric disorders most likely to co-occur, it is helpful to distinguish the healthy forms of anxiety and depression manifest in climate distress. Healthy climate anxiety can be identified when the following occurs:

- The distress is appropriate to the scale of threat or risk of an external problem
- The distress does not overwhelm the individual's ability to function
- The distress serves adaptive functions, including motivation, drive, information gathering, and problem-solving
- The distress leads to risk minimization
- The response to the distress solves the problem rather than reduces the upsetting feelings
- The distress ends when the precipitating event or problem is over

Healthy climate sadness has characteristics that include the following:

- Improving memory and attention to detail, which improves judgments and actions
- Decreasing risky independent behavior, preserving energy, and increasing proximity to safe groups
- Promoting protection and connection by eliciting compassion and generosity and contributing to moral development and psychological awareness
- Motivating reparative or transformative action

As will be familiar to clinicians, unhealthy anxiety and depression are associated with more impairment in function, avoidance of precipitating problems, distortions of threats and the ability to cope with them, longer duration, neurovegetative impairment, and decreased social connectedness.

Key Points

- Climate distress encompasses wide-ranging feelings that are normal and predictable responses to the climate emergency.
- The majority of adults and young people around the world express moderate to severe worry and other distress about climate change.
- Eco-anxiety may include healthy anxiety, existential terror, and pre-traumatic anticipatory stress and may reflect or coexist with clinical anxiety disorders, probably in proportion to their usual population prevalence.
- Eco-grief, eco-paralysis, and solastalgia are climate loss syndromes with empirical support.
- Cassandra syndrome is experienced by climate activists and scientists and carries psychiatric risks associated with traumatic invalidation, moral injury, and burnout.
- The ostrich effect and eco-rage are additional emotional responses with specific features.
- Aversion to nature and deficits in contact with nature are increasingly common in modern society and are associated with less pro-environmental behavior and adverse health effects.
- Climate distress coexists with psychological and developmental issues faced by all people and can stand in various relationships to these issues.
- Climate distress coexists with other psychiatric disorders; delineating healthy from unhealthy aspects of climate distress is therefore clinically essential.

References

Albrecht GA: Chronic environmental change: emerging psychoterratic syndromes, in Climate Change and Human Well-Being. Edited by Weissbecker I. New York, Springer, 2011, pp 43–56

Albrecht GA: Earth Emotions: New Words for a New World. Ithaca, NY, Cornell University Press, 2019

Albrecht G, Sartore G-M, Connor L, et al: Solastalgia: the distress caused by environmental change. Australas Psychiatry 15(1)(Suppl 1):S95–S98, 2007 18027145

American Psychiatric Association: Americans report mental health effects of climate change, worry about the future. Washington, DC, American

Emotional Reactions and Syndromes

Psychiatric Association, April 5, 2022. Available at: www.psychiatry.org/News-room/News-Releases/Americans-Report-Mental-Health-Effects-of-Climate. Accessed December 3, 2024.

American Psychiatric Association: More Americans say climate change is having an effect on their mental health now than in 2022, APA survey finds. Washington, DC, American Psychiatric Association, June 18, 2024. Available at: www.psychiatry.org/News-room/News-Releases/More-Americans-Say-Climate-Change-Is-Having-an-Imp. Accessed December 3, 2024.

Bell JF, Wilson JS, Liu GC: Neighborhood greenness and 2-year changes in body mass index of children and youth. Am J Prev Med 35(6):547–553, 2008 19000844

Berntsen D, Rubin DC: Pretraumatic stress reactions in soldiers deployed to Afghanistan. Clin Psychol Sci 3(5):663–674, 2015 26366328

Bodnar S: Wasted and bombed: clinical enactments of a changing relationship to the Earth. Psychoanal Dialogues 18(4):484–512, 2008

Clayton S, Crandon T: Climate distress among young people: an overview, in Climate Change and Youth Mental Health: Multidisciplinary Perspectives. Edited by Haase E, Hudson K. Cambridge, UK, Cambridge University Press, 2024, pp 3–20

Clayton S, Karazsia BT: Development and validation of a measure of climate change anxiety. J Environ Psychol 69:101434, 2020

Comtesse H, Ertl V, Hengst SMC, et al: Ecological grief as a response to environmental change: a mental health risk or functional response? Int J Environ Res Public Health 18(2):1–10, 2021 33467018

Conroy JO: A lawyer set himself on fire to protest climate change. Did anyone care? The Guardian, April 15, 2019. Available at: www.theguardian.com/environment/2019/apr/15/david-buckel-lawyer-climate-change-protest. Accessed December 7, 2024.

Conway MA, Loveday C, Cole SN: The remembering–imagining system. Mem Stud 9(3):256–265, 2016

Cunsolo A, Ellis NR: Ecological grief as a mental health response to climate change-related loss. Nat Clim Chang 8:275–281, 2018

de Pompignan N: Ecocide, mass violence and résistance. Paris, Sciences Po, November 3, 2007. Available at: www.sciencespo.fr/mass-violence-war-massacre-resistance/en/document/ecocide.html. Accessed December 7, 2024.

Fitzgerald KD, Schroder HS, Marsh R: Cognitive control in pediatric obsessive-compulsive and anxiety disorders: brain-behavioral targets for early intervention. Biol Psychiatry 89(7):697–706, 2021 33454049

Fromm E: The Heart of Man. New York, Harper & Row, 1964

Galway LP, Beery T, Jones-Casey K, et al: Mapping the solastalgia literature: a scoping review study. Int J Environ Res Public Health 16(15):2662, 2019 31349659

Golman R, Hagmann D, Loewenstein G: Information avoidance. J Econ Lit 55(1):96–135, 2017

Goral A, Feder-Bubis P, Lahad M, et al: Development and validation of the Continuous Traumatic Stress Response scale (CTSR) among adults exposed to ongoing security threats. PLoS One 16(5):e0251724, 2021 34043646

Griffin BJ, Purcell N, Burkman K, et al: Moral injury: an integrative review. J Trauma Stress 32(3):350–362, 2019 30688367

Griffith J: Wordsworth's great honesty that "trailing clouds of glory do we come." Freedom Essay 31. Sydney, Australia, World Transformation Movement, 2017. Available at: www.humancondition.com/freedom-essays/wordsworths-majestic-poem. Accessed December 7, 2024.

Grigg RW: Coral reef environmental science: truth versus the Cassandra syndrome. Coral Reefs 11:183–186, 1992

Hans S: Is eco-terrorism now self-defence? Inside explosive film How to Blow Up a Pipeline. The Guardian, April 17, 2023. Available at: www.theguardian.com/film/2023/apr/17/how-to-blow-up-a-pipeline-oil-extreme-action-eco-terrorism-self-defence. Accessed December 7, 2024.

Heneghan L: The ecology of Pooh. Aeon, March 5, 2013. Available at: https://aeon.co/essays/can-we-ever-return-to-the-enchanted-forests-of-childhood. Accessed December 7, 2024.

Herman J: Trauma and Recovery: The Aftermath of Violence—From Domestic Abuse to Political Terror. New York, Basic Books, 1992

Hickman C, Marks E, Pihkala P, et al: Climate anxiety in children and young people and their beliefs about government responses to climate change: a global survey. Lancet Planet Health 5(12):e863–e873, 2021 34895496

Higginbotham N, Connor L, Albrecht G, et al: Validation of an environmental distress scale. EcoHealth 3(4):245–254, 2006

Itzhaky L, Gelkopf M, Levin Y, et al: Psychiatric reactions to continuous traumatic stress: a latent profile analysis of two Israeli samples. J Anxiety Disord 51:94–100, 2017 28709689

Izak K: Is there a decline in ecoterrorism? Internal Security Review 14(26):394–431, 2022

Jones MK, Wootton BM, Vaccaro LD, et al: The impact of climate change on obsessive compulsive checking concerns. Aust N Z J Psychiatry 46(3):265–270, 2012 22391284

Kaplan EA: Climate Trauma: Foreseeing the Future in Dystopian Film and Fiction. New Brunswick, NJ, Rutgers University Press, 2015

Kaufman J: Completely unplugged, fully green. New York Times, October 17, 2008. Available at: www.nytimes.com/2008/10/19/fashion/19greenorexia.html. Accessed December 7, 2024.

Lee SSM, Keng S-L, Yeo GC, et al: Parental invalidation and its associations with borderline personality disorder symptoms: a multivariate meta-analysis. Personal Disord 13(6):572–582, 2022 34766788

Leiserowitz A, Carman J, Buttermore N, et al: International Public Opinion on Climate Change, 2022. New Haven, CT, Yale Program on Climate Change Communication and Data for Good at Meta, 2022

Lertzman R: The myth of apathy, in Engaging With Climate Change: Psychoanalytic and Interdisciplinary Perspectives. Edited by Weintrobe S. Hove, UK, Routledge, 2013, pp 28–45

Linehan M: Cognitive-Behavioral Treatment of Borderline Personality Disorder. New York, Guilford, 1993

Lingham G, Yazar S, Lucas RM, et al: Time spent outdoors in childhood is associated with reduced risk of myopia as an adult. Sci Rep 11(1):6337, 2021 33737652

Louv R: Last Child in the Woods: Saving Our Children From Nature-Deficit Disorder. Chapel Hill, NC, Algonquin Books of Chapel Hill, 2005

Mobbs D, Hagan CC, Dalgleish T, et al: The ecology of human fear: survival optimization and the nervous system. Front Neurosci 9:55, 2015 25852451

Naismith I, Zarate Guerrero S, Feigenbaum J: Abuse, invalidation, and lack of early warmth show distinct relationships with self-criticism, self-compassion, and fear of self-compassion in personality disorder. Clin Psychol Psychother 26(3):350–361, 2019 30715768

Pihkala P: Anxiety and the ecological crisis: an analysis of eco-anxiety and climate anxiety. Sustainability 12(19):7836, 2020

Pihkala P: Ecological sorrow: types of grief and loss in ecological grief. Sustainability 16(2):849, 2024

Schwartz SEO, Benoit L, Clayton S, et al: Climate change anxiety and mental health: environmental activism as buffer. Curr Psychol 28:1–14, 2022 35250241

Soga M, Gaston KJ, Fukano Y, et al: The vicious cycle of biophobia. Trends Ecol Evol 38(6):512–520, 2023 36707258

Stanley SK, Hogg TL, Leviston Z, et al: From anger to action: differential impacts of eco-anxiety, eco-depression, and eco-anger on climate action and wellbeing. J Clim Change Health 1:100003, 2021

Tam K-P, Chan H-W, Clayton S: Climate change anxiety in China, India, Japan, and the United States. J Environ Psychol 87:101991, 2023

Uppalapati SS, Ballew M, Campbell E, et al: The Prevalence of Climate Change Psychological Distress Among American Adults. New Haven, CT, Yale Program on Climate Change Communication, 2023

van Zomeren M, Spears R, Leach CW: Exploring psychological mechanisms of collective action: does relevance of group identity influence how people cope with collective disadvantage? Br J Soc Psychol 47(Pt 2):353–372, 2008 17697447

Weintrobe S: Living with our feelings about the climate crisis, in Psychological Roots of the Climate Crisis: Neoliberal Exceptionalism and the Culture of Uncare. New York, Bloomsbury Academic, 2021, pp 235–244

Wolf J, Salo R: Water, water, everywhere, nor any drop to drink: climate change delusion. Aust N Z J Psychiatry 42(4):350, 2008 18330779

Woodbury Z: Climate trauma: toward a new taxonomy of trauma. Ecopsychology 11(1):1–8, 2019

Wullenkord M, Toger J, Hamann KR, et al: Anxiety and climate change: a validation of the climate anxiety scale in a German-speaking quota sample and an investigation of psychological correlates. Clim Chang 168:20211022, 2021

Xu Y, Ramanathan V: Well below 2°C: mitigation strategies for avoiding dangerous to catastrophic climate changes. Proc Natl Acad Sci USA 114(39):10315–10323, 2017 28912354

Zamora AN, Waselewski ME, Frank AJ, et al: Exploring the beliefs and perceptions of spending time in nature among U.S. youth. BMC Public Health 21(1):1586, 2021 34425797

11

Assessment of the Patient

Climate-Related Vulnerabilities and Psychology

Climate-Informed Patient Assessment

A climate-informed assessment of an individual patient can range from a single question to several clinical hours in length. It can be incorporated into a general assessment or conducted as part of subsequent work. What matters is that it is done. In this chapter, I present first a full climate assessment and then a brief nine-question assessment at the chapter's end. The goal of these assessments is to understand the patient's climate-related risks as well as their level of climate awareness and capacity to think, feel, and act in a way that will lead them to live sustainably and thrive despite climate adversities. This patient evaluation can be divided into five general areas:

- Relationship to nature
- Ability to reckon with reality
- Emotional and psychological responses to climate change

- Capacities and difficulties related to climate adaptation and resilience
- Abilities and actions to mitigate climate-related harm

A complete climate assessment takes at least a full session to conduct and may be better divided over several sessions. It is focused on four core issues:

1. Is the patient connected emotionally to the natural world?
2. Does the patient understand how the climate crisis is affecting their life and their future?
3. What obstacles—emotional, cognitive, and practical—stand in the way of their transitioning to a way of life that will allow them to thrive through the climate crisis?
4. What is the patient's unique position in relation to climate-related stress?

This information can be used in formulating a treatment plan to help the individual person adapt optimally to their climate reality.

Assessing the Patient's Relationship to Nature and Pro-environmental Behaviors

The first and most important piece of the climate assessment reviews the patient's capacity for a secure and loving attachment to the natural world. This positive attachment, like any other, creates the conditions and motivation for concern and action for Nature's well-being and an understanding that their own well-being is interdependent with and dependent on the well-being of natural systems. In determining this, the clinician should assess for the following:

- General attachment style (secure, anxious/preoccupied, avoidant/dismissive, disorganized)
- Childhood and family experiences and attitudes toward animals and the outdoors
- Adult experiences in the natural world, including moments of awe and connection
- Traumatic or dangerous experiences outdoors or with animals
- View of the relationship between humans and nature in terms of how the relationship is conceived: the relatively more hierarchical

Assessment of the Patient

versus interdependent view of human-nature relationships that the patient holds, what an appropriate use of nature and animals for humans means to them, and what the patient feels about the duty to care for and protect nonhuman life

- Pro-environmental behaviors that reflect the capacity for concern, widely defined to include gardening, care of pets, environmentally conscious behaviors such as recycling or using electric cars and solar energy, participation in conservation groups or outdoor clubs, and other activities

The Environmental Identity Scale (revised) (https://evaluation.naaee.org/tools/environmental-identity-scale) may be helpful in this piece of the assessment (Clayton et al. 2021). Interpersonal characteristics that have been associated with more and less nature relatedness and pro-environmental behaviors are listed in Table 11.1.

Four *myths of nature* have been used in research studies (Adams 1995; Poortinga et al. 2003) and can be considered in assessing how the patient describes the relationship of humans to nature. These four myths of nature are

- Nature as benign—In this view, nature has the capacity to tolerate, adjust to, and recover from whatever humankind does.
- Nature as capricious—In this view, nature is dangerous and unpredictable and therefore is to be feared. This view is likely to gain prominence as climate change proceeds. It can also be part of a splitting process in the patient's relationship to nature in which nature is viewed either as an all-giving "breast and diaper" mother or in wrathful, punitive terms.
- Nature as ephemeral—In this view, nature is seen as fragile and vulnerable. This view is most closely correlated with pro-environmental behavior.
- Nature as tolerant but perverse—In this view, nature will put up with as much as it can and then suddenly and dramatically collapse.

Questioning these myths in lay language might include asking if the patient feels frightened of nature, thinks nature will get even for what is being done, and whether they believe nature will be able to recover from climate change.

After assessing the patient's relationship with nature more broadly, the clinician can ask whether the patient is aware of and concerned

Table 11.1 Factors associated with pro-environmental behavior and nature relatedness

Female gender

Younger age

Education

Environmental knowledge

Openness, agreeableness, and conscientiousness

High self-efficacy

Meta-personal sense of self as connected to living beings

Internal locus of control

Future orientation

Postmaterialism

Antiauthoritarianism

Exposure to nature

Habitual ecological worry

Higher climate distress

Vitality

Psychological well-being

Source. Gifford and Nilsson 2014; Verplanken and Roy 2013.

about climate change and whether it is having positive or adverse effects on their ability to function. This includes straightforward questions related to the following:

- The patient's awareness of what climate change is and its impacts, current and future
- The patient's level of worry about climate change and the environment, ranging from terrified or alarmed to disengaged or dismissive (Leiserowitz et al. 2018)
- Current symptoms the patient ascribes to climate distress, such as insomnia, anxiety, asthenia, somatic symptoms such as headaches, and symptoms of burnout

Assessment of the Patient 225

- Current symptoms the patient ascribes to direct climate impacts, most commonly heat illness, physical and mental impacts of air pollution, and psychiatric consequences of climate traumas due to extreme weather or natural disaster
- What practical problems the patient expects to have because of climate change, including limitations to quality of life, habitat, resources, safety, and capacity for future growth

Many patients may have, and want to share, the story of a moment when they awakened to concern about climate change, which can be an empowering entry point into understanding the values that guide them in climate concern.

Assessing the Patient's Cognitive and Emotional Reactions to Climate Change

The assessment now turns to psychological, cognitive, and social difficulties—and also strengths—that the patient is experiencing in relation to climate change. The emotions felt by the patient can range from positivity to fear, sadness, and anger (Climate Mental Health Network 2023).

In this part of the assessment, gentle confrontation is appropriate in order to see what defensive strategies the patient uses to push back against a greater reckoning with their feelings and actions in response to climate change. Issues to be understood during this part of the assessment should include the following:

- Cognitive reactions to climate change

  - Perceived adequacy of climate understanding

    - Ignorance
    - Uncertainty
    - Cognitive biases used by the patient to understand climate change

  - Perceived adequacy of climate response

    - Expectations for climate outcomes and solutions
    - Awareness of inconsistency, disavowal, or hypocrisy in their own and others' responses (ability to apply critical pedagogy to themselves and others)

- Social pressures on the patient in regard to sustainable behavior

  - Family attitudes, including differences in attitude and levels of interest with partners, parents, and other family members
  - Social norms in the patient's communities and friends
  - Awareness of social justice issues

- Shifts in identity that have arisen or will arise because of climate change directly or from actions taken in response to it

  - Likely changes to livelihood
  - Risk of forced displacement
  - Impact on childbearing
  - Impacts on legacy

- Ways of avoiding climate awareness

  - Climate denialism
  - Denial of climate impacts on the patient and their social groups
  - Disavowal of personal carbon footprint or importance of climate-aware feelings and reactions

- Growth and benefits that have or could result from climate change

  - Development of new capacities and roles
  - Strengthened social connections
  - Positive emotions such as feelings of empowerment, improved self-esteem, courage, grit, tenacity, and hope
  - Development of new ideals and dreams

As the clinician listens to this material, the individual predispositions, symptoms, and other psychological states and traits of the patient will be embedded in their self-report. In empirical studies, higher levels of climate distress have been associated with pro-environmental behaviors such as climate activism, resource conservation, and following a more sustainable diet (Tam et al. 2023). A formulation that considers these relationships in the patient and a general understanding of where climate change fits in the patient's personality structure and life choices can be considered at this point.

Psychiatric Disorders and the Climate Assessment

A task that runs throughout the assessment is to listen for other psychiatric and psychological problems that may be co-occurring with climate distress, as they do at approximately the same rate that they occur in the general population (Clayton and Crandon 2024), so that they can be evaluated and treated appropriately. The following common diagnoses can be expected in this population from the limited data so far:

- Generalized anxiety disorder
- Posttraumatic stress disorder
- Panic disorder
- Separation anxiety disorder
- Obsessive-compulsive disorder
- Persistent depressive disorder (formerly dysthymia)
- Major depressive disorder

High heat and air pollution exposures can be expected to elevate the frequency of suicidal and aggressive thoughts in patients and should not be overlooked. The clinician should also consider the trait anxiety sensitivity of the patient, their innate behavioral inhibition versus activation, and the Big Five personality traits of openness versus cautiousness, conscientiousness versus extravagance, extroversion versus introversion, agreeableness versus criticalness or judgmentalism, and neuroticism demonstrated by the patient. Because openness, agreeableness, and conscientiousness correlate with pro-environmental behavior, a quick assessment for these traits is worthy of the time investment and can be done easily with the Ten Item Personality Measure (TIPI; Gosling et al. 2003).

Assessing Social Equity and Neurobiological Risks

Regarding determining the unique position of a given patient in relation to the climate crisis, the clinician should assess for significant and likely direct impacts of climate change, including local threats to physical survival. A VESA (vulnerabilities, exposures, secondary or prolonged impacts, and adaptation capacities) framework has been proposed for this part of the assessment (Wang et al. 2024), which includes the following:

- Heat health and mental health risks to which they are physiologically and behaviorally vulnerable as individuals
- Heat risks for the neighborhood and home in which they live
- Air pollution exposure and health and mental health risks
- Access to clean water
- Adequacy of their local water supply and planning for future water shortages
- Local changes in infectious disease epidemiology
- Changes in food supply

  - Consistency and quality of food available for purchase
  - Access to plant-based foods
  - Predicted changes in their food supply, including likely local and global production shifts to which they will be vulnerable

The clinician can generate a list of the specific heat, fire, and flood risk predictions for a particular patient's personal address for the next 30 years from First Street Technology (2023) and county-specific risks for heat, drought, flooding, hurricanes, cold and ice, earthquakes, and hail events from the Federal Emergency Management Agency (FEMA; 2023). FEMA's website also shows county-level social vulnerability and community resilience that will aid in assessing the patient's vulnerability to climate effects. This vulnerability is greatly increased for disadvantaged populations. The climate-related social vulnerability assessment must therefore also include the following:

- Intersectional assessment to determine the unique cultural, racial, and socioeconomic heritage and position of the patient

  - Degree of socioeconomic privilege and personal factors contributing to ability to travel, change homes, or otherwise access safety with climate impacts
  - Vulnerability to structural racism
  - Victimization by climate injustice due to

    - Quality of residence
    - Quality of local habitat
    - Age

Assessment of the Patient

○ Membership in a vulnerable group (e.g., women, marginalized racial and ethnic groups, young people)

These social determinants of health can be evaluated in more depth through the use of clinical screening tools:

- Accountable Health Communities Health-Related Social Needs (AHC-HRSN) screening tool, an instrument developed by the Centers for Medicare and Medicaid Services in the United States (https://innovation.cms.gov/files/worksheets/ahcm-screening-tool.pdf)
- The Cross Ethnic-Racial Identity Scale-Adult (CERIS-A; Worrell et al. 2019)

Questioning how the patient perceives higher temperatures, air pollution, and local habitat to be contributing to their health will also help the clinician assess the patient's awareness of climate health risks and justice issues, lack of which can be a source of vulnerability in itself.

Assessing Capacity for Survival

The climate assessment can then move to the patient's ability to take effective action both to keep themself safe in response to climate impacts and to respond to the climate crisis. The first part of this is to query the patient's general capacity for resilience and climate-related growth. *Resilience* is the process of adapting well in the face of adversity. In individuals it is characterized by high levels of self-esteem, flexibility, openness, humor, sense of self-efficacy, capacity for gratitude, hope, bravery, kindness, and transcendence, as well as the ability to do hard work, keep high expectations, and seek and maintain connectedness and social support (Moore 2019; Southwick et al. 2014). Growth here is defined as posttraumatic growth, including finding new opportunities, building deeper and more empathic connections, having a sense of being a survivor, having a deeper appreciation for life, and having deeper spirituality. The Connor-Davidson Resilience Scale (CD-RISC; Connor and Davidson 2003), Brief Resilience Scale (Smith et al. 2008), and expanded Post-Traumatic Growth Inventory (Tedeschi et al. 2017) can be helpful for these assessments.

In the face of the rapid changes associated with global warming and the need for radical adaptation, it may also be useful to consider assessing the patient's capacity for, resistance to, and readiness for change and ability to imagine a range of possible futures (Lewis and Haase 2025). Instruments that can be used for formal change assessment include the Acceptance of Change Scale (Di Fabio and Gori 2016) and the Resistance to Change Scale (Oreg 2003). Patients more resistant to change are likely to demonstrate the following characteristics:

- Reluctance to lose control
- Cognitive rigidity
- Lack of resilience
- Intolerance of the adjustment period to change
- Preference for low stimulation and low novelty
- Reluctance to give up old habits or high preference for routines

Patients can be asked if they like routines, dislike changes in plans or surprises, expect that changes will be negative, take a long time to adjust to new situations, or resist even changes likely to benefit them. In contrast, those more able to embrace (accept) change are more likely to do the following:

- Be open to receiving information about change
- Participate in the change process
- Believe in their ability to change
- Gather social support during changes
- Perceive a positive personal impact of change

Patients may indicate that they are open to changing their opinions, making new plans, considering alternatives and multiple perspectives when assessing a change, taking advantage of opportunities and trusting those involved, seeking diversity and change in daily activities, and tolerating the stress of change.

Having established how capable the patient may be to enact resilient and transformational change, it is helpful to know what actions the patient has taken or would like to take to mitigate the impacts of climate change, both in their own lives and for larger goals. The following considerations can be addressed:

- What has the patient tried to reduce their impact on the environment and lessen their contributions to climate change? This can be an opportunity for education because most people do

Assessment of the Patient

not accurately identify the most impactful actions they can take individually, which are, in the following order:

- Having one fewer child
- Living car-free
- Avoiding one long-distance (>6 hours) flight
- Eating a plant-based diet and reducing food waste (Wynes and Nicholas 2017)

- What frustrations and difficulties has the patient experienced putting these changes into place?
- Does the patient know how to assess their own climate footprint? Good carbon footprint calculators include Greenly, CoolClimate, CarbonFootprint.com, Conservation International, and the carbon offset platform provided by the United Nations.
- Does the patient know how to access information about effective responses to climate change? Numerous resources are available for this, particularly Project Drawdown, as well as the websites of the United Nations, the World Economic Forum, the U.S. Environmental Protection Agency, and others.
- What is the adequacy of the patient's climate support systems? Are they connected to environmentally active groups such as the Sunrise Movement and Extinction Rebellion?

Finally, although office-based climate assessment is likely to focus more on psychological and long-term concerns, a climate safety assessment is imperative and may include questions about the following attributes:

- Response to high-stress situations, including the emotional and cognitive ability to identify and respond to rising danger, capacities for leadership, levelheadedness, courage, grit, and tenacity, as well as fight-or-flight patterns under extreme stress
- Training in personal safety, including military experience, outdoor training experience, history of disaster drills, education in safety during extreme weather and natural disasters, heat awareness and response, water safety and lifesaving skills, first aid, wilderness medicine, and emergency medical services or other first-responder experience
- Self-reliance: survival skills, including camping and other related experiences such as fire starting, water filtration, hunting

and fishing, shelter design, carpentry, gardening and farming skills, and bike and car repair, and knowledge base for relevant areas such as meteorology, edible plants, and food preservation

Shortening the Climate Change Assessment

For those who would like to conduct a more brief climate assessment interview, the full assessment can be summarized in a few open-ended questions that may elicit much of the same information. Some caution about countertransference must be given, however, in that good answers to the questions below do not relieve the treating professional from the obligation to think about what vulnerabilities, dangers, and risks the patient may have omitted in considering how to protect themselves and their loved ones. A shortened climate assessment might include the following questions:

- Tell me about your feelings and reactions to climate change.
- What role do animals and nature play in your life?
- Are there things that scare you about nature and climate change?
- What risks do you see for yourself because of climate impacts on the weather and the world?
- Do you feel any special personal vulnerability to climate impacts because of social disadvantage?
- What actions and preparations do you take with regard to climate change?
- Do you see yourself as able to adapt to new and challenging situations when needed?
- Have you had difficulty with anxiety, anger, depression, or similar emotions in other aspects of your life as well?
- What skills and resources do you have to keep yourself safe during these times?

Concluding the Assessment

Because climate material is inherently charged, it is likely that both patient and therapist will conclude the assessment in an emotionally vulnerable state. The patient may want to escape the anxiety generated by discussing real mortal threats by idealizing the therapist as immune to risk and able to (falsely) reassure or rescue them. The therapist may feel de-skilled by anxiety aroused by recognition of their shared vulnerability to these threats if they have not predated this work with their own reflection.

Assessment of the Patient 233

Two concluding actions are recommended for the clinician. First, it is important to recognize the difficulties of discussing climate change explicitly, as one does after any session focused on severe trauma. Second, the therapist should try to create an appropriate frame in which further conversations about climate change can occur. As discussed in detail in Chapter 12, "Psychotherapy Considerations and Approaches for Climate-Related Distress," it is important to validate the patient's concerns, acknowledge the shared reality of an uncertain climate future fraught with risk, and establish active hope that the patient's distress can be reduced through preparation and meaningful work with others engaged in solving the problem. These elements are geared toward reassuring the patient that they will not be struggling or suffering alone and toward demonstrating that the therapist is able to remain with reality even if they themselves are fearful or in danger.

At the conclusion of this climate evaluation, the clinician will have a good idea of how the patient relates to their natural world and the threats posed by climate change, as well as their psychological and practical resources and limitations in responding to them in a way that reduces anxiety and promotes survival. The groundwork will have been laid for deeper work on all aspects of the patient's climate response, having established a therapeutic framework that anticipates resilient change and a way of working with the uncertain interdependence of patient, therapist, and planet that offers containment and hope.

Key Points

- A climate-informed patient assessment can be done in less than a dozen questions or can span several hours and offers a chance to explore the patient's relationships and social determinants of health at a broad and deep level.
- Climate-informed assessment includes evaluation of the patient's neuropsychiatric, physical, and social risks from climate change; their attachment to nature; and their capacity for adaptive, resilient, and self-protective actions, including mitigation of emissions.
- Several screening instruments are available to support the assessment of climate-related attitudes and risks.
- The climate-informed assessment conveys the clinician's biological expertise and psychological depth, and it lays the groundwork for successful psychotherapeutic work.

References

Adams J: Risk. London, Routledge, 1995

Clayton S, Crandon T: Climate distress among young people: an overview, in Climate Change and Youth Mental Health: Multidisciplinary Perspectives. Edited by Haase E, Hudson K. Cambridge, UK, Cambridge University Press, 2024, pp 3–20

Clayton S, Czellar S, Nartova-Bochaver S, et al: Cross-cultural validation of a revised environmental identity scale. Sustainability 13(4):2387, 2021

Climate Mental Health Network: Climate emotions wheel. Los Angeles, CA, Climate Mental Health Network, 2023. Available at: www.climatementalhealth.net/wheel. Accessed December 12, 2024.

Connor KM, Davidson JR: Development of a new resilience scale: the Connor-Davidson Resilience Scale (CD-RISC). Depress Anxiety 18(2):76–82, 2003 12964174

Di Fabio A, Gori A: Developing a new instrument for assessing acceptance of change. Front Psychol 7:802–802, 2016 27303356

Federal Emergency Management Agency: National Risk Index. Washington, DC, Federal Emergency Management Agency, 2023. Available at: https://hazards.fema.gov/nri/map. Accessed July 24, 2023.

First Street Technology: The standard for climate risk financial modeling. New York, First Street Technology, 2023. Available at: https://firststreet.org. Accessed November 24, 2024.

Gifford R, Nilsson A: Personal and social factors that influence pro-environmental concern and behaviour: a review. Int J Psychol 49(3):141–157, 2014 24821503

Gosling SD, Rentfrow PJ, Swann WB: A very brief measure of the Big-Five personality domains. J Res Pers 37(6):504–528, 2003

Leiserowitz A, Maibach E, Rosenthal S, et al: Climate Change in the American Mind: December 2018. New Haven, CT, Yale Program on Climate Change Communication, 2018

Lewis J, Haase E: Futures thinking: the fifth mode is containment. Submitted to Psychodynamic Psychiatry, January 2025.

Moore C: Resilience theory: a summary of the research. PositivePsychology.com, December 30, 2019. Available at: https://positivepsychology.com/resilience-theory. Accessed July 24, 2024.

Oreg S: Resistance to change: developing an individual differences measure. J Appl Psychol 88(4):680–693, 2003 12940408

Poortinga W, Steg L, Vlek C: Myths of nature and environmental management strategies: a field study on energy reductions in traffic and transport, in People, Places, and Sustainability. Edited by Moser G, Pol E, Bernard Y, et al. Kirkland, WA, Hogrefe & Huber, 2003, pp 280–290

Smith BW, Dalen J, Wiggins K, et al: The brief resilience scale: assessing the ability to bounce back. Int J Behav Med 15(3):194–200, 2008 18696313

Assessment of the Patient

Southwick SM, Bonanno GA, Masten AS, et al: Resilience definitions, theory, and challenges: interdisciplinary perspectives. Eur J Psychotraumatol 5(1):25338, 2014 25317257

Tam K-P, Chan H-W, Clayton S: Climate change anxiety in China, India, Japan, and the United States. J Environ Psychol 87:101991, 2023

Tedeschi RG, Cann A, Taku K, et al: The Posttraumatic Growth Inventory: a revision integrating existential and spiritual change. J Trauma Stress 30(1):11–18, 2017 28099764

Verplanken B, Roy D: "My worries are rational, climate change is not": habitual ecological worrying is an adaptive response. PloS One 8(9):e74708, 2013 24023958

Wang RS, Seritan A, Hatcher A, et al: The climate formulation: addressing climate change in mental health practice. Acad Psychiatry, 2024 39285134 Online ahead of print

Worrell FC, Mendoza-Denton R, Wang A: Introducing a new assessment tool for measuring ethnic-racial identity: the Cross Ethnic-Racial Identity Scale-Adult (CERIS-A). Assessment 26(3):404–418, 2019 29214847

Wynes S, Nicholas KA: The climate mitigation gap: education and government recommendations miss the most effective individual actions. Environ Res Lett 12(7):74024, 2017

12

Psychotherapy Considerations and Approaches for Climate-Related Distress

Overview of the Psychotherapeutic Approach and Treatment Frame for the Climate-Distressed Patient

The current knowledge base for how to do psychotherapy work on climate distress is conceptual and practical, gained by consensus work by interested professionals and without study of psychotherapy patients (Seaman 2016). Many scientific questions remain about the patient characteristics that may benefit from climate therapy and the psychotherapy processes that are truly beneficial. Therefore, the recommendations in this chapter cannot be considered evidence-based but are, rather, derived from broad sociological knowledge and solid evidence from existing evidence-based therapies for similar techniques and approaches. Experience to date suggests that this psychotherapeutic work around climate change can facilitate tremendous growth in patients (and in therapists): at existential, social, and functional levels;

237

as an isolated exploration; and embedded in a broader psychotherapeutic process. To be successful in this process, however, both therapist and patient must withstand the many pressures to escape from difficult states of mind and frightening realities that will be inherent in what is discussed, and work to process them in a full and embodied way toward resilient change.

The three pillars of this process can be described as reckoning with reality, containment, and transformation. *Reckoning with reality* is a phrase that describes the ability to imagine and emotionally absorb the radically new situation that all people are in—the unprecedented scale and emotional experience of frightening global change, including mortality and extinction, and its implications for our own individual lives. *Containment* describes the work of the therapist, who must create a space where such feelings can be safely processed and discourage the myriad forms of dissociation and disavowal that most often arise in the individual and social climate response. Containment also describes the adaptations and actions by the patient that prevent overwhelm. *Transformation* describes the change and growth that emerge from the deep processing of climate realities and includes resilient, meaning-based personal change in both lifestyle and psyche. Models for transformation, including processes supporting posttraumatic growth, rites of passage, transformational resilience, deep adaptation, and others are described later in this chapter.

Therapists are reporting increased interest from patients wanting to work on climate distress, although as yet neither the prevalence with which they are seeking treatment, the content emerging from formal psychotherapy, nor the effectiveness of common interventions has been more than minimally researched. In a scoping review of which ecotherapy interventions have been suggested for working with climate-distressed patients, Baudon (2021) highlighted common general elements that include the following:

- Taking action
- Connecting to nature
- Seeking social support

Baudon also provided the following advice to practitioners:

- Do inner work
- Educate yourself
- Support client resilience

Psychotherapy Considerations and Approaches

Although adaptive actions are often reactive to climatic events, the longer-term and broader climate psychotherapy goal is anticipatory, planned, and autonomous alterations in decision-making and orientation of beliefs. The mental health professions need to do further work to determine how best to interact with patients in relation to climate material, including researching the outcomes of the different models proposed.

Therapeutic Preparation, Disclosure, and Authority

Therapists are themselves in the process of emerging from the pervasive disavowal of climate change that has been the modus operandi of the past century (see Chapter 10, "Emotional Reactions and Syndromes Associated With Climate Change"), and they are as prone as their patients to experiencing anxiety as they gain awareness of climate realities. Therapist training in climate change science and therapists doing personal work on their own reactions are thus critical elements for them to develop the understanding and emotional attitudes that will facilitate successful treatment. Lack of knowledge of climate change can contribute to psychological denial of grim scientific realities, and lack of knowledge of solutions and the creative emergent qualities of complex systems can equally lead to excessive hopelessness. Delineating irrational from rational climate worry also is complicated because of the unpredictable, complex, potentially existential, and evolving nature of the climate problem, the many different realities in which it is happening (see section "Pillar 1: Reckoning With Reality"), as well as the increasingly disinformed politics that surround its discussion. This requires therapeutic reflection on the important transferential aspects of the following:

- Attending to climate anxiety without contributing to hysterical exaggeration of the likely risks, in the therapist as well as in the patient
- Avoiding collusion with a patient's wish to avoid full exploration of climate fears, particularly avoiding or denying mortality questions
- Interpreting overlap with other life issues and developmental fears without invalidating the climate concern

Numerous psychological dynamics (more technically, transference/countertransference paradigms) between the patient and the therapist are possible in this scenario, including, but not limited to, the following:

- Therapist alarm about climate change that leads them to suppress, deny, or catastrophize frightening material brought by the patient
- Therapist disavowal of the climate situation, shared with the patient in proceeding with the status quo, that manifests in overly rigid adherence to traditional treatment frames and failure to innovate new treatment processes
- Therapist disavowal of the impacts of their own carboniferous lifestyle that leads them to fail to grapple with or acknowledge their own complicity in a system that has contributed to a patient's anger and darker reality
- Patient hidden protection of or even denigration of the therapist for being unable to handle the moral ghastliness or scientific realities of what is unfolding, leading them to enjoy the shock and masochistic triumph of showing off their capacity to be with the grisliness of climate effects; this can also be a countertransference of a therapist to a naive or climate-denying patient
- Patient highlighting of their climate distress as a sadistic punishing of parental figures who have failed them, enacting other parallel transferences to cultivate pity, rejection, dependency, or other motive
- The patient or therapist's subtle eroticization of or overexcitement in the relationship by being in the in-club of the climate-aware

The problem of how to remain in the climate reality without being too "into it"—staying with the acknowledgment that the problem is faced by the therapist as well as the patient, while protecting the privacy and authority of the therapist (transference boundaries)—is thus a difficult one. Nonetheless, therapists are encouraged to communicate their awareness of and engagement with climate change when working with climate-distressed patients. In a recent small thematic analysis, patients particularly valued four aspects of the therapist's response:

- Therapist understanding of climate change
- Therapist support for patients' competence in coping with climate change

Psychotherapy Considerations and Approaches

- Therapist validation of patient feelings
- Therapist assistance in seeking meaning-based responses

In this study and as reported elsewhere, patients did not speak as freely about climate fears if they did not feel their therapist was informed. This may suggest protectively wanting not to frighten or burden them, showing concern that it might destabilize the therapist and thus their treatment, and perhaps seeking the gratification and favoritism of being a "good child" by "sugarcoating it a bit" (Budziszewska and Jonsson 2022).

The recommendation for the therapist to affirm their climate knowledge and engagement differs from the usual therapy practices of avoiding personal disclosure and taking a position on an issue with which a patient is struggling. However, it falls within standards of good therapeutic practice in situations where there has been traumatic neglect of an important aspect of reality contributing to a patient's feeling of helplessness. Therapists routinely affirm their belief in the patient's reality and personal support for reparative or nondiscriminatory action even while being mindful of the potential distortions of recalled memory and perceived victimization, as in work with victims of childhood sexual abuse; persons discriminated against for their race, gender, or sexuality; or those who have experienced oppression. The therapist's knowledge of climate change establishes their professional ability to evaluate and stand up for truth and scientific information, as well as their capacity to consider their own and others' distortions in how it is being understood. Their engagement is part of the containing function for the patient's climate anxiety because it demonstrates that there are things that can be done and conveys an attitude of hope.

It is nonetheless somewhat problematic that in such overt disclosure the therapist presents themself as invested in and having the authority to understand climate change and the social forces that are shaping its response, as well as the authority to determine a right attitude to the problem. It is obviously impossible to know how to feel in response to a global problem in which up to two-thirds of humanity dies (Xu and Ramanathan 2017). But as the Buddha said when questioned who was he to be enlightened, "I am the one that is here." His recorded gesture, pointing to the ground, has been interpreted as a statement that the Earth was his witness: The work is worthwhile because the problem is here and therapy is something a clinician can do; the problem is one that must be addressed with immediacy, regardless of therapeutic authority. Together, therapist and patient can develop a new, more unfiltered mode of interacting over a shared situation: "setting up a camp together, then holding hands in the boat, bonding in a tribal way as they set out over new waters, dealing with shared threat together. This is our perennial ritual of what we can do, now in this new situation" (Lewis 2024). The willingness to stand together in difficulty is also an essential element of successful therapy, going to the mat with the patient despite uncertainty of complete understanding.

The sources of psychotherapeutic expertise that support mental health professionals presenting themselves as capable of providing guidance in this new realm of authority bear mention here. Mental health professionals have relevant authority and transferable skills to play this role vis-à-vis climate change (as well as to assist in the societal psychological struggle with climate responsiveness) as a result of the following:

- Their training in how to evaluate the statistics, strengths, and weaknesses of scientific studies
- Their training in how to evaluate personality structures, defenses, conscious and unconscious conflicts, and other factors that influence attitudes
- Psychotherapeutic knowledge of and skills for relating to others, including empathy, secure attachment, and capacity for concern, that facilitate an ability to understand what it means to be connected in a sustainable way to the natural world as well
- Daily immersion in processing communications while remaining neutral and nonjudgmental and returning this information to patients in a way that is fully inclusive of the multidetermined elements of a particular concern
- Self-analysis as an embedded element of practice

These skills are also the basis by which the therapist has authority over another listening ear in understanding the patient's life problems. They are not, however, inclusive of all the skills and transdisciplinary collaboration needed to alleviate climate distress or protect oneself from its impacts. Such humble collaboration might include staying connected to experts in planetary physiology, soil science, communication science, intersectionality, legal, sociological, and other related fields of response (Haase and Hudson 2024).

Pillar 1: Reckoning With Reality

Which Reality?

Part of both reckoning with climate realities and containing climate distress includes resisting the urge to deny, disavow, and otherwise emotionally escape difficult realities. Staying with reality is therefore something that keeps this work from spinning out of control. Freud introduced the reality principle to describe the need of the ego to mediate its internal states through operations that are consonant with external reality. In the case of climate change, however, there are two competing reality principles to follow. First, we can be realistic about the urgent need for rapid change called for by the science of global warming. Second, we can "be realistic" about our social and institutional reality, which is pulled by inertia and motivated biases to continue with business as usual. The cognitive dissonance of these two tends to lead both patient and therapist to collapse their mental experience onto one of these two reality-based positions to the exclusion of the other in order to have a stable frame of reference for feeling and belief. This collapse makes therapeutic neutrality, which stays with the conflictual validity of both realities, more difficult. Dialectic techniques are presented in the "Climate Dialectics" section below for avoiding this therapeutic pitfall. Additionally, reckoning with reality includes increasing appreciation for the interdependence of humans and nature to overcome the false separation and disorientation from nature of Western societies.

Climate Denial as a Psychic Retreat

The concept of the psychic retreat, developed by British psychoanalyst John Steiner (2003), can help illuminate the difficulties of staying with climate realities. Steiner saw psychic withdrawal as destructive—a temporarily protected space but without contact with reality. He described two processes that can occur when an anxiety-producing stimulus, such as climate change, breaks into consciousness. In the first, conflictual fragmentation and splitting occur, associated with high clinical drama, as we have seen in the dissolution of efforts and political polarization that have occurred when we have tried as a society to come into contact with climate realities. Second, there is what object relations theorists call the *depressive position*, which Steiner particularly subdivides into the denial of loss and the experience of loss. The person in denial of loss is unable to act because of their fear of recognizing and grappling with loss, as we see so often paralyzing climate efforts, whereas the person experiencing loss is able to mourn and emerge from their psychic retreat into new behaviors.

From the point of view of object relations theory, the reality-based fears of destruction, deprivation, and annihilation that underlie climate change are not far from the psychic fears of the paranoid position. In the paranoid position, there is not only the tendency to retreat but also the use of the more primitive defenses: omnipotence, denial or schizoid withdrawal, projection, projective identification, and splitting. The defenses of the paranoid position are called primitive because they emerge earlier in development and are not as functional when dealing with complex adult situations where compromise and acknowledging the needs and feelings of others must be taken into account to preserve social relations.

These defenses can be seen in the denial of climate realities that is visible everywhere, from beachfront developments to growth-oriented economic goals, often associated with the projection of vulnerability and the omnipotent defensive claim that the likely climate damage of these practices will happen to someone else. In parallel with this denial of personal vulnerability is the wish to project blame onto others, such as for responsibility for bad real estate sales when beachfront properties flood. Metabolizing climate realities in a meaningful way requires tolerating the frustration, guilt, vulnerability, and fear of acknowledging the harm we are doing, both to ourselves and to others. It also requires changing our way of life and calling out the primitive defenses by which such awareness is avoided.

Validation of Reality

Patients with climate distress often live in societies that invalidate, deny, or disavow their climate reality, the emotions they are feeling, the systems that harm the things they care about and worsen their future conditions, and the moral injury they experience from participation in society. Pushing back against this by continually aligning with climate science against the upstream pressures of disavowal becomes an anchoring activity that therapist and patient can do together, thus generating new realities and connecting to the current and future historical moments.

Climate uncertainties also complicate reckoning with climate realities. Although in many ways they are no different from other very

Psychotherapy Considerations and Approaches

similar uncertainties that worry patients—When and how will I die? How will my children turn out? Will those who claim to love me protect me when I need them?—there is more experience with the answers to these questions than with climate change. This combination of climate invalidation and climate uncertainty increases distress.

Validation is thus a critical element of the general therapeutic approach to a patient with climate-related concerns and part of the reckoning with reality work. Many reports show young people who have been turned off from therapy when they felt the therapist was not interested in their feelings about climate change, kept trying to change the topic or blame their feelings on something else, did not seem concerned about climate change, or had similarly dismissive reactions. Part of this validation of climate distress includes validating what is known of the scientific realities. The remainder includes validating that it is natural and normal to feel scared, angry, sad, and other strong emotions about the climate situation, and that anyone aware of the realities, including the therapist, would be expected to have such feelings.

Boundaries and Boundary Violations for Planet-Sized Distress

The concept of boundary violations in working with climate distress needs to be understood in a different way than is usual in psychiatry. Boundary violations occur when one person, usually in a position of strength or power, takes something from another person that does not belong to them. They are disrespecting the reasons for and rules of the interpersonal relationship and failing to recognize 1) that the thing taken is part of that person, or 2) that there is a relationship between the person and that thing: for example, a business colleague dates an ex-partner, a psychiatrist takes the patient's art in substitution for payment, a professor trades a top grade for sexual favors, a teacher makes a medical decision for a parent, an abuser violates the body of an individual. The thing that is stolen is often nonmaterial: the ability to trust that what is loved or integral to a person's body, mind, relationships, or talents will not be violated or exploited in a relationship.

Vis-à-vis climate psychotherapy, two ideas can be introduced:

- The boundary of self-concern is expanded to include the relationship of the self to all of the natural world and to future and past generations

- Because the boundary of the self includes all of the land and beings around it, what has been excessively taken from nature by dominant individuals violates the actual bodily integrity of other people who feel that pain

As has always been understood by Indigenous peoples, the boundary of the self when these ideas are fully appreciated is very large, and our understanding of what is inviolable for a particular individual must be large enough to acknowledge and encompass all of it. The Land is, from the perspective of boundaries, an individual to whom the patient is closely related as well as a part of the person. She cannot be violated, and when she is violated, it is a violation of the patient. All living beings, and even inanimate nature, are granted the same inalienable rights as well as encompassing continuity with the living bodies of humankind. As a result, the therapist must consider the patient's total relationship with the living world as an embodied and psychic part of the patient, and violations of that world through the destruction of nature or the excessive hoarding of resources as violations of the patient's self and valued relational parts. The distress of the patient who feels the chopping down of a tree as a stab in the gut, the loss of a species as the death of a child, or the destruction of the future healthy environment as the brutal murder of their family can be conceived of in this way. This may change the therapist's understanding of and approach to issues of bodily distress, personalization, terror, and identity associated with such reactions. It may also lead to an understanding of care of the Mother Earth as self-enrichment, familial love, and reciprocal nurturance in which there is compersion or joy in seeing nature thrive.

Pillar 1, the reckoning with reality pillar of climate psychotherapy, thus has several features that include opening up and supporting a rich attachment to the natural world and its current science-based situation, and creating a psychotherapeutic space that accomplishes the following:

- Validates the patient's reactions to climate change and respects the patient's relationship with the natural world
- Avoids a limited frame of cognitive and emotional reference for what is "real"
- Seeks to recognize and confront forms of denial and disavowal, as well as other psychic retreats from the terrifying possibilities of climate change

Psychotherapy Considerations and Approaches 247

- Creates a particularly large holding environment in which reality encompasses and contains the uncertainties of, the many actors in, and the scale of the climate crisis
- Creates particular room for the novel, the unexpected, and the creative that is part of emergent realities

Established Psychotherapy Techniques for Reckoning With Reality

Psychodynamically trained therapists will recognize the familiarity of the therapy orientation just described, which mirrors its own techniques: fully accepting any psychic reality, reducing resistances to the recognition of difficult or unpleasant mental experiences, avoiding flights into more intellectualized or otherwise defended points of view and relational modes, and creating a therapy space that has, as British psychoanalyst Wilfred Bion said, "neither expectation nor desire" of what will be found in the patient's unconscious and the creative possibilities of healing (Bion 1967). The psychodynamic concepts that parallel these elements of the climate approach and can be helpfully brought to bear in doing climate psychotherapy include the following:

- Nonjudgment and unconditional acceptance
- Free-floating attention
- Resistance interpretation
- Attention to transferences and signal anxiety
- Principle of multidetermination when making an interpretation
- Empathic alignment with the emotions that have led to psychic retreats

Other psychotherapies may also be useful as conceptual models for the reality processing of climate distress. For example, the principle of radical acceptance from acceptance and commitment therapy, the testing and arguing the validity of automatic thoughts from cognitive-behavioral therapy, and the techniques from feminist and intersectional schools of therapy of questioning what has been left out or misrepresented may be useful in discussing the climate reality with patients. The application of existing psychotherapies' techniques to climate distress requires further refinement and testing in the coming years.

Pillar 2: Containment

Coping With Overwhelm

When patients are able to make contact with their emotions about climate change, they often experience overwhelm. This sense of overwhelm arises from the full reckoning of the painful realities; the complex characteristics of climate change; the inadequacy of individual capacities to cope with a global problem; and the intellectual complexity, misinformation, and disinformation that make it more difficult to form a cohesive response. Psychological states associated with this overwhelm include fragmentation, emptiness, paralysis, withdrawal, and terror; these can evacuate the patient's capacity to think and feel. They can often be heralded by feelings of depletion, exhaustion, or boredom in the countertransference feelings of the analyst.

Such states can also set up a psychic resonance and overidentification with more catastrophic potential climate futures in a positive feedback loop both within the patient and between the patient and therapist, which further exacerbates the precipitating terror and shuts down the capacity for imaginative and productive therapy work. Some climate therapists have found it helpful to deliberately slow down at such moments of depletion. They can take a moment to rest together and wait because, often, a bit of humor, a Freudian slip, or some other emergence of unconscious processing will suddenly reveal what is going on.

The work of Bion (1962) can also be helpful in conceptualizing climate overwhelm. For Bion, all persons have both psychotic and nonpsychotic modes of functioning connected to their ability to tolerate contact with difficult realities such as climate change. In his view, psychotic functioning is characterized by delinking consciousness and perception from reality, followed by the violent expulsion of unwanted information through the defense of projective identification and a resultant loss of mental organization and clarity, analogous to the feelings of overwhelm just described. In Bion's way of thinking, unwanted bits of reality that are too toxic or frightening to take in, such as the worst climate projections, penetrate real objects and turn them into what he called *bizarre objects*, leading to the paranoid annihilation fears experienced by someone functioning in a psychotic way. From this perspective, climate overwhelm represents the unwanted expulsion of frightening information, delinking consciousness and perception. The annihilation threats and other difficult qualities of climate change are bizarre

Psychotherapy Considerations and Approaches 249

enough on their own that they do not require much theoretical elaboration through such projective identification. Their ability to worsen human psychic function derives from a similar process, however; our ability to take them in is not adequate to the scale of the task.

Forms of Containment

The containment function of the therapist becomes particularly important in response to climate overwhelm and its ability to evaluate the patient's capacity to think and feel. *Containment* refers to the process by which the therapist supports and protects the patient from overwhelming emotional chaos or breakdown through co-regulation, allowing the patient to lean on and borrow from the therapist's emotional stability at moments of distress. The therapist co-regulates patient distress by *metabolizing* it into a more manageable form: reflecting on it through a process of reverie, transforming it, and then giving it back to the patient in a form that can be tolerated. Containment makes the intolerable tolerable and initiates a process of adding new space to previously stuck perceptions. In connecting the patient's emotions to an outside reality, it has, like a transitional object, a developmental function that moves a patient forward in time, morphing a catastrophe into something creative and fresh, developing the futurizing thought function or "capacity to conjure something new" (Winnicott 1945) and stabilizing inchoate aspects of identity (Lewis et al. 2020). In addition to the therapist's containing activity, the regularity, confidentiality, and reliability of therapy provide containment. Other mental and emotional means to contain climate distress include the following:

- Transcendent containment—turning attention to an individual's belonging to something larger than themself, whether through spiritual reflection, contemplation of the deep history and size of the universe, or awareness of the larger complexities of physical systems
- Agentic containment—helping the patient cultivate productive and goal-oriented activity
- Relational and community containment—the therapist's engagement demonstrates that the patient is safely on shared ground, as do relationships in which they can work on climate emotions with others
- Narrative containment—using familiar stories or metaphors for great transformation, such as Jesus's time in the wilderness, to

help the patient conceptualize what is happening and write their own transformation story

- Cognitive containment—providing organizing information about climate processes or intellectual content about climate solutions that can ground the overwhelmed patient in a hopeful, reality-based perspective

Climate Dialectics

The concept of climate dialectics developed out of the long tradition of dialectical philosophy in an attempt to describe particular splits in the climate experience (Lewis et al. 2020) where the nature of climate change makes it necessary to hold two irreconcilable ideas at the same time. These include the following:

- Maintaining hope when the situation is hopeless
- Trying to take personal action to mitigate climate impacts when only collective work will be effective
- Trying to live in a way consonant with the climate reality when the social reality works entirely differently
- Using nature for sustenance when nature is the threat

People tend to collapse onto one pole of these dialectics in their emotions and actions in response to climate threats, increasing the rigidity of their views, behaviors, and interactions with society as well as their distress. For example, by trying to enforce programs consistent with the needs of climate realities ("No more bottled water"), people may not adequately plan for and incorporate a response to the social forces that will need to be addressed (e.g., providing for those for whom bottled water is the only safe supply because of drought, or buying needed water when unexpectedly dehydrated). Similarly, overfocus on hope can lead to vulnerability to coming dangers, whereas excessive hopelessness can prevent people from seeing possibilities for positive outcomes. Therapists can intervene by attending to the other pole of these dialectics, asking what would happen if the patient considered the antithesis to their thesis. In so doing, therapists can open space for the patient to find creative or transformative syntheses of both in their actions, decreasing the patient's cognitive fusion with a limited point of view and entering into what Georg Wilhelm Friedrich Hegel referred to as a "being at home with oneself in the whole" (Hofmann 2019). Table 12.1 lists common climate dialectics.

Psychotherapy Considerations and Approaches 251

Table 12.1 Dialectics contributing to climate distress

Social reality vs. climate reality

Individual agency vs. collective agency

Nature as comfort vs. Nature as threat (safety vs. lack of safety)

Hope vs. hopelessness

Uncertainty vs. certainty

Mitigation vs. adaptation

Grounding and Presencing Skills for Containment

Climate emotions can also be contained by general and familiar psychotherapy skills for lowering adrenergic hyperarousal physiologically and psychically. Many physical techniques can be relaxing, depending on a patient's attunement to their body and physical capabilities, but a basic repertoire should include psychoeducation, breathwork, grounding, muscle relaxation, mindfulness, and calming techniques, as presented in Table 12.2.

Table 12.2 Grounding and presencing skills for containment

Skill	Description
Psychoeducation	Teaching about the physiology of the stress response and calling attention to how it is manifesting in the patient's body.
Breathwork	Deep, slow abdominal breathing involves breathing in and out slowly for a count of five to seven for each, done through the nostrils and by allowing the lower belly to swell and the ribs to flare as the diaphragm drops, relaxing the upper and accessory muscles of breathing. A patient may benefit from doing this exercise lying down with knees bent to aid in activating the diaphragm or from imagining they are breathing into the bottom of a saxophone, bearing down for a bowel movement, or other visual images for expanding the lower abdomen. Controlled breathing can also be helpful—just slowing and varying the breath pace.

Table 12.2 Grounding and presencing skills for containment (*continued*)

Skill	Description
Grounding and tracking	Increasing bodily awareness of the present by attending to one part of the body at a time, sometimes with the verbal direction of the therapist, starting with the toes or fingers and moving slowly up one limb, across the midline, and down the other limb, or from the base of the spine to the top of the skull. Instructions can be given to pay attention to the feel of the air on the skin, the level of heat in each part of the body, the weight of the body part, any areas of tension or pain, and so on.
Progressive muscle relaxation	Tensing and then relaxing muscles one group at a time, often starting from the extremities and moving toward the larger muscles of the core. For example, tensing and then relaxing the fingers and toes, then calves, thighs, buttocks, belly, upper arms, shoulders, and neck. Each muscle group is contracted optimally for 20 seconds and then released. Holding a plank or a squat with the arms flexed for 90 seconds can substitute as a rapid exercise.
Presencing and mindfulness	Enhancing both attention to and awareness of the richness of the present moment, attending to one of the senses or to a repetitive task in a highly detailed way. Examples include focusing on a scent; examining something from nature in great detail, such as taking in a tree's bark or other texture with the eyes closed; cutting vegetables, gardening, or sweeping a room with no distractions from one's focus on the task; and eating slowly and carefully, perhaps with the eyes closed.
Resourcing	Increasing a sense of personal safety by listing strengths, resources, and social networks.
Group processes	Creating a sense of safety through dance, music, yoga, Qigong, or other modalities.

Pillar 3: Transformation

Conceptualizing What Will Be Transformed

Perhaps more often than with other therapy problems, patients seek help for climate distress because of something wrong with something outside themselves: the society they are part of, the world that they are watching die, or the family or friends whose lifestyles cause them moral pain and conflict. With the few exceptions of those living as off-grid childless vegans, they also come to treatment with the awareness of discordance in themselves because of their complicity and participation in the human world that has created the Anthropocene. Some of the manifest reasons they come to climate psychotherapy are presented in Table 12.3.

As with any psychotherapy work, then, a therapeutic process in which a therapeutic action effects change is needed to put the psyche right. What is perhaps a bit different with climate distress work is the degree to which the person must transform the rules of the external environment in which they live to make needed change.

As delineated in Chapter 10, "Emotional Reactions and Syndromes Associated With Climate Change," what is disrupted in psychic processes in climate distress can be organized by the type of trauma associated with it: acute traumas such as natural disasters, anticipatory trauma as in pretraumatic stress disorder, and chronic traumatic stress from accumulating climate impacts such as civil unrest, prolonged famine, and migration, as a problem of complicated bereavement or as one of disrupted attachment. The different core emotional disturbances associated with each model (shocked or overstressed, anxiously future-preoccupied, numb or dissociated, grieving, disconnected or alienated) may help the therapist formulate what kinds of interventions may be most helpful for a given patient. For example, stress reduction may be helpful for acute traumas, presencing skills for the dissociated or future-preoccupied, community action for those who feel paralyzed and numb, and nature and Indigenous therapies or values-based changes for those disconnected in their lifestyle.

Goal of Transformation in Climate Psychotherapy

Through the deep processing and relinquishment of the thoughts, feelings, and actions that are out of harmony in our current way of

Table 12.3 Presentations of climate distress

New awareness, future anxiety, PTSD, losses, and community disruption after natural disasters

Grief and empathy for lost species and landscapes and for the suffering of human and animal life

Betrayal and anger at older generations and institutions

Disenfranchisement, disillusion, or burnout over inadequate workplace or civic climate action

Conflicts about childbearing given the future world

Relationship failures due to differences regarding the climate crisis and how to live ecologically

Shame and guilt over living a carboniferous lifestyle

Bereavement over lost legacies and future potential

Moral injury and career conflicts over the lack of sustainable choices

Unease and anxiety as a manifestation of climate disavowal; knowing but living "as if" not

Existential and mortality terrors about the future for oneself and future generations

Victimization by climate injustice: environmental illness or discrimination, forced relocation

Eco-emotions: eco-paralysis, eco-hopelessness, eco-numbing, and others

Obsessive-compulsive symptoms related to sustainable practices such as recycling

Acting out rage or hopelessness through actions such as illegal eco-defiance, substance use, or promiscuity

Unfocused malaise and despair about the world

living, patients in climate psychotherapy undergo a process of personal growth. This process aligns with transcultural concepts that growth comes from the destruction of the old idea or order by the new. Common elements in this process include deep emotional processing of environmental degradation, developing a closer connection to the natural world, and cultivating new forms of hope, purpose, and new life narratives. These commonalities are also found in other

Psychotherapy Considerations and Approaches

psychotherapy models oriented toward growth through the processing of trauma, which typically involve phases of creating safety, stabilizing the acute emotional state of the patient and preparing them with the skills needed to navigate the coming work, confronting difficult truths, and mourning what has been lost. This trauma work may be followed by emotional renewal, social reconnection, and expansion of activities and personal satisfaction (Hudgins and Durost 2022).

A good conceptual foundation for the psychology of this transformation can be found in posttraumatic growth (PTG). Originally developed and studied by Tedeschi and Calhoun (2004), PTG refers to the personal strengths that emerge from successfully working through a time of difficulty or despair and can be assessed with the Post-Traumatic Growth Inventory, recently revised to enhance questions about existential and spiritual growth (Tedeschi et al. 2017) and widely available online. PTG has been studied in veterans, first responders, medical diagnoses, terrorism, and life stressors and has been validated to eliminate bias due to "creating positive illusion" after sudden negative change. The following strengths are associated with PTG:

- Finding new opportunities
- Building deeper and more empathic connections
- Having a sense of strength, of being a survivor
- Having an increased appreciation for life
- Deepening spirituality

PTG has been shown to occur particularly when certain conditions are met:

- A high level of distress
- The distressing event is central to a person's identity (high event centrality)
- The event forces a reappraisal of an individual's assumptions, expectations, and beliefs about their life (cognitive engagement)
- Deep and prolonged processing of the distressing emotions occurs (positive rumination)
- A turning point is reached where the person decides against continuing despair

High levels of personal resilience do not necessarily predict PTG and may, in fact, work against it by circumventing the process of deliberative or positive rumination. PTG has instead been associated with a multitude of personal characteristics, including being female, higher education, being young or a young-at-heart older person, and in some studies, being part of a stigmatized or marginalized group. Personality traits of higher narcissism (supporting positive self-appraisal) and agreeableness, extroversion, and openness are also associated. Growth has been seen more often when the patient accepts difficult realities and when an approach to them involves positive reappraisal, meaning finding, and seeking a coherent worldview that encompasses the difficult situation. Sharing negative emotions in a group that has gone through a similar experience or in a couple in which the partner is responsive can be helpful, although only if those involved have a deep knowledge of the person's distress or they feel a clear sense of belonging. Through these processes, a person begins to engage spiritually, creatively, and interpersonally with new immediacy, authenticity, and confidence (reviewed in Henson et al. 2021).

PTG has been associated with many kinds of coping, including acceptance coping, problem-focused coping, meaning-based coping, and even avoidant coping, which may help individuals by allowing them to take a break from their distress. Because each type of coping may be helpful in different circumstances, flexible coping may be considered a summary approach to personal growth. In terms of climate change, however, meaning-based coping has been shown to be more helpful than practical problem-solving or emotionally based coping strategies in young people (Ojala and Chen 2024), perhaps because it focuses on a values-based creation of new narratives for how to live, and meaning-based actions are central to a person emerging with PTG out of despair.

Opening Space for Transformative Change in Climate Psychotherapy

Just as the therapeutic action of climate dialectic work is hypothesized to emerge from opening empty space between two rigid poles for the patient and therapist to cocreate new ways of looking at the climate problem, imaginative approaches to uncertainty, emptiness, and unknowability may also contribute to transformative climate distress work. These approaches include the metaphor of the baby, radical hope, dark optimism, futures thinking, and others as listed in Table 12.4. Through them, the therapist creates the *emergent container* (Martinez Acobi 2023) for the patient's new ideas, transforming helplessness into possibility.

Psychotherapy Considerations and Approaches

Table 12.4 Novel techniques for individual climate psychotherapy

Metaphor of the baby
Radical hope
Dark optimism
Catastrophic thinking
Futures thinking
Psychedelic-assisted therapy
Rites of passage
Ecolinguistics

Metaphor of the Baby

The expression *metaphor of the baby* describes a state of attuned alertness to the climate crisis that can be suggested to a patient to improve acceptance of where they are and not be excessively burdened by past modes of living or guilt about their impacts in a way that impairs growth. Recognizing that all people are in uncharted waters responding to the climate crisis, the therapist acknowledges that we are all waking up to new and continually shifting climate realities and, like an infant, do not yet know what we need to know. Cultivating this attitude prevents unhelpful modes of self-attack for the moral failures of the carboniferous lifestyle in which we are all entrenched by offering forgiveness and a metaphor for the opportunity for rapid growth and change that is seen in an infant or young child.

Radical Hope

The idea of *Radical Hope* was developed by philosopher and psychoanalyst Jonathan Lear (2006) to describe the kind of hope that can be held when outcomes are unknown. Using the story of Chief Plenty Coups, a Crow (Apsáalooke) chief whose people faced certain destruction if he did not sign a treaty with the White man, Lear reported on how the chief betrayed their immediate future and placed himself and his people in a situation where the words and stories they would live by were unknown to them. He acted on the basis of his trust in his ancestors and the continuity of generations and a dream he did not fully grasp but understood to be prophetic. The form of hope he demonstrated—beyond the ability of current language to articulate and assuming the basic goodness of unknowable larger universal forces—has been called Radical Hope, and it can be presented to the patient along with encouragement to trust the hopeful aspects of emergent systems.

Dark Optimism

A concept associated with futurists Shaun Chamberlin and David Fleming, *dark optimism* is an approach similar to that of Deep Adaptation Forum and the Dark Mountain Project (see subsections "Deep Adaptation" and "Uncivilization and the Dark Mountain Project"). It seeks to look unwaveringly at the true and devastating consequences of our growth mindset while also holding with equal tenacity to a belief in human potential, challenging dominant societal myths of what a good life looks like. Dark optimism particularly acknowledges the need to grapple with such wicked problems as how to change economic models without economic collapse and how to change education without losing knowledge, and its proponents offer "surviving the future" courses for such different social problems. Susan Kassouf (2022) encourages the cultivation of this kind of dark contemplation, which she calls *catastrophic thinking*. She proposed that catastrophic thoughts come from *trauma sensibility*, defined as beneficial enhanced intellectual and emotional capacities for facing difficult truths associated with having experienced severe life trauma. Referencing Bion, she sees catastrophic thinking as a cure for climate disavowal and dissociation: in an example of an infant forming thoughts on the basis of the absence or presence of a breast for food, "If the capacity for toleration of frustration is sufficient the no-breast inside becomes a thought, and an apparatus for thinking it develops" (Bion 1962). This quote communicates the idea that thinking about the catastrophic end points of climate change develops the cognitive apparatus necessary to avert them.

Futures Thinking

Futures thinking is an imaginative process that has been developed in the context of the history of futurism to help individuals and organizations cultivate *futures literacy*, a competency in incorporating the role of the future in what is seen and done now. Distinguished from future thinking, a neuropsychological concept for that human capacity (Gilbert and Wilson 2007), futures thinking recognizes the existence of

Psychotherapy Considerations and Approaches

infinite possible futures and seeks to heighten our present consciousness, particularly of that multiplicity, bringing attention to how we are dynamically and continually creating different futures with present actions to overcome "failures of the imagination" (Cork et al. 2023; Inayatullah 2008). In terms of climate change, this "the future is now" mentality combats the projection of climate anxieties into the future and has been suggested as a means of making our possible climate futures more alive in the present moment (Cork et al. 2023).

Inayatullah (2008) and Horst and Gladwin (2022) have delineated modes of futures thinking that include the following:

1. Predictive/empirical—quantitative probability modeling, such as that done by the Intergovernmental Panel on Climate Change for climate risks
2. Cultural/interpretive—practicing with futures using participatory scenario modeling to conceptualize multiple plausible futures and responses to them
3. Experimental experiential co-creation—doing now what can be imagined to enhance the evolutionary power of experiments in living, such as ecovillages or living by the principles of Burning Man
4. Critical/deconstructive—taking apart expected futures by ferreting out the biases and false assumptions in how we imagine the future

Through these modes, futures thinking imagines a *cone of futures* widening in time to include those that are preposterous, possible, plausible, probable, and currently projected. All are necessary to consider for the most creative outcomes. They are organized along three horizons: where we are now, the future that we could aim for or could be, and the intermediate and imperfect structures that may be necessary to get there (Figure 12.1).

For institutional psychiatry, futures thinking is essential for modeling services under a range of possible climate conditions, as well as for experimenting now with new treatment modes that may or may not be useful under changing future circumstances. In psychotherapy work, futures thinking can serve a variety of functions. Most therapists ask their patients to practice the psychological skill of future thinking routinely when they suggest playing out the downstream consequences of a current choice. What is different here is the playful emphasis on multiplicity that can help patients find alternative channels to stuck,

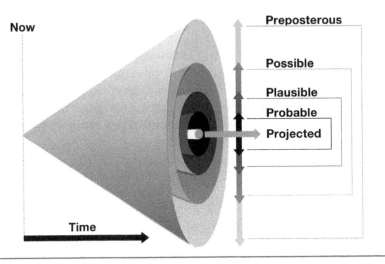

Figure 12.1 A futures cone.
Source. Used with permission from Mike Baxter, Goal Atlas, 2024.

obsessive, or ruminative mental processes and the creative backfilling of stages that will be necessary to reach the future goals identified.

Role of Psychedelics in Climate Distress and Transformation

Because most climate distress is not accompanied by a clinical level of functional impairment or a clear psychiatric disorder, medication approaches have not been considered or used for climate distress. Psychedelic treatments, however, may have an important role to play in augmenting the effectiveness of climate psychotherapy, particularly when combined with nature therapies. Both treatments decrease anxious rumination, enhance nature relatedness, elevate experiences of awe and interconnection to the natural world and universe, and increase openness to spiritual transformation and meaning-based life change that may contribute to PTG after climate traumas (reviewed in Gandy et al. 2020) when done in the appropriate setting.

Rites of Passage for Climate as a Transformative Technique

Rites of passage, as a category of ritual, facilitate transitions through important moments or stages of human experience. They can also be

Psychotherapy Considerations and Approaches 261

used in climate psychotherapy work to let go of unwanted modes of being and to embrace new behaviors. Rites of passage follow a defined pattern of three phases (van Gennep 1960):

- Separation—a phase marked by a clear break from usual forms of behavior, which often involves symbolically shedding some part or totem of the former self by cutting one's hair, burning a valued object, disrobing or donning a special form of dress, or performing behaviors such as crossing a physical threshold or going to a remote or isolated location
- Transition—entry into a liminal state characterized by dissolution of the ego, behavioral incoherence, and trance-like, chaotic, and hallucinatory states that contribute to fermenting change; this phase establishes a token or emblem of the new self that will often emerge; when done with others, a group process develops that follows a temporary and unusual set of rules that bond the group together
- Incorporation—transition back into society, having formed new behavioral norms

Van Gennep (1960) and Turner (1967) worked with primitive homogeneous groups in which dance and other body-based practices play important roles in these rituals. Janusz and Walkiewicz (2018) wrote that rites of passage may be a tool for fixing negative mental health processes that result when phases of the life cycle become disordered or disrupted, such as late teens derailed from the transition to college by drugs, and women losing fertility because of their age or those experiencing negative socioeconomic and health impacts from reversing the traditional progression from education to work, marriage, and children. From these perspectives, rites of passage may be particularly relevant for climate-related transformation for the following reasons:

- They open transformative spaces for deep shifts to sustainable identity and behavior
- They may cultivate embodied and community-based processes as an alternative to modern community breakdown and consumerist identities
- They connect inner transformation work to social processes
- They may realign the patient to the development stage and health needs of themselves and the planet, fixing unnatural cycles caused by modern lifestyles

Patients can be helped to develop a rite of passage for climate distress, ranging from a process in session to a retreat alone or with a small group. The rite should have a formal opening to process the patient's emotions in a novel or creative way through art, experience, or story, and then some ritual of closure that may contain a commitment to something meaningful explored in the process (Ray 2023). An object or a talisman of the new and old self may be included. Psychedelic drugs may increasingly play a role in rites of passage, as they do in Indigenous cultures, and can be considered as their approved use expands (Rodríguez Arce and Winkelman 2021).

Vignette

Sue, age 70, presented with protracted grief over the death of her husband and reported drinking excessively and rejecting her family. A traditional housewife, she saw no future for herself or her family or the world, highlighting the sense of lost legacy and eco-grief that comes with climate change. Elements of her therapy included honoring her grief (a therapeutic technique in the Work That Reconnects that exemplifies the positive rumination function of PTG), constructing a ritual to help her put away old roles (a rite of passage), and helping her imagine a range of possible outcomes for her later years (an exercise in futures thinking). Sue spontaneously decided to help groom wild horses at a conservation program and began to feel more grounded. This animal therapy helped her experience herself through nature metaphors and Indigenous ways of knowing as a wild young horse learning a new way of living.

Transformation Through Language and Metaphor

The creative use of language in climate psychotherapy can be both grounding and transformative. Metaphoric processing has been shown to be a neurophysiological process that both patterns and taps directly into emotional and sensory networks of the brain, circumventing cognition and only secondarily co-opted by the use of language (Modell 2009). For this reason, using natural metaphors, such as describing climate change as an earthquake or avalanche, or happiness in nature as oceanic or soaring, may particularly help patients in states of eco-paralysis, disavowal, or anxious dissociation to connect in an imaginative and embodied sensory way with what they are feeling.

Language can also be used to support ecological and cultural coherence in new narratives. For thousands of years, language has carried and inculcated an anthropocentric view of nature in how humankind is able to describe our world: Nature has been described as hierarchical (*scala naturae*), mechanistic (e.g., Newton's Cosmic Machine), or bioeconomic (as a factory or storehouse producing goods for higher species). More recently, the field of ecolinguistics and the accompanying use of biocentric language have emerged, building linguistic power into views of nature as web, mother, and measure (Verhagen 2008). Using words such as *community, web, ecology, alliance, unity, reverence, interconnection,* and *continuity*; verbs associated with harmonizing, flowing, and connecting instead of engineering or correcting (Rust 2020); and natural metaphors of transformation, such as the caterpillar to the butterfly or the mollusk or snake to a new shell or skin, can be grounding and can support a rewriting and rewiring of the metaphors that undergird the patient's perceived relationship with the natural world (Holmes and Matthews 2010; Mark 2023; Milstein 2016).

In shaping a new psychotherapy language of this kind, attention also needs to be paid to perverse, inaccurate, and fetishizing communication, particularly in relation to the people and institutions perpetuating climate change, to nature, and to solutions that simplify climate complexity. For example, language around nature may portray it as cute or anthropomorphized—"years of Shamu shows have conditioned the public to think of killer whales as pool toys," as one trainer aptly put it (Morton 2002, p. 190)—but animals do not operate by the same behavioral rules and ethics we do. Calling out inconsistencies, such as climate policy decisions that threaten tens of millions of lives made by politicians who rue single executives' homicides, corrects cultural distortions embedded in our cultural and value-based communications.

Group Models for Transformational Growth Through Climate Psychotherapy Work

The models for transformative growth around climate distress share features with the processes of PTG, placing a heavy emphasis on shattering old modes of belief and functioning and on embracing a new vision. For Bion (1962), the new idea is the contained, and the mind or the society is the container. These models (Table 12.5), then, seek

Table 12.5 Group processing models for climate distress

Deep adaptation

Uncivilization/Dark Mountain Project

The Work That Reconnects

Transformational resilience

Climate cafés

The Good Grief Network

to break the container and use new ideas to contain the emotions of climate distress. Because of the central importance of community in healing climate distress, all of these models are group processes. Their elements can, however, be adapted for individual work.

Deep Adaptation

The Deep Adaptation Forum (DAF) was developed by sustainability scholar Jem Bendell (2018, 2019) to support climate scientists because they are most aware of the degree of impending societal collapse due to climate change and are often, like Cassandra, ignored and alienated in their message. DAF is divided into professional and other interest groups, and it explores the psychosocial and spiritual implications of societal and environmental breakdown through a Socratic questioning process based on what it calls the four R's:

- Reconciliation—What do we want to make peace with as we awaken to our mortality?
- Relinquishment—What do we need to let go of to not make matters worse, both emotionally and environmentally, as we face this collapse?
- Resilience—What do we most value that we want to keep, and how?
- Restoration—What can we restore from the past to help with these difficult times?

Through this questioning, DAF seeks, without cultivating hope, to create collapse readiness (equitable plans for resource distribution) and collapse transcendence, fostering psychosocial and spiritual composure

Psychotherapy Considerations and Approaches

in the face of deep adversity. DAF is available online, but the four R's technique can also be useful for individual therapeutic exploration.

Uncivilization and the Dark Mountain Project

The Dark Mountain Project arose from a manifesto published by Paul Kingsnorth and Dougald Hine. The project attempts to overcome a split climate narrative that projects collapse into the future, thereby rendering it unmanageable then but allowing us to preserve business-as-usual optimism now (Randall 2009). Instead, the work focuses on facing unsolvable problems and losses now. It looks for new approaches to civilization, "uncivilizing" or deconstructing our current narratives for how to live. The attitudinal approach of Dark Mountain is one of humility, accepting chaos and the loss of meaning and master narratives, improvising, and "navigating with uncertainty" (Graugaard 2024). The Dark Mountain Project publishes a journal in which artists, seekers, and philosophers of all kinds, referred to as *mountaineers*, use narrative and other creative, playful, and improvisational formats to "re-story" ways of being in the world. The imaginative processes of finding new metaphors and writing new stories for how a person will live are useful climate psychotherapy techniques.

The Work That Reconnects

The Work That Reconnects describes itself as a transformational learning process (Hathaway 2017), arising from the work of Buddhist scholar Joanna Macy and incorporating aspects of deep ecology, ecopsychology, Buddhism, and activism. The work of transformation is described as the Great Turning, with a recent component focused on undoing colonial mindsets and cultivating equity called the Evolving Edge. The four steps of the Great Turning are as follows:

1. Cultivating gratitude
2. Honoring our grief for the world
3. Seeing with new eyes
4. Going forth

These steps involve dozens of group and individual exercises that cultivate attachment, appreciation, love, and gratitude for what we are given by the nonhuman world. They facilitate the mourning of what is being lost through grief rituals, song, fire, and other exercises; explore new stories and ways of relating to the planet and its systems; and build communities and courage for ongoing activism. This process is thought to lead to what is termed *Active Hope*, referring to hope from doing meaningful and necessary things without expectation regarding their outcome. Although preferably done in community, the Work That Reconnects exercises can also be used in climate-distressed patients.

Transformational Resilience

Transformational resilience (TR) is an approach developed by Bob Doppelt (2017) and the International Transformational Resilience Coalition, who also contributed to the first legislation proposed in the U.S. Congress to fund community climate mental resilience initiatives. The two foundational skills of this approach, *presencing* and *purposing*, are taught in TR workshops tailored to diverse groups and occupations. Presencing skills help participants understand and self-regulate the fight-or-flight response through education about its physical manifestations as well as its effects on communities in terms of greater aggression, distrust, and lack of concern for others and the environment. They also help with the grounding, mindfulness, and breathing techniques covered earlier (see subsection "Grounding and Presencing Skills for Containment" and Table 12.2). Purposing skills help participants cultivate an intentional and meaningful life and shift the organization of communities from trauma-bonded modes (fear, hierarchy, and rigid punitive approaches) to modes that enhance resilience over time. Examples of these new modes include cultivating appreciation for how others handle adversity, clarifying values, "harvesting hope" for the future through activities that promote the well-being of the self and the community, and developing more resilient social and resource-based infrastructure.

Climate Cafés

Among the more accessible group models for processing climate distress are climate cafés. As their name suggests, these are informal gatherings, free of charge, some led by laypersons and others by mental health professionals. The only goal is to provide a supportive space for sharing climate concerns and receiving feedback from other members. In facilitated groups, such as those organized by the Climate Psychology Alliance, leaders may identify group processes. Others,

Psychotherapy Considerations and Approaches

such as those facilitated by the Climate and Mind group, may provide support for how to take action.

The Good Grief Network

The Good Grief Network was founded by lay organizers LaUra Schmidt and Aimee Lewis Reau, who based their 10-step climate distress program on the Alcoholics Anonymous model and the belief that sitting in community with climate distress builds personal resilience. The 10 steps of the program emphasize accepting complicity and responsibility in climate processes and include elements of the other group models in this section as well. The program focuses on the following steps:

1. Accept the problem and acknowledge its severity
2. Acknowledge one's role and complicity in the problem and in the solution
3. Practice sitting with uncertainty
4. Confront one's own mortality and the mortality of all beings
5. Do inner work
6. Develop awareness of brain patterns and perceptions
7. Practice gratitude, seek beauty, and create connections
8. Take breaks and rest as needed
9. Show up
10. Reinvest in meaningful efforts

The Good Grief Network is easily relatable and can be a tool for organizing the stages of climate psychotherapy.

Using Existing Therapeutic Modalities to Work With Climate Distress

Clinicians may also find it useful to bring techniques from relevant existing therapies into the climate space (Table 12.6).

Techniques from acceptance and commitment therapy (ACT), for example, are likely to be generally useful for climate distress because ACT's emphasis on radical acceptance of difficult situations, transformation through cognitive defusion from previously fixed thoughts and beliefs, and meaning-based action overlaps significantly with many

Table 12.6 Established psychotherapies with relevance for climate distress

Acceptance and commitment therapy

Motivational interviewing

Existential therapy

Feminist therapy

Psychodynamic therapy

Nature therapy

Psychedelic therapy

climate-therapy suggestions. ACT is additionally similar in emphasizing that the patient and therapist are in the same boat in seeking a full, rich life despite the human condition.

The techniques of motivational interviewing, a treatment oriented toward contemplating and making change, may also help climate-oriented therapists support the transformation process in the following ways (Levounis et al. 2017):

- Noticing and responding to change talk
- Developing a discrepancy between current and desired selves
- Planning for and contemplating the pros and cons of considered changes
- Affirming the patient's intentions

Existential psychotherapy is particularly appropriate to bring to bear on climate fears. Developed around the time of the First and Second World Wars, existential psychotherapy sought to deal with the three existential anxieties identified by philosopher-theologian Paul Tillich in his seminal work, *The Courage to Be* (Tillich 1952):

- Anxiety about annihilation
- Anxiety about living an empty or meaningless existence
- Anxiety about not living up to our ethical or moral standards

Existential therapy calls attention to how each person can continually choose the reality they wish to create and live by, seeking freedom even within the most difficult and frightening situations. It can help patients

Psychotherapy Considerations and Approaches

269

confront their deepest climate fears in a safe setting, cultivate a sense of authentic self, live by their environmental ideals, and develop the kind of hope that emerges from the refutation of negative certainty (Solnit 2004).

Feminist therapy shares with climate psychotherapy an open encouragement for people to take social and political action, and it similarly makes explicit an egalitarian co-participant relationship between therapist and patient. Symptoms of patients in feminist therapy, like those in climate psychotherapy, are seen not as psychopathology but as an appropriate response to social conditions.

Finally, it may be possible to consider incorporating Indigenous practices into the climate psychotherapy setting. To date, literature on incorporating Indigenous practices in psychotherapy is minimal and is focused mostly on whether empirically studied therapies can be used effectively with Indigenous groups, for whom they are often poorly adapted. Rather than leaving therapists as "crypto-missionaries" of non-Indigenous views, some of these studies have looked at incorporating changes in wording or practices such as smudging or sweat lodges, but these studies have not tested the independent efficacy of these practices or their efficacy for non-Indigenous groups (Wendt et al. 2022). It is suggested that the environmental awareness of Indigenous peoples has much to offer non-Indigenous practices for climate-related transformative change (Cianconi et al. 2023; Katz 2012), cultivating the Seventh Generation Principle of the Haudenosaunee (Iroquois) to support personal action as well as continuity with and gratitude for nature.

Nature Therapy for Climate Distress

Including nature-based interventions in treating climate-related distress specifically is so intuitive that it is surprising that it was only formally considered in 2023, when a global consortium of scholars proposed a new "nature-based biopsychosocial resilience theory" (White et al. 2023). In this overview, as elsewhere as of 2024, neither contact with nature nor nature-based therapies had been formally studied for climate distress. At the same time, ecotherapists have been using nature therapies to support patients' environmental distress for decades, and a robust literature (Kaplan and Levounis 2025) details the positive effects of nature and nature therapies on mental health, physical health, and pro-environmental behavior (Table 12.7).

Extremely limited study exists about the effect of nature therapies on people with mental illness. A scoping review of international work

Table 12.7 Mental and physical benefits of contact with nature and nature therapies

Greater positive emotions, including joy, self-esteem, and well-being

Decreased rumination and loneliness

Decreased scores on measures of anxiety and depression

Faster autonomic recovery and improved cardiac outcomes from stress

Decreased salivary cortisol

Improved immune function; fewer proinflammatory cytokines, improved natural killer cell number and activity

More prosocial and less aggressive behavior in both adults and children

Lower amygdalar activity

Improved attention and working memory

Improved social function and motivation

Improved musculoskeletal function (balance, pain levels)

Decreased cardiovascular mortality and stroke

Improved parameters in diabetes, hypertension, obesity, and pulmonary disease

Improved social cohesion and perceived social support

Source. Summarized from White et al. (2023) and Thomas et al. (2022).

on green prescribing for those with mental illness retrieved only seven studies but demonstrated improvements in skills, confidence, and positive affects and decreased anxiety and depression. In this work, patients particularly emphasized that their sense of social connection and self-confidence improved and also reported large increases in nature relatedness (Thomas et al. 2022). Horticulture therapy (Tu 2022) and animal therapy (Spattini et al. 2018) have a greater but still limited evidence base, and positive effects have clearly been demonstrated.

The benefits of nature contact and nature therapy are thought to accrue from biophilic reactions, stress reduction, and restoration of attention. The biophilia hypothesis, originally proposed by E.O. Wilson in 1984, states that humans have an innate need to form attachment relationships with other living things. Biophilia is demonstrated by human attraction to animals, nature, and nature-based activities (Kellert and Wilson 1993; Vining 2003) and experiences of sublime

Psychotherapy Considerations and Approaches

emotions and vitality in response to nature (Bethelmy and Corraliza 2019). Biophobic, sadistic, and alienated responses to the natural world also occur and have some evolutionary advantages (Vining 2003), yet biophilic affiliation is found even in ruthless dictators and is central to some of the happiest experiences of most children and adults.

Nature attachment is increased by experiences in natural environments as well as through visual imagery of nature, and it mediates a significant portion of nature-protective behavior (Kals et al. 1999; Nisbet et al. 2009). Nature relatedness is a construct that describes this human-nature relationship; it is a trait-based appreciation for interconnectedness with living things, including both positive and dangerous or unappealing aspects of nature. Nature relatedness correlates with time in nature, pro-environmental actions, agreeable and open personality traits (Nisbet et al. 2009), lower levels of anxiety, more vitality, happiness and positive emotion, higher psychological functioning, and greater perceived meaning in life.

On the basis of these relationships between nature and mental health, nature and attachment, and nature and pro-environmental functioning, we can formulate an approach to nature therapy for climate distress that is broken into the following:

1. Using nature-based therapies to cultivate nature attachment, perhaps particularly for those with nature phobias or minimal natural access
2. Using nature-based therapies for alleviation of climate distress
3. Using nature-based therapies for transformative change

Co-benefits of nature therapies might also be expected to accrue, including improved general physical and mental health and improved social cohesion around the importance of caring for nature. Nature therapies may include the following types:

- Horticulture therapy
- Contact with nature through mindful hiking, fishing, and other outdoor activities
- Wilderness therapy
- Forest bathing (immersing oneself in the forest, popular in Japan)
- Keeping pets
- Conservation activities
- Blue mind therapy (attuning to water environments)

Horticulture therapy, or gardening, can be conducted in individual settings (gardening), groups, or inpatient units and includes such activities as planting, cultivating and harvesting vegetables, making meaningful art with flowers and natural elements, and cooking and sharing meals using plant foods. Conservation therapy work might include cleanup weekends, trail-making, campouts to assess resources in a particular area, or activist work with a compatible group. Wilderness therapy, a full consideration of which is beyond the scope of this work, is less well defined and has been associated with both controversy and death, as well as benefits for adolescents, persons with substance abuse, and those with other mental disorders. It generally includes at least several days in a remote setting and practicing survival and backpacking skills.

Forest bathing (Shinrin-yoku) is a well-researched treatment that is compatible with climate distress goals of reducing stress and cultivating nature attachment. It is done by

- Preparation to prevent discomfort and collect baseline data, such as applying anti-allergens and sunscreen, taking vital signs, and mood assessments
- Marking entry into the forest with 15–20 minutes of standing still, cultivating awareness of the body and its surroundings
- Moving slowly through and sitting in a forest or similar environment with all electronic and interpersonal distractions removed for 2 hours
- Deeply breathing in the aromatics of forest air with an extended exhale
- Quietly observing natural details with the five senses while slow walking or sitting
- Creating a slow exit ritual, such as drinking tea

Forest bathing has been associated with numerous robust physical health benefits, including decreased cortisol, glucose, adrenergic markers, and pro-inflammatory markers; lower heart rate and blood pressure; and improved heart rate variability and natural killer function. Mental health improvements are robust and include decreased depression, hostility, fatigue, and anxiety and increased vigor (Wen et al. 2019).

For many people, their most intimate experiences with nonhuman beings in nature come from pet ownership. For this reason, pet therapy is an accessible treatment for climate distress: Approximately 60%–70% of households in Western countries have a pet, most often a dog, but also a cat, horse, fish, snake, or others (Pew Research Center 2023).

Psychotherapy Considerations and Approaches

Establishing a felt connection to a pet is associated with emotions that strengthen a loving and empathic connection to the natural world and to others, including emotions of love, peace, and joy (Aragunde-Kohl et al. 2020), as well as greater empathy and less delinquency (Jacobson and Chang 2018).

Relationships with animals are also shown to connect humans to nature more broadly (Myers and Saunders 2002; Vining 2003) and to have pro-environmental benefits on behavior (Vining 2003). Although pet ownership does not consistently improve mental health or establish a beneficial emotional connection, particularly when owners are depressed (Scoresby et al. 2021), the health and mental health benefits of pet ownership predominate. These benefits include improved cardiovascular parameters and post–myocardial infarction survival, social support, changes in cortisol and oxytocin associated with improved stress responses and more interpersonal relaxation, improved physical activity, and improved social connections across nations in both those with disabilities and those without (McCune et al. 2014). Other animal therapies include the use of a trained service animal to lower anxiety or assist with disabilities and sessions with animals such as horses and dolphins, but these may be less relevant for climate distress.

In addition to these therapies, there is a panoply of other creative means of engaging connection to the natural world, including participating in seed banks, animal mimicry, regenerative farming and reforesting, river mapping, writing new myths and holiday narratives, restorative justice efforts toward the Earth and Indigenous peoples, plant consciousness study, elevation of the divine feminine to enhance Mother Earth awareness, and myriad others. Readers may find the past programs on the website of the Bioneers organization particularly fruitful in this regard. The most important thing is for the patient to engage in something embodied, personally meaningful, and restorative in a lifestyle honoring interdependency with the natural world.

Key Points

- Therapists working with climate distress should be informed about climate change and willing to work with more personal openness and flexible boundaries and to incorporate novel approaches compared with traditional therapy settings.
- Successful work with climate distress requires the therapist to deeply process their own role in and reactions to the climate crisis.

- Climate psychotherapy can be organized under the three pillars of reckoning with reality, containment, and transformation.
- The model of posttraumatic growth is particularly applicable for moving from climate-related trauma and distress to transformation.
- Therapeutic techniques for climate distress often involve creating and working with unknowability and liminality to promote change.
- Group processes may be particularly helpful for climate distress and have been developed in the lay setting.
- Existing therapies, including acceptance and commitment therapy, motivational interviewing, and nature therapies, may be useful for climate distress work.

References

Aragunde-Kohl U, Gómez-Galán J, Lázaro-Pérez C, et al: Interaction and emotional connection with pets: a descriptive analysis from Puerto Rico. Animals (Basel) 10(11):2136, 2020 33212986

Baudon P: A scoping review of interventions for the treatment of eco-anxiety. In Analysis 5(1):82–85, 2021

Bendell J: Deep adaptation: a map for navigating climate tragedy. Institute for Leadership and Sustainability (IFLAS) Occasional Papers Vol 2. Ambleside, UK, University of Cumbria, 2018. Available at: http://insight.cumbria.ac.uk/id/eprint/4166/1/Bendell_DeepAdaptation.pdf. Accessed December 1, 2024.

Bendell J: Hope and vision in the face of collapse: the 4th R of deep adaptation. Prof Jem Bendell blog, January 9, 2019. Available at: https://jembendell.com/2019/01/09/hope-and-vision-in-the-face-of-collapse-the-4th-r-of-deep-adaptation. Accessed December 1, 2024.

Bethelmy LC, Corraliza JA: Transcendence and sublime experience in nature: awe and inspiring energy. Front Psychol 10:509, 2019 30918493

Bion WR: The psycho-analytic study of thinking: a theory of thinking. Int J Psychoanal 43:306–310, 1962 13968380

Bion WR: Notes on memory and desire. Psychoanal Forum 2:272–278, 1967

Budziszewska M, Jonsson SE: Talking about climate change and eco-anxiety in psychotherapy: a qualitative analysis of patients' experiences. Psychotherapy (Chic) 59(4):606–615, 2022 35758982

Cianconi P, Hanife B, Grillo F, et al: Eco-emotions and psychoterratic syndromes: reshaping mental health assessment under climate change. Yale J Biol Med 96(2):211–226, 2023 37396973

Psychotherapy Considerations and Approaches

Cork S, Alexandra C, Alvarez-Romero JG, et al: Exploring alternative futures in the Anthropocene. Annu Rev Environ Resour 48:25–54, 2023

Doppelt B: Transformational Resilience: How Building Human Resilience to Climate Disruption Can Safeguard Society and Increase Wellbeing. Abingdon, UK, Routledge, 2017

Gandy S, Forstmann M, Carhart-Harris RL, et al: The potential synergistic effects between psychedelic administration and nature contact for the improvement of mental health. Health Psychol Open 7(2):2055102920978123, 2020 33335742

Gilbert DT, Wilson TD: Prospection: experiencing the future. Science 317(5843):1351–1354, 2007 17823345

Graugaard J: Perspectives from creative spaces: transforming climate distress through creative practice and re-storying, in Climate Change and Youth Mental Health: Multidisciplinary Perspectives. Edited by Haase E, Hudson K. Cambridge, UK, Cambridge University Press, 2024, pp 367–384

Haase E, Hudson K: Climate Change and Youth Mental Health: Multidisciplinary Perspectives. Cambridge, UK, Cambridge University Press, 2024

Hathaway MD: Activating hope in the midst of crisis: emotions, transformative learning, and "the Work That Reconnects." J Transform Educ 15(4):296–314, 2017

Henson C, Truchot D, Canevello A: What promotes post traumatic growth? A systematic review. Eur J Trauma Dissociation 5:100195, 2021

Hofmann C: Being at home with oneself in the whole—Hegel's philosophy of freedom as actuality, in Concepts of Normality: Kant or Hegel? (Critical Studies in German Idealism Series, Vol 24). Edited by Krijnen C. Leiden, The Netherlands, Brill, 2019, pp 9–25

Holmes EA, Matthews A: Mental imagery in emotion and emotional disorders. Clin Psychol Rev 30(3): 349–362, 2010 20116915

Horst R, Gladwin D: Multiple futures literacies: an interdisciplinary review. Journal of Curriculum and Pedagogy 21(1):42–64, 2022

Hudgins K, Durost SW: Experiential Therapy From Trauma to Post-traumatic Growth: Therapeutic Spiral Model Psychodrama. Singapore, Springer, 2022

Inayatullah S: Six pillars: futures thinking for transforming. Foresight 10(1):4–21, 2008

Jacobson KC, Chang L: Associations between pet ownership and attitudes toward pets with youth socioemotional outcomes. Front Psychol 9:2304, 2018 30534102

Janusz B, Walkiewicz M: The rites of passage framework as a matrix of transgression processes in the life course. J Adult Dev 25(3):151–159, 2018 30174383

Kals E, Schumacher D, Montada L: Emotional affinity toward nature as a motivational basis to protect nature. Environ Behav 31:178–202, 1999

Kaplan Y, Levounis P (eds): Nature Therapy. Washington, DC, American Psychiatric Association Publishing, 2025

Kassouf S: Thinking catastrophic thoughts: a traumatized sensibility on a hotter planet. Am J Psychoanal 82(1):60–79, 2022 35165366

Katz R: Synergy and empowerment: renewing and expanding the community's healing resources, in Synergy, Healing, and Empowerment: Insights From Cultural Diversity. Edited by Katz R, Murphy-Shigematsu S. Calgary, AB, Canada, Brush Education, 2012, pp 21–48

Kellert SR, Wilson EO (eds): The Biophilia Hypothesis. Washington, DC, Island Press, 1993

Lear J: Radical Hope: Ethics in the Face of Cultural Devastation. Cambridge, MA, Harvard University Press, 2006

Levounis P, Arnaout B, Marienfeld C (eds): Motivational Interviewing for Clinical Practice. Arlington, VA, American Psychiatric Association Publishing, 2017

Lewis JL: Personal communication, February 2024

Lewis JL, Haase E, Trope A: Climate dialectics in psychotherapy: holding open the space between abyss and advance. Psychodyn Psychiatry 48(3):271–294, 2020 32996850

Mark B: The power of language: here's how nature metaphors can help process feelings about climate change. Psychology Today, August 9, 2023. Available at: www.psychologytoday.com/intl/blog/psychiatrys-think-tank/202308/the-power-of-language. Accessed December 1, 2024.

Martinez Acobi A: The Emergent Container in Psychoanalysis: Experiencing Absence and Future. Abingdon, UK, Routledge, 2023

McCune S, Kruger KA, Griffin JA, et al: Evolution of research into the mutual benefits of human-animal interaction. Anim Front 4(3):49–58, 2014

Milstein T: The performer metaphor: "Mother Nature never gives us the same show twice." Environ Commun 10(2):227–248, 2016

Modell A: Metaphor—the bridge between feelings and knowledge. Psychoanal Inq 29(1):6–11, 2009

Morton A: Listening to Whales: What the Orcas Have Taught Us. New York, Ballantine Books, 2002

Myers OE Jr, Saunders CD: Animals as links toward developing caring relationships with the natural world, in Children and Nature. Edited by Kahn PH, Kellert SR. Cambridge, MA, MIT Press, 2002, pp 153–178

Nisbet EK, Zelenski JM, Murphy SA: The Nature Relatedness Scale: linking individuals' connection with nature to environmental concern and behavior. Environ Behav 41(5):715–740, 2009

Ojala M, Chen X: Coping with climate change among young people: meaning-focused coping and constructive hope, in Climate Change and Youth Mental Health: Multidisciplinary Perspectives. Edited by Haase E, Hudson K. Cambridge, UK, Cambridge University Press, 2024, pp 269–286

Psychotherapy Considerations and Approaches

Pew Research Center: Survey of U.S. adults, April 10–16, 2023. Available at: www.pewresearch.org/short-reads/2023/07/07/about-half-us-of-pet-owners-say-their-pets-are-as-much-a-part-of-their-family-as-a-human-member. Accessed December 1, 2024.

Randall R: Loss and climate change: the cost of parallel narratives. Ecopsychology 1(3):118–129, 2009

Ray B: Remaking rites of passage to change your mindset—and your life. Better Humans, September 25, 2023. Available at: https://betterhumans.pub/remaking-rites-of-passage-to-change-your-mindset-and-your-life-7c4923edd3a. Accessed December 1, 2024.

Rodríguez Arce JM, Winkelman MJ: Psychedelics, sociality, and human evolution. Front Psychol 12:729425, 2021 34659037

Rust M-J: Towards an Ecopsychotherapy. London, Confer Books, 2020

Scoresby KJ, Strand EB, Ng Z, et al: Pet ownership and quality of life: a systematic review of the literature. Vet Sci 8(12):332, 2021 34941859

Seaman EB: Climate change on the therapist's couch: how mental health clinicians receive and respond to indirect psychological impacts of climate change in the therapeutic setting. Master's thesis, Northampton, MA, Smith College, 2016. Available at: https://scholarworks.smith.edu/theses/1736. Accessed December 1, 2024.

Solnit R: Hope in the Dark: Untold Histories, Wild Possibilities. New York, Nation Books, 2004

Spattini L, Mattei G, Raisi F, et al: Efficacy of animal assisted therapy on people with mental disorders: an update on the evidence. Minerva Psichiatrica 59(1):54–66, 2018

Steiner J: Psychic Retreats. London, Routledge, 2003

Tedeschi RG, Calhoun LG: Posttraumatic growth: conceptual foundations and empirical evidence. Psychol Inq 15(1):1–18, 2004

Tedeschi RG, Cann A, Taku K, et al: The Posttraumatic Growth Inventory: a revision integrating existential and spiritual change. J Trauma Stress 30(1):11–18, 2017 28099764

Thomas T, Aggar C, Baker J, et al: Social prescribing of nature therapy for adults with mental illness living in the community: a scoping review of peer-reviewed international evidence. Front Psychol 13:1041675, 2022 36562055

Tillich P: The Courage to Be. New Haven, CT, Yale University Press, 1952

Tu HM: Effect of horticultural therapy on mental health: a meta-analysis of randomized controlled trials. J Psychiatr Ment Health Nurs 29(4):603–615, 2022 35000249

Turner VW: Betwixt and between: the liminal period in rites de passage, in The Forest of Symbols. Ithaca, NY, Cornell University Press, 1967, pp 93–111

van Gennep A: The Rites of Passage. Chicago, IL, University of Chicago, 1960

Verhagen FC: Worldviews and metaphors in the human-nature relationship. Language and Ecology 2(3):1–19, 2008

Vining J: The connection to other animals and caring for nature. Hum Ecol Rev 10:87–99, 2003

Wen Y, Yan Q, Pan Y, et al: Medical empirical research on forest bathing (Shinrin-yoku): a systematic review. Environ Health Prev Med 24(1):70, 2019 31787069

Wendt DC, Huson K, Albatnuni M, et al: What are the best practices for psychotherapy with indigenous peoples in the United States and Canada? A thorny question. J Consult Clin Psychol 90(10):802–814, 2022 36190756

White MP, Hartig T, Martin L, et al: Nature-based biopsychosocial resilience: an integrative theoretical framework for research on nature and health. Environ Int 181:108234, 2023 37832260

Winnicott DW: Primitive emotional development. Int J Psychoanal 26:137–153, 1945

Xu Y, Ramanathan V: Well below 2°C: mitigation strategies for avoiding dangerous to catastrophic climate changes. Proc Natl Acad Sci USA 114(39):10315–10323, 2017 28912354

PART IV

Community, Institutional, and Global Psychiatry for Climate Change

13

Coordinating the Climate Psychiatry Response

Global, Institutional, Educational, and Research Agendas

Overview of Global Climate Mental Health

Existing studies suggest that about 60% of the U.S. population is already moderately to extremely anxious about climate change (American Psychiatric Association 2020; Leiserowitz et al. 2023). Studies of natural disasters, one of the most easily delineated climate effects to study, have shown cumulative rates of mental disorders around 40% (with a wide range and higher in some studies). Research on population-level psychiatric needs in response to specific climate effects is limited (reviewed in Corvetto et al. 2023), but one study found that sea level rise combined with intermittent storm surges in two counties of Florida alone could increase the number of people with a psychiatric disorder by about 4.2 million—almost 100% of the population, by dint of the cumulative effects of multiple disaster traumas and their associated rates of psychiatric disorders (Monsour et al. 2022). In an unpublished study of the kinds of compound disasters that are increasing with climate change, a county that had three disasters in 3 years had a surge in case management needs of 700% and an increase in mental health line calls of 400% from the second disaster alone (Bernstein 2021). These findings suggest that mental health needs related to climate change will significantly exceed current institutional capacity.

Large programmatic responses will be required of psychiatric education, research, and global mental health organizations to address this need. Mental health institutions and their leaders will have to plan for increases in service needs that are difficult to imagine in advance, investigate new phenomena and treatments, educate trainees on evolving climate impacts, and bring their institutions into alignment with national and international climate emissions policies. They face vexing hurdles. Trillions of dollars have been allocated toward climate resilience, including all aspects of infrastructure, food security, technological development, health, and disaster and community planning, yet, remarkably, without allocating any funds specifically to address climate mental health impacts, let alone the psychological adjustments to such rapid social developments.

Institutional leaders must also face a central conceptual uncertainty: whether climate change will create new and unique psychiatric and psychological problems that require novel forms of treatment and service delivery, or whether climate mental health concerns can be handled by expanding existing mental health treatment practices and service-delivery structures. Most climate-aware mental health professionals exploring these questions feel that the scale of climate impacts, as well as the heavily unjust distribution of impacts in disadvantaged and marginalized groups, will require fundamental shifts in the approach to mental health care delivery, particularly given the global scarcity of services. The core elements of this shift are thought to be the following:

- Increased role of public and global health in mental health care
- Transition to population-level delivery of care in the community
- Change to embedding mental health services in other climate adaptation programs
- Increased coordination of interventions with outside agencies and lay organizations
- Change of institutional practice to meet health care sustainability targets

Coordinating the Climate Psychiatry Response **283**

- Alignment of research with this agenda
- Education and socialization of psychiatrists and psychiatric trainees into these new climate-informed ways of delivering care

Considerations for how organized psychiatry can make these transitions are explored throughout the remainder of this chapter.

Governmental Climate Mental Health Advancement Around the Globe

As a first step in responding to climate health and mental health service preparation, countries need to assess their climate health vulnerabilities and designate an agency for the response. As of 2021, about half of all countries had made this general climate health assessment, and most of these had established a climate health department and process for engaging stakeholders in it. A range of specific climate health efforts are underway globally, as detailed in Ansah et al. (2024). Mental health, however, has been grossly neglected and is included in the climate health plans of only 19% of those countries that have begun preparations (World Health Organization 2021). In the United States, efforts to establish climate mental health plans have been hampered by the complete absence of funding for mental health support in the Inflation Reduction Act, the lack of environmental or climate mental health funding in the Strategic Plan for 2023–2026 of the Substance Abuse and Mental Health Services Administration, and similar funding issues at the Office of Climate Change and Health Equity and other agencies, as well as hostility toward such efforts in the two Trump administrations. Putting mental health on the map and in the minds of stakeholders planning comprehensive climate responses is a critical need and has recently been recognized as such by the World Health Organization (2022). The Community Mental Wellness and Resilience Act and the Green New Deal for Health Act are hard-won legislative efforts that were awaiting committee action in the U.S. Congress at the end of 2024.

Vignette

Dr. P, a psychiatrist attending a United Nations Conference of the Parties (COP) meeting, became concerned that the cultural and behavioral pressures on women were not being addressed in a climate resilience platform that included water management. She was able to network with global psychiatry leaders through the Connecting Climate Minds (CCM) research collaborative and implement a small study showing alcohol use and domestic violence increases in response to the initiative. Her work led to more sensitivity to emotional pressures on women and integration of an integrative community therapy (ICT) (Sabina et al. 2023) component into the COP climate resilience platform with follow-up study by the CCM group she had energized showing ICT benefit.

Transitioning to Population-Level Care Based in Community Institutions

Country-level climate mental health programs will need to decentralize the mental health response away from traditional treatment models and toward community-wide interventions to respond adequately to the scale and pervasiveness of climate-related distress. Governments can support community-based efforts by providing psychoeducational tools to label the experiences people are having and teach them how to cope. Resilience programs labeling climate mental health impacts and how to grow from them will be important and can be distributed through internet-based platforms and public health campaigns as well as in educational and civic settings. Governments can also develop hubs to network community organizations with each other and link them to mental health services, training peer supports, and lay mutual help groups. Psychiatrists and other mental health professionals can serve as liaisons in these efforts and be available as consultants should more serious needs arise.

There is an inherent tension in moving the source and structure of authority for promoting mental health to nonprofessionals and their communities, who know best how to care for themselves, and away from existing mental health institutions and their well-earned treatment expertise. Community organizational structures tend to follow the model of organic organizations, which are less formal, less standardized, more flexible, more creative, and integrated into their culture, but they can be subject to role confusion, overwhelm, disorientation, a lack of mentoring, and failure of continuity planning. More formal psychiatric treatment structures typically operate in a more mechanistic organizational model, excelling at role clarity, stability, and productivity, but

Coordinating the Climate Psychiatry Response

at the risk of being inflexible and having too long a chain of command to respond to evolving needs.

Communities are most likely to experience climate distress in response to environmental crises in food and water availability, community traumas such as fires or flooding, and increased strain on first-responder systems. Community institutions are more likely than outside professionals to be able to empathize with and respond to the emotional needs of their members in response to these local conditions and to provide the first point of access to mental health support before entry into formal psychiatric and psychological care. Participation in community institutions is also by its nature empowering and promotes the resilience of those undergoing these strains. It may have sustainability and psychotherapeutic co-benefits if their activities involve food systems, animals, or the outdoors. Working with community groups to identify their strengths and needs and how mental health care can emerge from and be provided within this lived experience will be a critical part of scaling up the climate mental health response.

Remaining flexibly within this institutional authority–community decentralization dialectic can be promoted through coproduction of services. The concept of coproduction refers to the design of mental health plans through shared and equitable contributions from service users, providers, and professionals. It is thought to be more contextually specific, generate greater total engagement, promote creativity and collaboration, and bridge the translational gap between academic knowledge and real-world implementation (Hanlon et al. 2023). Coproduction and the related methods of peer support, mutual help groups, and other forms of paraprofessional mental health activity have all been shown to have significant benefits, such as the following (Durlak 1979):

- Improved quality of care overall, including symptom improvement, medication adherence, sobriety, and control of automatic thoughts
- Subjective benefits of feeling cared for, identity and life narrative clarification, and spiritual benefit
- Improved everyday living skills, job retention, and relationships and reduced delinquency

It must also be noted, however, that meta-analyses have revealed bias and neutral or mixed results in a few of thousands of positive outcome studies for community interventions meeting optimal research criteria, particularly in terms of specific improvements in the symptoms of mental illness (Baskin et al. 2021; Grant et al. 2018; Pistrang et al. 2008; White et al. 2020). An important role for psychiatrists will be to monitor and research whether national and international interventions for nonclinical climate-related distress are meeting their target goals and adequately identifying people with more severe psychiatric symptoms who may need professional care.

Structuring National and Global Responses to Climate Mental Health Needs

Many practical questions remain about how to set up national and global structures to provide broad, cost-effective, and accessible mental health support, whether through professional or community distribution networks. U.S. psychiatry, for example, could organize its response through the district branches of the American Psychiatric Association, the National Institute of Mental Health, and/or the Substance Abuse and Mental Health Services Administration. Each of these organizations has particular advantages in terms of the likelihood of continuity, local relevance, and engagement without participant burnout. In the absence of governmental support, most climate mental health work has been conducted by self-organized professional groups listed in the Appendix. These groups collaborate with each other to contribute to climate-aware therapist trainings, educational presentations, media communications, lobbying and policy development, legal testimony, and other efforts.

Under the auspices of the Race to Resilience and the United Nations Framework Convention on Climate Change (UNFCCC) Sharm-El-Sheikh Adaptation Agenda of COP27, there is now a first global initiative to provide a worldwide platform for groups allied around reducing climate distress. The initiative, Care of People and Planet (COP²), aims to grow capacity for community-wide psychological resilience in 4 billion people. COP² embodies the ideal of a flexible network of local organizations supported by institutional expertise. It is organized into five regional hubs, one for each involved continent, that aim to produce road maps and shareable resilience tools for broad distribution within UNFCCC and other climate adaptation initiatives. Hubs support tools that are organized as follows:

Coordinating the Climate Psychiatry Response

- Care—skills for bolstering mental strengths and alleviating distress
- Change—transformational skills that underpin participatory climate action

The model for scaling the delivery of those tools is based on the following:

- Anchors—expert organizations that provide content and skills training, planning, distribution and implementation, measuring, and formal care if needed
- Paths—content channels such as social media, trusted groups, and places of support and learning such as churches and schools

The COP[2] initiative presented its first road map at COP28 in Dubai and launched several Race to Resilience Early Adopter initiatives, including programs for peer-to-peer counseling in slums and informal settlements, and an insurance conglomerate effort to place a value on climate emotional distress and its associated monetary costs (Belkin 2023).

The Climate Mental Health Research Agenda

The climate research agenda supporting such a large global effort will require a full spectrum of studies, including investigation of the social and psychological aspects of climate distress, its effects on psychiatric epidemiology, the effectiveness of new global initiatives and treatments to address it, and the more formal neurobiology of climate change for the brain. The CCM initiative is based at Imperial College London and is building a global network of researchers to collaborate on these issues, negotiate financial support, and develop a research agenda. A suggested climate research agenda (Haase 2021) is summarized in the following lists, organized by category.

Neurobiology

- Heat impacts on the brain
- Central and peripheral neurobiology of thermoregulation in patients with mental illness

- Heat-related effects on transport, storage, and individual metabolism of medications
- Brain impacts of particulate matter and other greenhouse gases for all age groups
- Impact of climate-related nutritional shifts on brain disorders
- Neurobiology of new infectious diseases

Epidemiology

- Emergent patterns in psychiatric epidemiology, environmental toxicology, and infectious and nutritional illness
- Definition and measurement of the prevalence and symptoms of new psychological states associated with planetary decline (eco-anxiety, solastalgia, psychology of social collapse), with particular attention to cross-cultural differences
- Outcome differences between single, compound, and prolonged natural disasters
- DSM modification to reflect emergent states

Psychology and Sociology

- Differentiation of normal from functionally impairing climate distress
- Clarifying impacts of factors such as race, culture, age, and sex/gender on climate distress
- Application of existing distress and trauma models to understanding climate distress (e.g., is it better conceived as a form of bereavement, attachment difficulty, continuous traumatic stress, PTSD or pretraumatic stress disorder, or existential or spiritual problem?)
- Identifying preexisting psychological vulnerabilities that worsen climate adaptation
- Understanding the interactions between climate change, social determinants of health, and mental health outcomes
- Understanding the psychological trajectories of those who are forced to become climate migrants or experience climate-related human rights violations at the hands of others
- Understanding the psychology and trajectory of voluntary climate migration

Coordinating the Climate Psychiatry Response

- Understanding the impacts of disinformation, fearmongering, politics, coping styles, and group and individual identities on climate adaptation
- Studying climate impacts on life trajectory and adult developmental pathways

Treatment

- Testing the efficacy of techniques for therapeutic management of negative affect states; existential threats on distress reduction; and negative outcomes such as isolation, burnout, and suicidality
- Testing the large-scale deployment of psychological change strategies, positive psychology, and related work to climate adaptation
- Testing climate-related interventions in populations with mental illness
- Testing population modes of treatment delivery in terms of the following:

  - Means (internet vs. in person; lay, peer, or professional)
  - Circumstances (in the field, acute vs. delayed)
  - Adaptability to change (inclusion and effectiveness of techniques to modify treatments to the setting and population)
  - Scalability, including across cultures

- Evaluating nature-based treatments, social prescribing, and other sustainable and nature-based interventions compared with traditional treatment delivery
- Defining and measuring community resilience in response to treatments
- Evaluating the equity of treatment and resource distribution
- Evaluating the outcomes of climate mitigation practices (e.g., development of green spaces, coal plant closures, increased active transport) on health and mental health

Service Delivery

- Predicting the scale of need on the basis of large datasets for heat and other impacts
- Testing the efficacy of curricular and other educational measures to improve provider responsiveness to climate impacts

- Measuring the impact of climate exposures on emergency, hospital, and outpatient visits
- Measuring the relationship between specific climate exposures and subsequent psychiatric presentations
- Studying the impact of psychiatric sustainability practices on greenhouse gas emissions and patient outcomes

Climate change is thus making significant demands on psychiatric services and research priorities. The scale of what is needed can be balanced at the institutional level by the groundswell of layperson activity and psychiatric activism that has paved the way for a large institutional response. For the researcher accustomed to working carefully toward the highest standards of evidence, the qualities of rapidity, uncertainty, scale, and global diversity of climate effects may benefit from a different idea of excellence than has been traditional in the past century: a more emergency mindset that is creative and willing to take risks. Asking the questions "What is important to do now?" and "What will the impact of this be in 10 years?" may direct projects at the institutional and research levels that are meaningful and responsive to evolving conditions.

Climate Mental Health and Psychiatric Education

Organizations providing medical and psychiatric education have a responsibility to teach trainees about the health and mental health effects of the climate crisis as the health challenge of this century (Lancet 2024; Wortzel et al. 2022a). Recognizing this, Columbia University's Mailman School of Public Health established the Global Consortium on Climate and Health Education, and George Mason University Center for Climate Change Communication established the Medical Society Consortium on Climate and Health. These serve as repositories of educational material, including recorded lectures, slideshows, and case studies. The National Institute of Environmental Health Sciences also has a Climate Change and Human Health Literature Portal, a curated database of peer-reviewed research and gray papers. These sites host numerous educational resources on climate change and mental health. In 2022, the journal *Academic Psychiatry* devoted an issue to climate mental health education, highlighting that climate mental health impacts were being taught in only 13% of psychiatric training programs (Wortzel et al. 2022b) and exploring obstacles to this education (Seritan et al. 2022). These obstacles include the following:

- A lack of expert teachers in the field
- Insufficient space in the curriculum
- A lack of agreed-on competencies
- A lack of means to evaluate learning (e.g., on board exams)
- Postulated defensive resistance to engaging with this topic

The special issue also provides a case-based teaching module (Haase 2022) and suggestions for overcoming curricular space constraints and lack of experts by offering material about climate effects for established lectures (e.g., adding heat effects to a lecture on aggression), which has the co-benefit of increasing teachers' learning (Cooper and Li 2022). Further work is underway to validate a 1-hour climate mental health curriculum and establish test questions for trainees and postgraduate psychiatrists through the American Board of Psychiatry and Neurology. Teaching equity awareness (Kaslow et al. 2021) is essential to ensure trainees can adequately address climate injustice.

Key Points

- Global and institutional responses are essential to climate mental health and must encompass programmatic responses by international, governmental, educational, professional, and scientific organizations.
- New models of treatment and institutional organization are required to address the global scale of climate-related mental distress, emphasizing flexibility, innovation, community-wide programming, and lay involvement.
- The gross under-recognition and underfunding of climate mental health require urgent redress.
- Psychiatrists bear the responsibility of educating future mental health care providers to address the climate mental health impacts of the coming century.

References

American Psychiatric Association: APA public opinion poll—annual meeting 2020. Washington, DC, American Psychiatric Association, September

2020. Available at: www.psychiatry.org/newsroom/apa-public-opinion-poll-2020. Accessed November 4, 2023.

Ansah EW, Amoadu M, Obeng P, et al: Health systems response to climate change adaptation: a scoping review of global evidence. BMC Public Health 24(1):2015–2023, 2024 39075368

Baskin C, Zijlstra G, McGrath M, et al: Community-centred interventions for improving public mental health among adults from ethnic minority populations in the UK: a scoping review. BMJ Open 11:e041102, 2021

Belkin G: Roadmap for care and change. COP2, December 2023. Available at: www.cop2.org/roadmap. Accessed November 23, 2024.

Bernstein D: Unpublished data, December 2021

Cooper R, Li D: Preclinical curricular changes to address sustainable healthcare education in psychiatry. Acad Psychiatry 46(5):582–583, 2022 35486366

Corvetto JF, Helou AY, Dambach P, et al: A systematic literature review of the impact of climate change on the global demand for psychiatric services. Int J Environ Res Public Health 20(2):1190, 2023 36673946

Durlak JA: Comparative effectiveness of paraprofessional and professional helpers. Psychol Bull 86(1):80–92, 1979 377356

Grant KL, Simmons MB, Davey CG: Three nontraditional approaches to improving the capacity, accessibility, and quality of mental health services: an overview. Psychiatr Serv 69(5):508–516, 2018 29334876

Haase E: Climate change and mental health: research gaps and priorities. Presentation to the American Psychiatric Association, Atlanta, GA, 2021

Haase E: Using case-based teaching of climate change to broaden appreciation of socio-environmental determinants of mental health. Acad Psychiatry 46(5):574–578, 2022 36109425

Hanlon CA, McIlroy D, Poole H, et al: Evaluating the role and effectiveness of co-produced community-based mental health interventions that aim to reduce suicide among adults: a systematic review. Health Expect 26(1):64–86, 2023 36377305

Kaslow NJ, Schwartz AC, Ayna DK, et al: Integrating diversity, equity, and inclusion into an academic department of psychiatry and behavioral sciences. Focus Am Psychiatr Publ 19(1):61–65, 2021 34483770

Lancet: The Lancet Countdown on health and climate change. London, Lancet, 2024. Available at: www.thelancet.com/countdown-health-climate. Accessed November 23, 2024.

Leiserowitz A, Maibach E, Rosenthal S, et al: Climate Change in the American Mind: Beliefs and Attitudes, Fall 2023. New Haven, CT, Yale Program on Climate Change Communication, 2023

Monsour M, Clarke-Rubright E, Lieberman-Cribbin W, et al: The impact of climate change on the prevalence of mental illness symptoms. J Affect Disord 300:430–440, 2022 34986372

Pistrang N, Barker C, Humphreys K: Mutual help groups for mental health problems: a review of effectiveness studies. Am J Community Psychol 42(1–2):110–121, 2008 18679792

Sabina C, Perez-Figueroa D, Reyes L, et al: Evaluation of integrative community therapy with domestic violence survivors in Quito, Ecuador. Int J Environ Res Public Health 20(8):5492, 2023 37107774

Seritan AL, Coverdale J, Brenner AM: Climate change and mental health curricula: addressing barriers to teaching. Acad Psychiatry 46(5):551–555, 2022 35314961

White S, Foster R, Marks J, et al: The effectiveness of one-to-one peer support in mental health services: a systematic review and meta-analysis. BMC Psychiatry 20(1):534, 2020 33176729

World Health Organization: WHO Health and Climate Change Global Survey Report. Geneva, Switzerland, World Health Organization, 2021

World Health Organization: Mental Health and Climate Change: Policy Brief. Geneva, Switzerland, World Health Organization, 2022. Available at: https://iris.who.int/bitstream/handle/10665/354104/9789240045125-eng. pdf?sequence=1. Accessed November 5, 2023.

Wortzel JR, Guerrero APS, Aggarwal R, et al: Climate change and the professional obligation to socialize physicians and trainees into an environmentally sustainable medical culture. Acad Psychiatry 46(5):556–561, 2022a 35879599

Wortzel JR, Haase E, Mark B, et al: Teaching to our time: a survey study of current opinions and didactics about climate mental health training in US psychiatry residency and fellowship programs. Acad Psychiatry 46(5):586–587, 2022b 35804189

14

Community Psychiatry and Its Role in Climate Mitigation and Adaptation

Role of the Community Psychiatrist in the Climate Mental Health Response

Like disaster psychiatrists, community psychiatrists will be at the forefront of climate-related mental health impacts in the United States and around the world. Their importance in mitigating and helping their populations adapt to these impacts will be related to their particular expertise and public roles in the following areas:

- Understanding and planning system responses to community-wide mental health issues
- Supporting disadvantaged populations, who bear a vastly increased burden of climate change on their health and mental health
- Supporting and advocating for people with severe mental illness, who carry greater mental health risks from high temperatures and other climate factors

- Ensuring that substance use outcomes, which are worsened by heat and other climate impacts, are not omitted from planning
- Implementing community-based group psychological support to build mental resilience
- Planning for and executing needed shifts in psychiatric service delivery, where service demands and changing circumstances will favor group and public health interventions over individual treatment

Overlapping Values of Community Mental Health and Climate Responsiveness

Community psychiatry is grounded in ethical pillars and competencies that overlap with the approach and tools necessary to support climate-related mental health (Sullenbarger et al. 2022). The shared concerns of climate responsiveness and community psychiatry that can be brought to bear on the climate situation include the following:

- An interest in empowering individuals and communities to take ownership of outcomes and recovery
- An interest in communal goals of prevention, population health, and universal benefits
- An emphasis on being nimble, flexible, and practical rather than adhering to elite practice principles and treatment frames
- A focus on collaboration rather than hierarchy
- Strategies for recovery-focused care that reduce social stress and strife, including promoting hope, community, respect, cultural integrity, diversity, and forgiveness
- A basis in efficient, standardized, comprehensive integrated system management, essential for the multisystemic interdependent nature of climate effects and recovery
- An emphasis on diversity, equity, and inclusion and on social justice and advocacy work with marginalized populations, including those with chronic and severe mental illness
- An understanding of the role of individual and community trauma and social determinants of health in all outcomes
- An understanding of the psychiatrist's role that focuses on collaboration with communities and institutions and on policy and public health actions

Community Psychiatry

297

Table 14.1 Agenda for the community psychiatry response to the climate crisis

Educate behavioral health stakeholders about climate impacts on emotional and psychiatric health

Engage communities in mitigating climate effects, including effects on mental illness and well-being

Incorporate climate-protective measures in clinical and clinic practice, including system-wide protections for patients and measures that lower the clinic's carbon footprint

Protect people with mental illness from neglect and stigma in climate efforts

Advocate for sustainable, resilient health and community systems and policies at the state, national, and international levels

---

- A familiarity with working in complex environments requiring evolving and imperfect solutions

All of these skills prepare the community psychiatrist with the optimal mindset for dealing with the evolving and complex impacts of climate change on communities and mental health across the globe, as well as the ability to implement strategies for the three pillars of the climate response: mitigation, adaptation, and resilience. Already accustomed to systems work and their public health role, community psychiatrists are likely to work even more in these domains as climate effects deepen. The agenda that can be set for this work is shown in Table 14.1.

Tasks of the Community Climate Psychiatrist

Community Psychiatry Climate Advocacy

The core values of community psychiatry, including recovery, population health, prevention, and collaboration, align well with the advocacy goals of climate action to recover planetary health and prevent further harm by living in a more collaborative way with nature. The focus on person-centered care in community psychiatry also emphasizes the ethical value of individual lives, regardless of stature, that must underlie climate justice efforts to adequately compensate and care for groups disproportionately affected by climate harm. The American Association for Community Psychiatry strategic plan specifically includes advocacy work to "influence health and social policies...guided by principles of social justice." Skills and areas for climate activism are covered in more detail in Chapter 3, "Psychiatric Ethics, Climate Justice, and Climate Advocacy and Activism," with a list of climate mental health groups involved in advocacy available in the Appendix.

Preparing for Climate-Related Community Mental Health Needs at the Planning and Policy Level

Climate change poses threats to mental health service delivery because of the magnitude of traumatic distress when whole communities are affected (Augustinavicius et al. 2021). Assessing and making a plan for the impact of climate change on the mental health needs of the community and its community psychiatric clinic is thus one of the most valuable ways community psychiatrists can participate in climate action. Climate adaptation planning includes four steps (Figure 14.1):

- Awareness
- Assessment
- Planning
- Implementation, monitoring, evaluation, and readjustment

These steps of adaptation planning are conducted in a reiterative way to continually reassess and improve outcomes. The scope of these steps includes the following:

- Objective measures of community well-being, such as green space, services, schools, air quality, and other assets
- Objective measures of individual well-being, such as health, income, and social capital
- Subjective community and individual well-being (satisfaction with and perceived quality of the objective elements by community stakeholders)
- Capacity to withstand and recover from climate stressors such as extreme weather, heat-related infrastructure demands, and so on

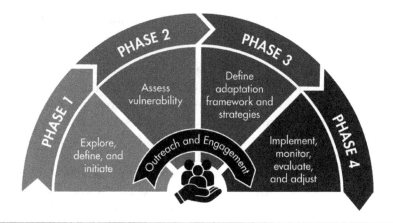

Figure 14.1 Stages of climate adaptation planning.

Source. Reprinted from California Adaptation Planning Guide. Sacramento, California Governor's Office of Emergency Services, 2020. Available at: https://resilientca.org/apg. Used with permission.

Accurate data about local risks are essential for a strong adaptation plan. Numerous tools have been developed to assess such climate risks to communities at the county or district level. These include the following:

- The National Risk Index in the United States
- Climate and disaster risk screening tools provided internationally by the U.S. Agency for International Development, World Health Organization (WHO), and World Bank, among others
- The WHO checklist for climate-related vulnerability for health care facilities (World Health Organization 2021)

These powerful tools integrate large datasets from weather, census, economic, and other monitoring sources. They provide the capacity to evaluate a district or community for each of 18 or more natural hazards. Additionally, they provide discrete scores for social vulnerability, health institution vulnerability, and community resilience based on assessments of the economic, infrastructure, sociodemographic, and health-related weaknesses and strengths of a particular region or facility, which can be used to plan improvements to infrastructure and community systems affected by climate change.

Risk assessment tools can be the beginning step of a community mental health needs assessment. Mental health facilities can take the following risk-mitigating actions in response to the climate threats that are identified:

- Setting up surveillance for and chains of communication to alert patients and community members during climate risk events such as heat waves, wildfire smoke, tornadoes, and flooding
- Training and coordinating with local first responders regarding special emergency needs and likely behaviors of people with mental illness in these situations
- Preparing evacuation plans that are responsive to the limited capacities of patients with severe mental disorders for negotiating transportation and other needs in complex and fearsome circumstances
- Planning for continued access to supplies and medications in the event of restricted supply chains and disaster-related availability
- Ensuring that clinic and hospital infrastructure, particularly including information technology, has a backup system for maintaining function

A core part of such planning for climate-related emergencies includes asset mapping. Asset mapping is the practice of taking an inventory of the strengths and resources of a community and mapping their locations. This process helps to highlight potential solutions to threats and promotes community involvement, ownership, and empowerment in responses to climate threats. An asset is often thought of as an entity, but it can also include the strengths and abilities of the community and its members. Community assets that should be mapped in this process include the following:

- Physical structures with group potential such as churches, libraries, and recreation centers
- Private, public, and nonprofit organizations
- Social service agencies
- Disaster response agencies
- Government and military agencies
- Providers of food (grocery stores and restaurants), medications (pharmacies), and other basics (gas, essential goods)
- Natural assets, including water, food, and geographical advantages
- Spaces with resilience co-benefits, such as green and blue spaces, and community hubs
- The strength and abilities of the community and its members

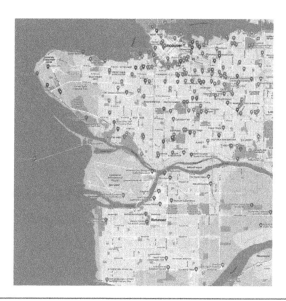

Figure 14.2 Example of an asset map.

This asset map focuses on community gardens and orchards, seed libraries, and other garden programs. Asset maps can be broad or narrow in the scope of institutions they identify.

Source. Used with permission from Vancouver Food Bank.

Examples of a community asset map and its use are provided in Figure 14.2 and the following vignette.

Vignette

Smithville is a town of 100,000 residents that is prone to fires in the summer and flash floods during the rainy season. Over a 2-year span, a flood downed power lines and wiped out the supplies of insulin and long-acting injectable antipsychotics for half the town's pharmacies, and a fire destroyed the town-supported group housing for residents with severe mental illness. In improving their climate resilience, the town conducted an asset map that identified a large hotel on higher ground, which could be repurposed for housing, and a solar-powered food refrigeration plant, with which they were able to contract for backup storage of essential medications.

Planning for such large-scale interventions can make even seasoned managers feel overwhelmed and de-skilled. Starting small and taking care not to reinvent the wheel are effective ways to combat overwhelm.

The Climate Adaptation Knowledge Exchange (CAKE), the Adaptation Clearinghouse associated with the Georgetown Climate Center, and COP[2] regional hubs are three examples of hubs where communities have shared case examples of how they attempted to solve a particular problem. Best practices for community psychiatric programs starting to address climate impacts are presented in Table 14.2. These practices encourage community adaptation and promote the mitigation goals of reducing exposure, sensitivity, and damage from climate change.

Using the Skills of Community Psychiatrists to Build Climate Resilience for Communities and Vulnerable Groups

Participating in Community-Based Climate Mental Health Education, Training, and Initiatives

Community psychiatrists can also use their unique psychological skills to help vulnerable populations and communities deal with accumulating climate stresses. Climate planning increasingly incorporates change theory and empirically supported climate communication strategies to cope with resistance to action. This latter aspect, however, is significantly underdeveloped and needs greater help from mental health professionals. Community psychiatrists, who are trained to work with undermotivated groups, to see and respond to emotional issues percolating through group processes that create group dysfunction or may represent preconscious or symbolized concerns, and to tolerate and improve the slow pace of change, may be particularly helpful in removing obstacles to climate action. Reviews have also shown that community outcomes are undermined by inadequate attention to the lived psychological experience of community members—the intangible aspects of cultural heritage, local realities, social inequalities, intergenerational relationships, and local histories—the inclusion of which will improve community mental health efforts (Atkinson et al. 2017). Attending to these relational, cultural, and equity issues may require alternative forms of data collection, such as focus groups, deliberation,

Community Psychiatry 303

Table 14.2 Best practices for community psychiatry climate resilience programs

Mainstream climate change into all aspects of community psychiatry planning and practice

Pursue actions that address multiple community goals, including climate change, in one program, such as developing green space

Hire adequate professional staff and gain official approval specifically for climate resilience, mitigation, and adaptation efforts

Engage diverse and disenfranchised individuals in community plan development

Develop regional collaborations and teams or networks for action on specific goals

Obtain adequate funding, demonstrating cost-benefit in reduced crime and health expenditure

Structure implementation and follow-up with integrative monitoring, reassessment, and revision

and narrative analysis, to which community psychiatrists can contribute, as described in the following vignette.

Vignette

The town representative of Coleman asked their local psychiatrist, Dr. L, to lead the discussion at a community forum to introduce their new sustainability plan, which included a transition to solar energy for all new development and electric transportation. Noting the nonverbal behavior of numerous tense men, Dr. L drew them out, eliciting their anger and fear of losing their jobs as mechanics and propane fuel technicians. Dr. L decided to lead the whole audience in an exercise to increase empathy for the personal emotions of losing a job and then facilitated a group process that empowered the men to become core members of the planning committee. There, he and the affected men worked together to add adequate funds for retraining and preservation of their incomes through the transition, while also setting up a distribution system for part of the taxes from the new plan to go to members of the town, bonding them to the new behavior and improving perceived fairness.

In addition to the above tasks, community psychiatrists should advocate that climate resilience planning attend to the direct mental health needs of the climate situation:

- Educating patients and the community on the health and mental health effects of climate change, including climate-related emotional distress and seemingly unrelated phenomena such as rising conflict and violence
- Conducting community-wide training in strategies to support emotional resilience
- Providing adequate access to the natural world in town planning
- Training therapists and lay and peer counselors in the management of climate distress, with particular emphasis on young people
- Providing forums for the community to process difficult aspects of the transition to a clean energy society, such as loss or transition of employment, fears of the new and unknown, or presumed loss of beloved traditions (e.g., around car culture)
- Considering possible mental health co-benefits of climate decisions, such as increased access to green and blue spaces, exercise-related benefits from biking and walking, and the emotional improvements associated with cleaner air, as well as the potential adverse mental health impacts of poor decisions such as loss of landscapes to development
- Preparing first responders and other health systems for the expected increase in violence and suicide, particularly during heat waves and poor air conditions
- Adequately considering the special needs of people with mental illness in their ability to adapt

The need to transition to new and more sustainable ways of living, and of practicing psychiatry, is unfamiliar and may be regarded with suspicion and resistance. Many questions about how service delivery can be adapted to these challenges need to be answered, both practically and through systematic research. In particular, questions may touch on the following topics:

- Overcoming organization and individual inertia and resistance to change
- Scaling up existing treatments for community-wide interventions

Community Psychiatry

Table 14.3 Errors in climate resilience planning

Assumed stationarity (that things will be and feel the same in the future)

Equality of interventions

Excessive focus on current rather than long-term variability in conditions

Emphasis on recovery from recent events rather than proactive planning

Lack of comprehensiveness

Failure to include the additional cost of material climate risks in financial assessment of community needs

- Delivering treatments under novel, temporary, or rapidly changing circumstances
- Identifying and responding to new states of mind in group processes
- Incorporating sustainable interventions and more sustainable ways of practicing, such as nature-based therapies and social prescribing, into existing practices
- Incorporating knowledge from psychology, social sciences, communication, and information technology, including artificial intelligence, into interventions to help humankind keep pace with the scale of climate changes

In planning for community intervention, it is important to recognize that something new is required of us in response to the climate situation and therefore to avoid the pitfalls of a short-term and conventional view. Common inaccurate assumptions and limitations that worsen climate resilience planning are shown in Table 14.3.

To overcome these tendencies, it may be helpful to work backward from desired outcomes using the processes of *futures thinking*. This is an envisioning process (covered in Chapter 12, "Psychotherapy Considerations and Approaches for Climate-Related Distress") that considers a range of futures—probable, possible, plausible, and preferred—and then works backward to consider the supporting facts and trends that could divergently reach each. The emphasis is not on solving a problem to find one correct answer but on having a creative exploration of options that acknowledges uncertainty. This way of working facilitates *transformational adaptation* rather than efforts that are reactive, incremental, palliative, or siloed.

Climate-Related Group Work in Communities

Group work with communities is likely to become increasingly important as climate impacts become more evident and pervasive. Group therapy practices can be embedded in other community climate initiatives to ensure they are more inclusive and address community emotional issues that may otherwise destabilize their progress and outcomes, such as social isolation and loneliness (Bagnall et al. 2017). These group interventions do not necessarily need to be climate-specific. Community training of laypeople in peer counseling skills, anger management, conflict resolution, restorative justice, Psychological First Aid, trauma-sensitive care, and other techniques may help a community's ability to weather many climate-related adversities, including rising rates of social conflict, violence, weather disasters, and emotional distress, without incurring the political costs of a climate focus. Several group practices more specific to climate change, covered in Chapter 12, have been developed for processing climate-related distress and can be implemented in the community-psychiatry setting or by the community psychiatrist in the community. Those most appropriate for general community work include climate cafés and integrative community therapy.

Vulnerable Populations in Climate Community Psychiatry

By virtue of their work with marginalized groups, community psychiatrists have a particular responsibility for understanding and representing the mental health needs of vulnerable populations. Specific populations affected more by climate impacts include those experiencing homelessness, those with severe and chronic mental illness, marginalized racial and ethnic groups, rural and Indigenous communities, climate migrants, children, women, and older adults.

Homeless persons, particularly those with mental illness, are at high risk of climate health and mental health damage. They are particularly vulnerable to heat exposure and more likely to die or experience significant morbidity during heat events. Use of alcohol, methamphetamine, and other substances increases their risk, as does the primary risk factor of mental illness itself. Homeless encampments lack access to any cooling and are often built in urban heat islands, where temperatures can be up to 15°F higher than surrounding areas, and conditions are often

Community Psychiatry 307

further worsened by poor air quality. Limitations in cognition, physical ability, and perceptual limitations and distortions may limit the ability of unhoused persons to respond to heat warnings and take precautionary measures, if they are warned at all. Those on the margins of homelessness are also at higher risk of becoming unhoused as the rising costs of air conditioning with higher temperatures lead to unpaid bills, power cutoffs, and evictions (Bezgrebelna et al. 2021). Natural disasters also threaten to increase homelessness for displaced persons and to threaten homeless populations more than those with shelter.

Marginalized racial and ethnic groups are also disproportionately affected by climate impacts. African Americans live in greater proportion near fossil fuel refineries, making up 16%–54% of the population in these counties compared with their 13% representation in the population (Fleischman and Franklin 2017). Redlined communities, the result of racist real estate practices, have been associated with higher rates of traffic-related air pollution (TRAP), lesser green space, greater flood risk, and higher proportional temperatures (Katz 2021; Tessum et al. 2021). For African Americans, the risks of living with elevated heat risk or high TRAP are 52% and 56% higher than for control subjects; these risks are also higher for Asian and Hispanic groups, on the order of 20%–50% (Jessel et al. 2019; Tessum et al. 2019). These injustices should be remediated.

Climate migrants are another group with as yet poorly defined mental health needs. Migrants have been shown to face social marginalization, discrimination, and violence and to have adverse health and mental health outcomes linked to loss of social ties, lack of prior mental health treatment, inadequacy of health resources such as medications, and even relocation to worse conditions than those they were forced to leave (Herrán and Biehler 2020). As climate migration increases, these stresses can be expected to worsen, complicating the already fraught sociopolitical landscape of international immigration.

Indigenous communities have entered the climate crisis already carrying the legacy of colonization, which destroyed their way of life—which is rooted in deep connection to land, animals, and elements—both practically and spiritually. Their access to natural resources has been marginalized through the industrialization of natural resources on their lands, and this industrialization has carried heavy consequences for their mental and psychosocial well-being.

The consequences of these practices for Indigenous mental health are multiple, encompassing broad psychosocial and psychiatric impacts, and are magnified by the climate crisis. These impacts include the following:

- Experiences of loss, including grief, sadness, and solastalgia, from lost lands covered by hydroelectric dams or petroleum spills
- Stress, distress, fear, and anxiety related to their own fate, as well as the fate of animals and fish on the land and in surrounding water
- Hopelessness and powerlessness related to being stripped of self-determination, with disenfranchisement and lack of remediation
- Increased suicidal ideation, self-harm, and suicides
- Increased teen pregnancies
- Increased alcohol and other substance abuse
- Increased violence against women, including sexual and domestic violence
- Increased anger

Psychosocial impacts also include the following (Ninomiya et al. 2023):

- Increased conflict related to short-term, high-income jobs for some people and increased costs of living and housing
- Disruption of community networks (e.g., from placement of children in residential schools, relocation, and out-migration)
- Food insecurity related to lost land for hunting and fishing because of pollution, extreme weather, and drought, mediating other psychological effects such as lost transmission of intergenerational knowledge; disruption of social ties; and the adverse consequences of food insecurity for learning, negative affect, and externalizing behaviors (Banerji et al. 2023)
- Loss of access to areas used for harvesting traditional and spiritual foods and medicines
- Loss of access to burial grounds and inability to conduct spiritual practices at sacred sites
- Disruption of the relationship between the people and the land, which is central for emotional and spiritual well-being
- Inability to transfer cultural knowledge to younger generations

The arrogance, foolishness, and lack of appreciation and gratitude underlying the mistreatment of Indigenous people is even more transparent when we consider the critical role of Indigenous peoples as stewards of our planetary past and future. The approximately 475 million Indigenous peoples who occupy a quarter of Earth's lands are caretakers to 80% of planetary biodiversity. They understand better than the rest of us the interdependence of humankind and Nature: the degree

Community Psychiatry 309

to which we are literally the land, air, and water and our dependence on other beings and ecosystems for life. They therefore offer our greatest hope for rediscovering and embracing a mindset that could reverse the course of our current climate-related decline. That Indigenous people are often disempowered from protecting their practices and way of life by settler colonial, legal, and industrial forces that deny them their rights to occupy, control, and use their lands represents one of the most illustrative examples of the psychological misguidedness of the Anthropocene.

The psychology of this relationship of non-Indigenous to Indigenous cultures is thus worthy of psychological and perhaps therapeutic attention in community healing. The primacy of the autonomous self in non-Indigenous cultures makes it difficult to understand the fused nature of self and land in these cultures—what it really means to say "I am Eagle" or "I am the Water and the Water is me"—and therefore to provide what would be required to sanctify this relationship. There can be a tendency to split reactions to the Indigenous relationship with the land and its beings, either idealizing or denigrating it, both of which polarize the out-group rather than promoting community unity. Various forms of othering, including pity, idealization, intellectualization, devaluation, and projection of vulnerability in depending on Indigenous peoples and their knowledge, are in truth self-harm and are part of a dysfunctional group process in our planetary community to which community psychiatrists have much to contribute.

Key Points

- Community psychiatry will be at the forefront of climate mental health mitigation and adaptation.
- The roles and values of community psychiatry align with the values and needs of the climate response.
- Community psychiatry expertise in group function is critical to community processing of climate impacts and adaptation.
- Available tools and processes for asset mapping and resilience planning can serve now to establish mental health systems for mitigating and adapting to climate risks.
- The needs of people with mental illness and other marginalized groups have not been and must be adequately included in the climate and health response.

- An embrace of the psychological strengths of Indigenous and other disenfranchised groups is critical for community psychological health in the coming decades.

References

Atkinson S, Bagnall A-M, Corcoran R, et al: What is community wellbeing? Conceptual review. Bristol, UK, What Works Wellbeing, 2017

Augustinavicius JL, Lowe SR, Massazza A, et al: Global climate change and trauma: an International Society for Traumatic Stress Studies Briefing Paper. Brentwood, TN, International Society for Traumatic Stress Studies, 2021. Available at: https://istss.org/wp-content/uploads/2024/09/ISTSS-Briefing-Paper_Climate-Change-Final.pdf. Accessed February 10, 2024.

Bagnall AM, South J, Di Martino S, et al: What works to boost social relations and community wellbeing? A scoping review of the evidence. Eur J Public Health 27(Suppl 3):ckx187.157, 2017

Banerji A, Pelletier VA, Haring R, et al: Food insecurity and its consequences in indigenous children and youth in Canada. PLOS Glob Public Health 3(9):e0002406, 2023 37756390

Bezgrebelna M, McKenzie K, Wells S, et al: Climate change, weather, housing precarity, and homelessness: a systematic review of reviews. Int J Environ Res Public Health 18(11):5812, 2021 34071641

Fleischman L, Franklin M: Fumes across the fence-line: the health impacts of air pollution from oil and gas facilities on African American communities. Baltimore, MD, National American Association for the Advancement of Colored People, 2017. Available at: www.catf.us/wp-content/uploads/2017/11/CATF_Pub_FumesAcrossTheFenceLine.pdf. Accessed November 23, 2024.

Herrán K, Biehler D: Analysis of environmental migrants and their mental health in strengthening health systems. F1000 Res 9:1367, 2020

Jessel S, Sawyer S, Hernández D: Energy, poverty, and health in climate change: a comprehensive review of an emerging literature. Front Public Health 7:357, 2019 31921733

Katz L: A racist past, a flooded future: formerly redlined areas have $107 billion worth of homes facing high flood risk—25% more than non-redlined areas. Redfin, March 14, 2021. Available at: www.redfin.com/news/redlining-flood-risk/. Accessed February 15, 2024.

Ninomiya MEM, Burns N, Pollock NJ, et al: Indigenous communities and the mental health impacts of land dispossession related to industrial resource development: a systematic review. Lancet Planet Health 7(6):e501–e517, 2023 37286247

Sullenbarger J, Schutzenhofer E, Haase E: Climate change: implications for community mental health, in Textbook of Community Psychiatry, 2nd

Edition. Edited by Sowers WE, McQuistion HL, Ranz JM, et al. Cham, Switzerland, Springer, 2022, pp 427–442

Tessum CW, Apte JS, Goodkind AL, et al: Inequity in consumption of goods and services adds to racial-ethnic disparities in air pollution exposure. Proc Natl Acad Sci USA 116(13):6001–6006, 2019 30858319

Tessum CW, Paolella DA, Chambliss SE, et al: PM2.5 polluters disproportionately and systemically affect people of color in the United States. Sci Adv 7(18):eabf4491, 2021

World Health Organization: Climate change and health toolkit. Geneva, Switzerland, World Health Organization, 2021. Available at: www.who. int/teams/environment-climate-change-and-health/climate-change-and-health/capacity-building/toolkit-on-climate-change-and-health/vulnerability. Accessed November 4, 2023.

15

Sustainable Psychiatry

Reducing the Carbon Footprint of Mental Health Care

Negative Health Impacts of the Carbon Footprint of Health Care

Actions to limit the progression of global warming dwarf any other measures to mitigate the mental health and health impacts of climate change, which threatens the existence of more than half of the people alive today and 90% of species over the coming century (Xu and Ramanathan 2017) and is arguably fundamental to providing conditions necessary to work productively on any other mental health needs, given this level of threat. Decreasing global greenhouse emissions at the personal, local, national, and international levels is thus the most important intervention for climate mental health that any psychiatrist can make. In this chapter, I cover how health care greenhouse gases are measured, their health consequences, and actions psychiatrists can take to mitigate the harm they are causing.

Health care emits approximately 4.5% of the world's greenhouse gases, and the emissions of U.S. health care account for 8%–10% of U.S. total annual emissions and a quarter of the health care emissions of the world (Chung and Meltzer 2009; Eckelman and Sherman 2016). These emissions can be calculated for any part of the health care we deliver: for countries, individual facilities, or modes of production. They are broken down into the following:

- Those emitted directly by facilities (referred to as scope 1, 7%)
- Those from purchased electricity (scope 2, 11%)
- Those emitted in the supply chain of goods and services used by health care systems (scope 3, 82%); pharmaceuticals and chemicals comprise 20% of scope 3 emissions

Across all three divisions, the electricity sector is responsible for 29% (Tennison et al. 2021). Health care emissions include particulate matter, sulfur oxides (particularly sulfur dioxide), methane, and anesthetic and other gases that have long atmospheric lives, affecting ozone production and depletion, smog, and ecotoxicity, among other impacts.

We can be explicit about the medical consequences of these health care greenhouse emissions by analyzing the medical impacts of these scope 1–3 emissions. This analysis involves three steps:

- Translating the money spent on a particular health care activity into the emissions associated with conducting that much business in that sector
- Breaking down these emissions into the particular gases associated with a particular activity
- Translating those gases into their environmental health impacts and the known health consequences associated with them

Scope emissions analysis relies on three well-established models that are used across industries to assess greenhouse gas impacts. These tools can be applied to any product or aspect of care:

1. The 2012 U.S. Bureau of Economic Analysis dataset
2. The U.S. Environmentally Extended Input-Output (USEEIO) model (Environmental Protection Agency 2023b; Yang et al. 2017)
3. The Tool for the Reduction and Assessment of Chemicals and other Environmental Impacts (TRACI; Bare 2011; Environmental Protection Agency 2023a)

Training in scope emissions analysis has been available from the National Academy of Medicine and Health Care Without Harm organization.

Sustainable Psychiatry 315

When we analyze the health impacts of the greenhouse gas emissions of the health care industry in the United States in this way, we learn that the annual respiratory, cardiovascular, and other illnesses that result from human-made emissions are responsible for morbidity and mortality that rival those of annual medical errors: around 200,000 direct disability-adjusted life years (DALYs) per year in the United States alone and 244,000–531,000 additional DALYs from their climate effects over time (Eckelman et al. 2020). The mental health consequences of climate change are likely to increase the need for psychiatric services (Corvetto et al. 2023), creating an adverse positive feedback loop in which greenhouse gases lead to mental health damage, increasing services that require more greenhouse gases to function with even further worsening of mental health. Decreasing the carbon footprint of health care is therefore not only a priority for the control of climate change but is essential to remain true to the Hippocratic oath, so that physicians are not harming patients through the emissions generated by the way we conduct our work. In recognition of this priority, 60 countries, including the United States, committed to low-carbon sustainable health care systems at the 26th United Nations Climate Change Conference in 2021, and 20 countries committed to net-zero health care system emissions by 2050.

The Carbon Footprint of Psychiatry

The carbon footprint of psychiatric practice, independent of other specialties, has been calculated only for the National Health Service (NHS) in the United Kingdom (Figure 15.1) and is likely to vary in different cultures.

The NHS analysis, however, paired with a general analysis of the breakdown of health care emissions overall (Figure 15.2), can provide some guidance for where psychiatry should focus to reduce its carbon footprint and bring itself in line with national and international emissions targets. As can be appreciated in Figures 15.1 and 15.2, the major sources of carbon emissions for psychiatry are buildings, including the electricity and gas they use; the business services, equipment, and products required to run psychiatric facilities and offices; psychiatric pharmaceuticals; and the provision of food. For psychiatrists, then, the most important ways to improve the carbon footprint of their work are as follows:

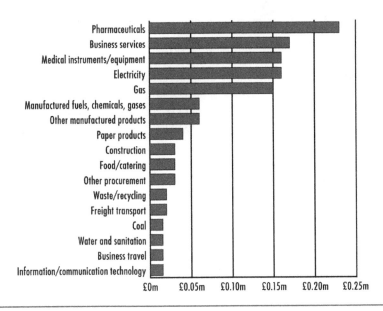

Figure 15.1 Carbon hotspots in mental health care.

Source. Maughan D: Sustainability in psychiatry (Occasional Paper 97). Oxford, UK, Centre for Sustainable Healthcare, 2015. Used with permission.

- Reducing the size and materials usage of their physical plant
- Reducing energy used for keeping facilities open
- Reducing energy usage for the transportation of staff and patients
- Reducing the number and quantity of the medications prescribed
- Improving food services and food waste

Although each of these interventions can reduce the psychiatric carbon footprint by a meaningful percentage, it is the carbon cost of individual patient visits and hospital stays that is by far the most significant input, through the transportation of patients to and from appointments and the energy needs of the visit space. As an example, a small study of the carbon benefits that could be achieved by improved prescribing of single long-acting injectable antipsychotics demonstrated that overprescribing of medication increased carbon footprints by about 170 kg CO_2e per patient per year, but the total carbon costs of this overprescribing derived almost entirely from appointment-related emissions in terms of staffing and facilities rather than the pharmaceutical footprint of the medication itself (Maughan et al. 2016).

Sustainable Psychiatry

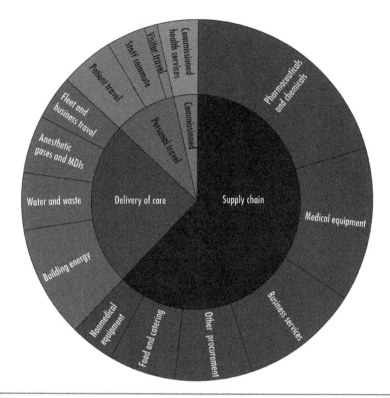

Figure 15.2 Contribution of different sectors to the greenhouse gas emissions of the U.K. National Health Service, 2019.

MDIs=metered-dose inhalers.

Source. Modified and reproduced from Tennison et al. 2021. Data available in Appendix 1 (p. 39). Permission is available at https://creativecommons.org/licenses/by/4.0.

System Shifts to Decrease the Carbon Footprint of Psychiatric Practice

Telepsychiatry

In light of the carbon costs described in the previous section, "The Carbon Footprint of Psychiatry," preventative care is the most sustainable action to decrease health care emissions, and changes in how and where appointments are conducted if they do become needed, as well as improved efficiency of psychiatric interventions, may be of second greatest benefit in meeting sustainability targets. In this context, telepsychiatry, particularly done from the practitioner's home, has a great likelihood of reducing psychiatry's carbon footprint. Telemedicine visits use a small fraction (1%–2%) of the greenhouse gases necessary for an in-person appointment, which are dominated by patient transport to the office. For situations such as helicopter transport or where traveling long distances is necessary to see a specialist, the savings are particularly magnified (Dullet et al. 2017; Penaskovic et al. 2022).

Telepsychiatry can be considered environmentally worthwhile for any patient coming to their appointments from more than 4 miles away (Purohit et al. 2021). Telepsychiatry visits decrease wait times and missed appointments (Kruse et al. 2017). They have been estimated to save 4 hours of time and $150 in childcare, lost work wages, and fuel costs per visit for the average patient, which contributes to patient sustainability and resilience by improving their ability to maintain financial stability and care of themselves and their families. Telepsychiatry also decreases stigma about mental health care, perhaps particularly for men, children, and teens (Substance Abuse and Mental Health Services Administration 2021). In addition to these clinical benefits, telepsychiatry includes the following climate-specific co-benefits:

- Addressing the root cause of neuropsychiatric damage related to fossil-fuel particulates (see Chapter 5, "Air Pollution Impacts on the Brain")
- Improving climate justice by better serving patients in rural settings, disabled patients, and those from socioeconomically disadvantaged groups who are most affected by climate change
- Allowing for the delivery of services during disasters, which decreases emergency department congestion during these events (Grover et al. 2020)
- Allowing psychiatrists to serve as health ambassadors for overseas climate impacts in the natural disaster setting

Like telepsychiatry, artificial intelligence (AI) is an advancing technology that may play a significant role in decreasing the carbon footprint of health care intervention and energy usage (Cho 2023), although it has significant carbon footprint challenges of its own. AI can decrease the time spent collecting health care information and improve diagnostic accuracy, eliminating the need for diagnostic tests and decreasing

Sustainable Psychiatry

energy space requirements for staff. Particularly in developing nations, it can identify illness without the environmental costs of human travel (Krishnan et al. 2023). These technologies decrease the carbon costs of in-person contact but must be balanced against the carbon footprint of AI and the emotional effects of less intimate human engagement, discussed further in the section "Relational Aspects of Change to Telepsychiatry."

Professional Conferences

The carbon footprint of professional travel to attend professional conferences and interview for residency and fellowship positions is another area where significant emissions reductions are possible by switching to virtual technologies (Young 2009). The American Psychiatric Association meeting, one of the largest psychiatric conferences in the world, generates approximately 20 metric tons of CO_2 in annual travel, the equivalent of burning 22 million tons of coal. This impact can be reduced to near zero by holding conferences virtually or reduced by 30%–160% by locating the conference at optimized locations to minimize total participant flight distance (Wortzel et al. 2021). The carbon footprint of residency interviews was estimated in two studies at 0.43–0.47 metric tons per candidate, which becomes highly substantial when multiplied by 39,000 residency candidates interviewing per year (Bernstein and Beshar 2021; Domingo et al. 2023). Candidates, programs, and conference-goers also benefit both financially and practically from not having to travel to these events, particularly during early career years when child-rearing and paying back high student loans are significant priorities. The stresses of in-person attendance contribute to gender and financial inequity and injustice in career development. At the same time, the opportunities to network, socialize, collaborate, and understand new science, technologies, health care opportunities, and treatments at these events are also critical for professional development and well-being.

Relational Aspects of Change to Telepsychiatry

In assessing the use of telepsychiatry with patients and for professional exchange, psychiatrists should balance what is sustaining for relationships with patients and colleagues with environmental concerns.

Mentalizing, mirror neuron, and social reward systems are activated by in-person (second-person) social interactions, leading to coordination of nonverbal behaviors such as eye contact, synchronous movement, and mimicry of facial expressions. These activations promote turn-taking and agreement about what to call things, and they guide linguistic learning (Redcay and Schilbach 2019). Video exchange may promote a third-person stance of observation that does not engage these affective, cognitive, and motoric connections. Creating a sustainable society includes supporting the social systems that keep people positively connected to each other, which is an important aspect of climate resilience. The three-dimensional experience of being in a room with someone also activates the senses and carries a greater sense of presence. For some, this is too overstimulating, making remote technologies advantageous. However, overuse of remote means may change social, presencing, and mindfulness capacities that are also part of the resilient response (Lewis et al. 2021).

Education

Medical student and psychiatric education offer additional opportunities for program leadership to acculturate trainees into sustainable attitudes and practices. Providing a sustainable format for educating students models professionalism and ethical integrity and also facilitates the recruitment of top candidates (Wortzel et al. 2022). Moral injury can be inflicted by insisting that trainees participate in unsustainable practices that violate their oath to do no harm. In recent years, medical students are demanding environmentally responsive health care education (Navarrete-Welton et al. 2022), and they are grading training programs on the quality of their climate health education with a Planetary Health Report Card to achieve these goals (Hampshire et al. 2022). Sustainable education can also be achieved by conducting interviews remotely, creating eco-friendly office spaces, and providing climate mental health lectures that include training in advocacy, public health, and the best practices to slow the root causes of climate change.

Health Care Systems

Mental health professionals can also enact emissions reductions as advocates and experts for sustainable change in their health care system. Hospital admissions are responsible for the bulk of health care energy use, given their requirement for maintaining large facilities; therefore, same-day or outpatient approaches to care are preferable. An ICU bed is extremely energy-intensive, consuming 178 kg of CO_2 per day, so getting patients more rapidly to the regular floors through good treatment of delirium and similar measures is also a sustainability action. Some medical specialties have unique points of intensive greenhouse gas production that can be quite easily modified. For example, anesthetic gases have very high greenhouse gas potential and extremely long half-lives, with marked differences in negative climate effects between clinically equivalent gases. The anesthetic gases desflurane, isoflurane, and sevoflurane have 6810×, 1800×, and 440×, respectively, the warming potential of CO_2 over their first 20 years in the atmosphere. Changing to sevoflurane, increasing the use of regional anesthesia (Kuvadia et al. 2020), and limiting anesthesia time have been shown to significantly lower emissions. As demonstrated by the anesthesia department of the University of British Columbia, greater use of sevoflurane reduced emissions from 13.4 million kg CO_2e to 4.5 million kg over 4 years, a reduction the equivalent of 1,700 cars each driving 14,000 miles per year (Alexander et al. 2018).

Similarly, aerosolized inhalers (Fulford et al. 2022) and antibiotics (Taylor et al. 2024) are other areas of pharmacology that have an outsized carbon footprint, with many familiar powder-inhaler substitutes easily available. Information about the carbon footprint of other medications, including the relative carbon footprint of specific antidepressants, antipsychotics, and other psychiatric medications, is under development (Taylor et al. 2024) and suggests that there will be sustainability benefits to prescribing certain therapeutically equivalent medications over others. For those wishing to make comprehensive changes to their clinic or institution but unsure or overwhelmed by how to proceed, My Green Doctor is a program developed by Dr. Todd Sack (2021) that provides guidance for small interventions that are initiated in the clinic setting every week over a year. My Green Doctor has been shown to save about $1,500 per doctor per year and to improve morale, save resources, and model sustainable behaviors for patients. Health Care Without Harm (www.noharm.org) is a leading organization providing guidance to hospitals to address sustainability needs, and the National Academy of Medicine (https://nam.edu/programs/climate-change-and-human-health/action-collaborative-on-decarbonizing-the-u-s-health-sector) and American Hospital Association (www.sustainabilityroadmap.org) offer other excellent resources.

Table 15.1 Putting the relative benefits of pro-environmental behavior in perspective

Action	Kilograms of CO_2e saved
One hour of telepsychiatry (electricity used)	0.5
One tree's carbon absorption for the year	24
One pound of beef not eaten	60
Eliminating one long drive to a specialist	60–180
Eliminating one trip to an APA meeting	1,200–1,600
One set of virtual residency interviews	5,400
Two weeks of clinic visits conducted remotely	54,000

Source. Bernstein and Beshar 2021; Domingo et al. 2023; Dullet et al. 2017; Purohit et al. 2021; Wortzel et al. 2021.

Psychiatrists and other mental health professionals could benefit from greater leadership from national organizations in providing targets for emissions cuts for individual practices and health care facilities, as well as more and better information about the emissions associated with different medications, materials, and other elements specific to psychiatric work. In pursuing the clear ethical mandate to mitigate their health care–associated footprint, psychiatrists can find guidance in the meantime by reaching an understanding of the intertwined nature of mitigation, adaptation, and sustainability. If mitigation efforts decrease the ability to adapt, for example, by decreasing social well-being and thereby resilience, the response will not sustain the needs of both the planet and those who inhabit it. Sustainable psychiatry must support the triple bottom line, wherein sustaining the environment, sustaining people and society, and sustaining financial viability must each be adequately addressed. In seeking to achieve these goals, Table 15.1 delineates concrete personal and professional approaches to meaningful sustainable action.

Pharmaceutical Companies

Pharmaceuticals play a significant role in health care emissions and can be a focus of sustainable intervention. More than half of medications are never consumed (Law et al. 2015), and one study modeled the

Sustainable Psychiatry 323

possibility of recovering and recycling up to 50% of unwanted medication in a large-scale program. This work did, however, acknowledge the need for government sustainability subsidies as well as incentives for consumers, large pharmaceutical companies, and drugstores in order for the program to succeed (Luo and Wan 2022). Big pharmaceutical companies themselves can also be a focal point for emissions reduction. They have a carbon footprint greater than that of the automotive industry and have been associated with additional adverse environmental practices, such as releasing large amounts of medication into the environment, thus damaging wildlife and contributing to antimicrobial resistance. Lobbying to withdraw large contracts from companies that have violated environmental law, or those that have the highest normalized relative intensity of emissions (particularly Eli Lilly and Proctor & Gamble, but also others) (Belkhir and Elmeligi 2019) is an effective way of mitigating the carbon footprint of the pharmaceuticals associated with psychiatric prescribing. Changes to prescribing practices for individual psychiatrists are described in the section "Prescribing" later in the chapter.

Actions to Decrease Carbon Footprint in Personal Behavior and in Solo and Clinic-Based Practice

Vignette

Dr. R became alarmed about the influence of fossil fuel–based microplastics and particle pollutants on the brain and the long half-life effects of anesthetic gases on global warming. Attempts to reduce plastic use in clinic were met with obstacles to a rational response, including complaints about the length of the meetings and the difficulty of minor changes. The anesthesiology chair, Dr. M, mocked him by posting pictures of his large diesel truck on the doctor chat line, reinforcing American values. Dr. R changed his approach, limiting discussion in clinic to 5 minutes per week (My Green Doctor) and focusing on the health benefits and solutions for clinic families, optimizing climate communications. Dr. R used multidisciplinary collaboration by forging an alliance with a clinic receptionist who was also an artist to update the common area with colorful mugs and dinnerware, saving plastic use. Patients noticed this physician modeling, and the artist's work became a local trend, improving community sustainability. Dr. R posted a funny poster in the surgical suite that said, "Use sevoflurane and Dr. M can keep his truck!"—a recognition of the climate reality–social reality dialectic. Anchoring and relative benefit cognitive biases were evident in the distaste for change, but the size of the sevoflurane benefit surprised people used to media urging them to put aside their emotional attachment to American car culture and stop using gas cars, and sevoflurane use increased 90%. The joke led to better rapport between Dr. R and Dr. M. They bonded over their mutual love of the wilderness and worked together to enact system change by supporting greater telemedicine, online continuing medical education (CME), and waste reduction across their health care system.

Personal Action

Physicians are one of the most trusted voices on climate change in the public domain (Maibach et al. 2021). Whether in homes, offices, institutions, or advocacy work, the sustainability actions that we take and the importance we place on taking them have effects beyond themselves, motivating changes in patient behavior and increasing recognition of the climate emergency. At a personal level, the most potent actions to decrease an individual's carbon footprint include

- Having one fewer child or encouraging someone else to do so
- Living car-free
- Avoiding one transatlantic flight per year
- Buying green energy
- Eating a plant-based diet

Actions in the Clinic

Actions to improve the carbon footprint of solo practices and clinics should focus on the emissions associated with facilities, pharmaceuticals, business materials, transportation, and energy (see Figure 15.1). They include the following:

- Limiting the size of offices and inpatient unit areas
- Sharing offices and using common areas for multiple purposes in inpatient and outpatient programs
- Improving energy efficiency and contracting for clean energy for buildings and offices
- Working from home where able
- Reducing consumption of office and medical supplies

Sustainable Psychiatry 325

- Using telepsychiatry
- Reducing unnecessary and redundant care, including advocating for payment plans that reimburse telephone management and non-fee for service interventions

The following actions may decrease use of fuel for work-related transportation and heating:

- Living close to work; using active and public transport (walking, biking, bus) as able
- Using telepsychiatry
- Decreasing in-person attendance at conferences, particularly those that are far away
- Increasing use of online CME and conference attendance
- Advocating for virtual interviews of trainees and job candidates
- Coordinating attendance at conferences and other professional events (speakerships) with vacation planning and visits to family
- Traveling by car, train, or bus instead of by plane when possible

To decrease the institutional footprint, it is necessary to work with food services, administration, the utilities department, and so on, and this will involve culture change. Actions to decrease the consumption of materials include the following:

- Switching to electronic record systems, faxes, and other insurance communications
- Centralizing access to office supplies
- Limiting the number of garbage cans, paper towel dispensers, staff areas, and other redundancies that encourage the increased use of plastic bags and other supplies and energy
- Switching to green supply companies
- Decreasing food waste by reducing portion sizes and the number of items on trays, donating excess food, and increasing plant-based foods
- Deliberating before building or refurbishing

Prescribing

Finally, reducing the number, mass, and packaging of pills taken is a significant pro-environmental action with ramifications across sectors of society (Adeyeye et al. 2022). Actions to decrease the carbon footprint of pharmaceuticals include the following:

- Reducing polypharmacy
- Giving smaller initial prescriptions
- Increasing interventions to improve compliance, which also decreases waste
- Developing state programs for recycling unused medication
- Avoiding and eliminating unnecessary prescriptions
- Testing if existing medications are necessary and effective by vigilant trial discontinuation of those with a high number needed to treat or potentially completed course
- Lobbying for accurate bioavailability and expiration dates to avoid excess dosing or unnecessary disposal of expired medications
- Using sustained-release formulations or larger doses divided over 2 days to reduce the total pill count
- Increasing use of light boxes and neuromodulatory therapies (although their energy use has not been studied)
- Increasing use of nature therapy, exercise, meditation, and social prescribing
- Increasing use of symptom-targeted psychotherapy techniques such as iRest, cognitive-behavioral therapy for insomnia, or breathing practices for panic disorder
- Preventing illness: a good target is 72% prevention and 28% treatment

Choosing Wisely is a website that advises about low-quality prescribing, such as antipsychotics in older adults and for delirium, antipsychotics in children, and using two antipsychotics, as well as the benefits of avoiding cholinesterase inhibitors and benzodiazepines (Levinson et al. 2015).

Reducing Emissions Through Action on the National and Global Stage

In addition to these changes in their own habits of practice, mental health professionals can take action through advocacy work for organized health care, countries, and the global community. At a national

Sustainable Psychiatry 327

and an international level, many effective strategies can change the course of global warming. These were comprehensively reviewed by Paul Hawken and his associates in Project Drawdown, a project that evaluated the capacity of particular big actions to change emissions between 2020 and 2050. The top actions they found include the following (Hawken 2017):

- Improving refrigeration
- Using onshore wind power
- Reducing food waste
- Eating a plant-rich diet
- Sustaining tropical forests
- Educating girls
- Providing universal access to family planning
- Increasing solar farms
- Increasing rooftop solar
- Practicing silvopasture

It is worth noting that the top actions supported by this research are both counterintuitive and 20–160 times more impactful than many common pro-environmental recommendations. For example, changes to refrigeration have the capacity to remove 89.74 gigatons (GT) of CO_2e from the atmosphere over the next three decades, whereas increased use of trains and ride-sharing measure at 0.52 and 0.32 GT, respectively. Project Drawdown solutions are also organized by sector, offering the ability to compare advocacy and investment opportunities. For example, in considering measures to maintain forest and plant canopy, a donation to preserve the rainforest supports a climate mitigation process that is 10 times more effective than a donation to a local forest protection effort (61.23 vs. 6.20 GT of CO_2e). The climate solutions found by Project Drawdown (https://drawdown.org/solutions) offer useful entry points for discussions with patients about personal environmental action, not only because of their scientific importance but also because of their psychological aspects, such as the following:

- Identifying meaningful action
- Reducing guilt and over-dedication regarding individual behaviors that may be less effective and overly stressful
- Directing investment of personal energy and finance in ways that reduce burnout

328 Handbook of Climate Psychiatry and Psychotherapy

Table 15.2 Top effective individual actions to reduce personal annual carbon footprint

Action	CO_2e in tons saved (1 ton~900 kg)
Have one fewer child (United States)	58.6
Live car-free, per year	2.4
Avoid one transatlantic flight	1.6
Eat a plant-based diet and reduce food waste	0.8–1.6
Do not buy a new car	6–35
Do not construct a new home	15–100

- Developing patient strength in how to remain cognitively and emotionally clear-sighted in conversations containing misinformation and emotional targeting
- Educating younger patients on how to assess effective versus ineffective types of habit change and to identify cognitive biases in what they consider sustainable that may adversely affect the outcomes of their decisions

Tables 15.1 and 15.2 are also provided to help both psychiatrists and patients understand how disproportionately beneficial some actions are compared with others (Wynes and Nicholas 2017).

Key Points

- U.S. health care generates 10% of U.S. greenhouse gas emissions, contributing significantly to global warming and patient disability; reducing health care emissions is therefore an ethical imperative.
- The most carbon-intensive aspects of psychiatric practice are patient and provider travel, maintenance of facilities, and prescribing; telepsychiatry, shared space, and changes to prescribing are meaningful sustainable practices.
- Reducing the frequency of in-person attendance at conferences and screening training applicants remotely can make a large difference in the greenhouse gas emissions of nonclinical professional activity.

Sustainable Psychiatry

- Psychiatric educators have an ethical obligation to train and acculturate future psychiatrists in sustainable practices.
- Understanding the most impactful personal and societal changes to reduce emissions can direct meaningful action in ways that reduce stress and allow psychiatrists to work with patients on identifying distorted and masochistic patterns of thought in relation to sustainable living.

References

Adeyeye E, New BJM, Chen F, et al: Sustainable medicines use in clinical practice: a clinical pharmacological view on eco-pharmaco-stewardship. Br J Clin Pharmacol 88(7):3023–3029, 2022 34779524

Alexander R, Poznikoff A, Malherbe S: Greenhouse gases: the choice of volatile anesthetic does matter. Can J Anaesth 65(2):221–222, 2018 29119467

Bare J: TRACI 2.0: the tool for the reduction and assessment of chemical and other environmental impacts 2.0. Clean Technol Environ Policy 13:687–696, 2011

Belkhir L, Elmeligi A: Carbon footprint of the global pharmaceutical industry and relative impact of its major players. J Clean Prod 214:185–194, 2019

Bernstein D, Beshar I: The carbon footprint of residency interviews. Acad Med 96(7):932, 2021 34183479

Cho R: AI's growing carbon footprint, State of the Planet. New York, Columbia Climate School, 2023. Available at: https://news.climate.columbia.edu/2023/06/09/ais-growing-carbon-footprint. Accessed November 23, 2024.

Chung JW, Meltzer DO: Estimate of the carbon footprint of the US health care sector. JAMA 302(18):1970–1972, 2009 19903917

Corvetto JF, Helou AY, Dambach P, et al: A systematic literature review of the impact of climate change on the global demand for psychiatric services. Int J Environ Res Public Health 20(2):1190, 2023 36673946

Domingo A, Singer J, Cois A, et al: The carbon footprint and cost of virtual residency interviews. J Grad Med Educ 15(1):112–116, 2023 36817522

Dullet NW, Geraghty EM, Kaufman T, et al: Impact of a university outpatient telemedicine program on travel time, costs, and environmental pollutants. Value Health 20:542–546, 2017 28407995

Eckelman MJ, Sherman J: Environmental impacts of the U.S. health care system and effects on public health. PLoS One 11(6):e0157014, 2016 27280706

Eckelman MJ, Huang K, Lagasse R, et al: Health care pollution and public health damage in the United States: an update. Health Aff (Millwood) 39(12):2071–2079, 2020 33284703

Environmental Protection Agency: Tool for Reduction and Assessment of Chemicals and Other Environmental Impacts (TRACI). Washington, DC,

Environmental Protection Agency, 2023a. Available at: www.epa.gov/
chemical-research/tool-reduction-and-assessment-chemicals-and-other-
environmental-impacts-traci. Accessed October 25, 2023.

Environmental Protection Agency: US Environmentally-Extended
Input-Output (USEEIO) Models. Washington, DC, Environmental
Protection Agency, 2023b. Available at: www.epa.gov/land-research/
us-environmentally-extended-input-output-useeio-models. Accessed
November 23, 2024.

Fulford B, Mezzi K, Aumônier S, et al: Carbon footprints and life cycle
assessments of inhalers: a review of published evidence. Sustainability
14(12):7106, 2022

Grover JM, Smith B, Williams JG, et al: Novel use of telemedicine by
hurricane evacuation shelters. Prehosp Emerg Care 24(6):804–812, 2020
32011202

Hampshire K, Islam N, Kissel B, et al: The Planetary Health Report Card:
a student-led initiative to inspire planetary health in medical schools.
Lancet Planet Health 6(5):e449–e454, 2022 35461572

Hawken P (ed): Drawdown. New York, Penguin, 2017

Krishnan G, Singh S, Pathania M, et al: Artificial intelligence in clinical
medicine: catalyzing a sustainable global healthcare paradigm. Front
Artif Intell 6:1227091, 2023 37705603

Kruse CS, Krowski N, Rodriguez B, et al: Telehealth and patient satisfaction:
a systematic review and narrative analysis. BMJ Open 7(8):e016242, 2017
28775188

Kuvadia M, Cummis CE, Liguori G, et al: 'Green-gional' anesthesia: the non-
polluting benefits of regional anesthesia to decrease greenhouse gases
and attenuate climate change. Reg Anesth Pain Med 45(9):744–745, 2020
32546552

Law AV, Sakharkar P, Zargarzadeh A, et al: Taking stock of medication
wastage: unused medications in US households. Res Social Adm Pharm
11(4):571–578, 2015 25487420

Levinson W, Kallewaard M, Bhatia RS, et al: Choosing Wisely International
Working Group: 'Choosing Wisely': a growing international campaign.
BMJ Qual Saf 24(2):167–174, 2015 25552584

Lewis J, Mark B, Haase E, et al: Fostering human connection in a sustainable
virtual world (commentary). Psychiatric Times, May 4, 2021

Luo Y, Wan Z: An optimal system of recycling unwanted medicines
by sustainable synergy of drugmakers, drugstores, customers and
governments. Journal of Cleaner Production 376:134304, 2022

Maibach E, Frumkin H, Ahdoot S: Health professionals and the climate crisis:
trusted voices, essential roles. World Med Health Policy 13(1):137–145, 2021

Maughan D, Lillywhite R, Cooke M: Cost and carbon burden of long-acting
injections: a sustainable evaluation. BJPsych Bull 40(3):132–136, 2016
27280033

Navarrete-Welton A, Chen JJ, Byg B, et al: A grassroots approach for greener education: an example of a medical student-driven planetary health curriculum. Front Public Health 10:1013880, 2022 36225779

Penaskovic KM, Zeng X, Burgin S, et al: Telehealth: reducing patients' greenhouse gas emissions at one academic psychiatry department. Acad Psychiatry 46(5): 569–573, 2022 35997996

Purohit A, Smith J, Hibble A: Does telemedicine reduce the carbon footprint of healthcare? A systematic review. Future Healthc J 8(1):e85–e91, 2021 33791483

Redcay E, Schilbach L: Using second-person neuroscience to elucidate the mechanisms of social interaction. Nat Rev Neurosci 20(8):495–505, 2019 31138910

Sack T: My Green Doctor. Jacksonville Beach, FL, My Green Doctor Foundation, 2021. Available at: https://mygreendoctor.org/#. Accessed November 7, 2023.

Substance Abuse and Mental Health Services Administration: Telehealth for the Treatment of Serious Mental Illness and Substance Use Disorders (SAMHSA Publication No PEP21-06-02-001). Rockville, MD, Substance Abuse and Mental Health Services Administration, 2021

Taylor H, Mahamdallie S, Sawyer M, et al: MCF classifier: estimating, standardizing, and stratifying medicine carbon footprints, at scale. Br J Clin Pharmacol 90(11):2713–2723, 2024 39284639

Tennison I, Roschnik S, Ashby B, et al: Health care's response to climate change: a carbon footprint assessment of the NHS in England. Lancet Planet Health 5(2):e84–e92, 2021 33581070

Wortzel JR, Stashevsky A, Wortzel JD, et al: Estimation of the carbon footprint associated with attendees of the American Psychiatric Association Annual Meeting. JAMA Netw Open 4(1):e2035641, 2021 33507255

Wortzel JR, Guerrero APS, Aggarwal R, et al: Climate change and the professional obligation to socialize physicians and trainees into an environmentally sustainable medical culture. Acad Psychiatry 46(5):556–561, 2022 35879599

Wynes S, Nicholas KA: The climate mitigation gap: education and government recommendations miss the most effective individual actions. Environ Res Lett 12:74024, 2017

Xu Y, Ramanathan V: Well below 2°C: mitigation strategies for avoiding dangerous to catastrophic climate changes. Proc Natl Acad Sci USA 114(39):10315–10323, 2017 28912354

Yang Y, Ingwersen WW, Hawkins TR, et al: USEEIO: a new and transparent United States environmentally extended input-output model. J Clean Prod 158:308–318, 2017 30344374

Young SN: Rethinking scientific meetings: an imperative in an era of climate change. J Psychiatry Neurosci 34(5):341–342, 2009 19721843

Appendix

Climate Mental Health Organizations and Resources for Professional Engagement and Patient Support

This appendix includes many of the larger organizations and resource structures available for climate and mental health, as well as climate and health information. It is not, however, exhaustive and is likely to be in frequent flux. Almost every medical university, many states, and almost all national governments additionally have climate and health initiatives that have not been included here, nor have the affiliated resources of the World Health Organization (www.who.int/health-topics/climate-change#tab=tab_1) and United States government (www.climate.gov). Finally, treatment-related resources (climate group therapies such as climate cafés, the Good Grief Network, the Work That Reconnects, and Deep Adaptation Forum) have not been included because access may change from year to year.

Resource	Website	Description	Type of entity and location
Associazione Italiana Ansia da Cambiamento Climatico (AIACC)	https://aiacc.it	Psychologists concerned with the climate crisis	No funding, offer fee-for-service psychotherapy, Italy
Care of People and Planet (COP²)	www.cop2.org	A United Nations–backed global network of organizations generating tangible mental health–related policies and actions to strengthen mental resilience, endurance, innovation, and adaptation to the climate crisis	Nonprofit, international
CIRCLE	https://circle.sites.stanford.edu/	An initiative at Stanford Psychiatry for research and action to advance Community-minded Interventions for Resilience, Climate Leadership, and Emotional wellbeing (CIRCLE)	Nonprofit, California, United States
Climate & Mind	www.climateandmind.org	An internet-based site for cataloging groups and resources in the climate and mental health online space	Self-funded, United States
Climate Cares Centre	www.imperial.ac.uk/climate-cares	Climate mental health education and tool kits, policy and implementation, and design of interventions	Nonprofit, United Kingdom
Climate Cares Collaborative (CCC)	www.climatecarecollaborative.com	Support for people from diverse backgrounds to develop a response to the climate crisis by using resources and models for care, addressing systemic inequities, and moving beyond the individualist model of care	Funding information unavailable, United States

Resource	Website	Description	Type of entity and location
Climate Mental Health Network	www.climate mentalhealth.net	An organization dedicated to supporting young people, parents, and educators, in particular, to navigate the difficult climate emotions that impede responses to the climate crisis	Fiscally sponsored by the Mockingbird Incubator, a nonprofit, United States
Climate Psychiatry Alliance (CPA)	www.climate psychiatry.org	A forum to educate and provide resources to mental health professionals and the public about climate mental health and advocate for change in climate policies to mitigate and adapt to climate change	Nonprofit, United States
Climate Psychology Alliance (CPA)	www.climatepsychol ogyalliance.org	Psychological support, outreach, professional development, and educational and community activities in response to the psychological states and needs of the climate crisis	Nonprofit, United States
Climigration Network	www.climigration.org	An organization dedicated to advancing transformative, psychologically sensitive, community-led climate migration	Fiscally sponsored by Multiplier, a nonprofit, United States
Connecting Climate Minds (CCM)	www.connecting climateminds.org	A global network of climate mental health researchers	Funded by the Wellcome charitable foundation, a nonprofit, United Kingdom
Ecopsi	www.ecopsi.org/en/ sobre-ecopsi	A group seeking to strengthen the exchange of information and best practices and coordinate international efforts in the context of climate emergency, particularly for activists and vulnerable groups	Funding unknown

Resource	Website	Description	Type of entity and location
Ecopsychepedia	https://ecopsyche pedia.org	A Wikipedia-like collaborative encyclopedia of climate mental health information	Funded by private donations, international
Gen Dread	https://gendread. substack.com	A newsletter for managing climate distress for young people	Funded by grants and private donations, international
Global Consortium on Climate and Health Education	www.publichealth. columbia.edu/ research/programs/ global-consortium-climate-health-education	Global coalition of health educators, nonprofits, and their institutions aimed at being a clearinghouse for climate health educational resources and promoting climate health education at all levels, including in licensing exams and through distribution of materials to laypersons	Funded by Columbia University, a nonprofit, New York, United States
Grand Challenge on Climate Change, Human Health, and Equity	https://nam.edu/ programs/climate-change-and-human-health	A global initiative to communicate the climate crisis as a crisis of health and equity, develop a road map for system transformation, enable the health sector to lower its carbon footprint, accelerate research on all goals, and reduce climate health inequity	A project of the National Academy of Medicine, a nonprofit, United States
Green Psychology	https://greenpsychol ogy.ru	Psychologists, coaches, and eco-activists offering tools for psychological support, burnout, and education	Funding unknown, Russia
Health Care Without Harm	https://noharm.org	Health care professionals working to transform health care worldwide so that it reduces its environmental footprint, becomes a community anchor for sustainability, and leads in the global movement for environmental health and justice	Nonprofit, international

Resource	Website	Description	Type of entity and location
Klimaatpsych	https://klimaatpsy chologiealliantie.com	Dutch psychologists spreading practical knowledge about sustainable change	Pro bono group, some private donations for tasks, the Netherlands
Medical Society Consortium on Climate and Health	https://medsocietiesfor climatehealth.org	An organization for building alliances between medical societies for different specialties around climate health impacts and amplifying the voices of doctors addressing climate change	Funded by the George Mason University Foundation, a nonprofit, Washington, D.C.
Medicine for a Changing Planet	www.medicinefora changingplanet.org	Repository of case studies provided by Stanford University and the University of Washington	Funded by Stanford University and the University of Washington, both nonprofits, United States
Mental Health and Climate Change Alliance (MHCCA)	https://mhcca.ca	Climate mental distress monitoring, climate mental health education, intervention development, and resource sharing	Nonprofit, Canada
Physicians for Social Responsibility	https://psr.org	A long-standing group focused on physician advocacy on climate change and health vis-à-vis clean energy and environmental health	Nonprofit, United States
Psychology for a Safe Climate (PSC)	www.psychologyfora safeclimate.org	Psychologists and other helping professionals promoting engagement with and help for psychological impacts of climate change	Nonprofit, Australia

Resource	Website	Description	Type of entity and location
Psychozaklimu	www.facebook.com/ psychozaklimu	Psychologists and psychology students informally organized to support the climate movement and provide information	Nonprofit, Slovakia
PsyFuture	https://psyfuture.org	An organization to bring together climate mental health groups for support, solidarity, advocacy, collection and sharing of resources, gathering, medicolegal advice, and enhanced voice	Unfunded organization of organizations, international
Sustainable Development Solutions Network	www.unsdsn.org	A global initiative under the United Nations to mobilize universities, laboratories, and think tanks for action on sustainable development goals, offering information, courses, and other support across a wide range of disciplines	Funded by international government contributions

Index

Page numbers printed in **boldface** *type refer to tables or figures.*

2005 Global Air Quality Guidelines
(World Health Organization), 75

Acceptance and commitment
therapy (ACT), 267
Acclimatization, 62–64
CDC recommendations for, 63
protocols for older adults, 64
Accountable Health Communities
Health-Related Social Needs,
229
ACT. *See* Acceptance and
commitment therapy
Acute disasters
mental health support, 159,
159–161
response techniques, 154, 156
calm and shift, 157
combat breathing, 157
denial and deliberation, 154
emotional support, 159
rehearsal, 156
scripting, 156
Acute psychological disturbances
associated with natural
disasters, **153**
Agenda for the community
psychiatry response to the
climate crisis, **297**
Air pollution, 3, 75, 80
acute health effects of, 77
Alzheimer's disease and 88
anxiety and panic due to, 84
autism spectrum disorder and, 79
brain pathologies and, 82
cardiovascular damage and, 77

climate change and social
behavior, 82
cytokine activation and, 78
dementia and 87–88
health effects of on children vs.
adults, 78
impacts on adults 87–88
impacts on children, 79
individual actions to reduce
exposure to, 90
mental health, 80–81, 161
neuropsychiatric illnesses, 78
physical impacts of, 84
psychiatric advocacy and, 85
respiratory distress, 84
schizophrenia or psychotic
exacerbation due to 87
strategies against, 82
structure of an air pollution
particle, **83**
Air quality, 86
advocacy for, 88
organizations for improving, 87
psychiatric advocacy to improve,
85
American Psychiatric Association, 14
Caucus on Climate Change and
Mental Health, 14
climate mental health, 12
American Psychological Association,
11
Anthropocene, 3
Arrhenius, Svante, 172
Artificial intelligence, 14
role in decreasing carbon
footprint, 329

Benefits of pro-environmental
behavior, **322**
Best practices for community
psychiatry climate resilience
programs, **303**
Bion, Wilfred, 247
Biophilia, 9, 270
Biophobia, 211
Bush, George H.W., 13

Callendar, Guy, 172
Carbon footprint, 315
actions for clinics to reduce,
324–325, 325
actions to decrease
pharmaceutical companies',
326
emission reductions in health care
systems, 320
inhalers and antibiotics, 321
national/international actions to
reduce, 327
personal actions to reduce, 324,
339
professional conference
emissions, 319
psychiatric practice and, 315, 317
residency interviews', 319
sustainable health care education
to reduce, 320
sustainable medications, 321
use of artificial intelligence in
reducing, 318
ways to improve, 315–316
Care of People and Planet (COP²), 286
regional hubs, 286
Characteristics of emergent systems,
177
Clean Air Act Amendments (1990),
85
Clean Air Act of 1970, 79
Climate action, 19, 28, 179, 181, 192,
297–298, 302
roles of, 25
unethical action, 19
Climate activism, 26
actions for mental health
professionals, 26–27
depression and burnout, 26

emotional regulation and, 26
medical professionals, 28
mitigation strategies for, 28
positive mental health benefits, 26
tips for effective activism, **31**
Climate advocacy, 17, 24, 26, 26–27,
28, 30, 86, 104, 298, 324, 327
community psychiatrist role in,
296–297, 298
Climate anxiety, 201, 202. *See also*
Eco-anxiety
clinical psychiatric symptoms, 202
Generalized Anxiety Disorder
(GAD-7), 203
Climate awareness, 190, 193
disavowal of, 190
mortality salience theory, 193
Climate-based social injustice, 24
Climate change, 4, 17, 28, 281
assessment and mitigation of food
impacts due to, 113–114
books on psychological effects
of, 4
as a complex and emergent
system, 176
definition of, 21
denialism tactics and techniques,
181–182
effects on human rights, 22
emotional reactions to, 194, 195
environmental information
numbing, 182
human action or inaction, 21
human rights, 21
as a hyperobject, 174–176
impacts, 22
on the Global South, 17
on pathogens, 123
projected health impacts, 14
on youth, 23
mental health and, 11, 54–55, 62
mental health consequences of,
315
mental health needs due to, 282
new health risks of, 20
plant-based diet and, 94
plant toxins and their impacts,
104–106
tragedy of the commons, 19

Index

as a wicked problem, 176–178
World Health Organization
   predictions, 17
Climate Change and Human Health
   Literature Portal, 290
Climate Change and Human Well-
   Being: Global Challenges and
   Opportunities (Weissbecker), 11
   climate mental health and, 11
Climate Change Anxiety Scale
   (CCAS), 202
Climate change losses, **205**
Climate change policy, 173
   Reagan administrations of
      1981–1989, 173
   Trump administration of
      2017–2021, 173
Climate communication, 29
   psychiatrists and, 28
   techniques of, 29
Climate denial and denialism, 181,
   209–210
   Cooler Heads Coalition, 173
   fossil fuel industries, 173
Climate dialectics, 250
   climate vs. social reality, 250
   hope vs. hopelessness, 250
   institutional authority vs.
      community decentralization,
      285
   personal vs. collective action, 250
Climate distress, 199
   anxiety and depressive disorders,
      215
   climate sadness, 215
   eco-paralysis, 206
   emotions and emotional
      syndromes related to, 199
   psychiatric disorders, 202
   surveys on, 199
   Yale Program on Climate Change
      Communication, 199
Climate health and mental health
   coalitions, 14, 15
   Care of People and Planet (COP²),
      15
   ecoAmerica, 14
   Medical Society Consortium on
      Climate and Health, 14

Social Climate Leadership Group,
   14
Yale Program on Climate Change
   Communication, 14
Climate inaction, 22, 191
   children's mental health, 23
   intergenerational injustice, 22
   perverse defenses, 191
   tyranny of the contemporary, 23
Climate-informed assessment of the
   patient, 221, 221–222
   acceptance of change
      characteristics, 230
   capacity for survival, 229–232
   climate change awareness,
      224–225
   cognitive reactions, 225–226
   Connor-Davidson Resilience
      Scale, 229
   Post-Traumatic Growth Inventory,
      229
   pyschiatric disorders, 227
   relationship to nature, 222–223, 224
   Resistance to Change Scale, 230
   social equity and neurobiological
      risks, 227–229
Climate injustice, 19, 30, 194, 228, 291
Climate justice, 23
   advocacy and activism actions, 23,
      25, 25–26
   citizen, 25
Climate mental health, 11, 15, 282,
   290–291
   Academic Psychiatry (journal on),
      290
   adaptation and planning, 298–302
   advancement by the government,
      283–284
   climate health plans, 283
   community asset mapping, 300
   community based education,
      302–305
   community group work, 306
   Community Mental Wellness and
      Resilience Act and the Green
      New Deal Health Act, 283
   community psychiatrist role in,
      295, 296–297
   community psychiatry, 306–309

Climate mental health (*continued*)
elements of, 282
equity awareness education, 291
Inflation Reduction Act, 283
national and global responses,
286–287
obstacles to education on, 291
Office of Climate Change and
Health Equity, 283
psychosocial and psychiatric
impacts, 307–308
risk-mitigating actions, 300
service delivery, 289–290, 298
Strategic Plan for 2023–2026 of
the Substance Abuse and
Mental Health Services
Administration, 283
Climate mental health programs, 284
population level care, 284–286
Climate mental health research
agenda, 287
epidemiology, 288
neurobiology, 287
psychology and sociology, 288
service delivery, 289–290
treatment, 289
Climate overwhelm, 248
bizarre objects, 248
Climate Psychiatry Alliance, 14
awareness about climate health
impacts, 14
Committee on Climate Change
and Mental Health, 14
Climate psychotherapy, 9, 237–239
boundary violations, 245–246
dark optimism, 258
established psychotherapies, 277
feminist therapy, 269
metaphor of the baby, 257
Radical Hope, 257
techniques, 247
therapist skills, 242
transformation goals, 253
transformative change in, 256
Climate-related distress, 3
Climate-related food and water
changes with mental health
impacts, **94**

Climate-related migration, 148
bird migration patterns, 122
human migration patterns, 125
Climate-related roles for the
psychiatrist, **24**
Climate responsiveness, 184
capitalism as a barrier to, 188–189
community psychiatry concerns,
296
European/Asian vs. American
cultures, 188
exploitation of free resources, 190
national ethos as a barrier to,
187–188
socio-cultural barriers to, 184–187
tragedy of the commons, 190
Climate therapy, 237, 239–242
ecotherapy interventions, 238
pillars of, 238
psychological dynamics between
therapist and patient, 240
recommendations for therapists,
241
therapist and patient relationship,
242
transferential aspects, 239
Climate uncertainty, 179
categories of, 179
defensive optimism, 190
volatility, 180
Clinebell, Howard, 9
Cognitive biases
influence on climate-related
decision-making, 191–192
preservation of preexisting views,
192
relevance for climate change,
193
Communication skills for talking
about climate change, **29**
Community Mental Wellness and
Resilience Act, 13
Community psychiatric programs
Adaptation Clearinghouse, 302
Climate Adaptation Knowledge
Exchange (CAKE), 302
for climate migrants, 307
for homeless persons, 306

Index

Indigenous communities and, 307, 309
marginalized racial and ethnic groups and, 307
Community psychiatry, 304, 306–309
climate resilience planning, 304
forms of othering, 309
patients' mental health needs, 304
service delivery adaptation, 304
Containment, 248, 249–250
Convention on the Rights of the Child, 22
Cooper, Robin, 14
COP28 in Dubai, 287
Courage to Be, The (Tillich), 268
CPA. *See* Climate Psychiatry Alliance
Cross Ethnic-Racial Identity Scale-Adult, 229

DAF. *See* Deep Adaptation Forum
Dark Mountain Project, 265, 265
Decision Point Systems, 145
Deep Adaptation Forum (DAF), 264
reconciliation, 264
relinquishment, 264
resilience, 264
restoration, 264
Deep Transition theory, 189
Denialism
Cassandra syndrome and, 217
factor impeding human climate response funded by Exxon, 181
tactics and techniques, 189–190
therapeutic highlighting of, 190
Dialectics contributing to climate distress, **251**
Disaster response systems in the United States, **160**
Distress, climate-related, 269, 286, 306
animal therapy, 270, 273
climate cafés, 266
conservation therapy, 272
existential issues, 213
forest bathing, 272
horticulture therapy, 270, 272
importance of community in, 264
nature-based interventions, 269

nature therapy, 271
nature therapy benefits, 270
pet therapy, 272
psychedelic treatments, 260
psychiatric syndromes and, 214–215
wilderness therapy, 272

Eco-anxiety, 200–201, 201
continuous traumatic stress model, 201
existential dread, 202
global dread, 202
insecure attachment, 201
Eco-grief. *See* Ecological grief
Ecological debt, 19
Ecological ego, 10
Ecological grief, 204
climate apathy, 205
elements of, 204
Eco-necrophilia, 212
ecocide, 213
examples of 221
Ecopsychology movement, 9
Eco-rage, 210
Eco-sabotage. *See* Ecotage
Ecotage, 210
Ecoterrorism. *See* Eco-sabotage
Ecotherapy, 9
EDS. *See* Environmental Distress Scale
Education and advice related to extreme weather and disasters, **157**
Emerging crisis vocabulary, **143**
Emotional syndromes associated with climate change, **200**
Endemophilia, 212
Environmental amnesia, 184
Environmental damage, 21
demonstrable individual harm, 21
telepsychiatry and, 320
Environmental Distress Scale (EDS), 206
Environmental Identity Scale, 223
Environmental injustice, 18
Environmentally Extended Input-Output (EEIO) model, 314

Environmental Protection Agency's Environmental Justice Screening and Mapping Tool, 27
Epistemic challenges to understanding climate change, 174, 178, 183–184
capitalist fantasy, 192
human optimism, 183
ontological barriers, 179
ontological difficulties, 174
preservation of preexisting views, 183
profit-based capitalism, 192
psychological/emotional difficulties, 174
recycling fantasy, 192
with relevance for climate change, 185
scientific solution fantasy, 191
secret weapon fantasy, 192
socioecological difficulties, 174
suprahuman power fantasy, 192
technological solution fantasy, 191
Errors in climate resilience planning, **305**
Existential anxieties, **268**
Existential therapy, 268
Extreme heat, 3
Extreme weather, 3, 139
Hurricane Maria, 140

Factors that impede the human climate response, **175**
Federal Emergency Management Agency, 228
Food insecurity, 93–94, 95
adverse health effects of, 96
medical outcomes, 95
migrants and refugees, 100
nutrition management recommendations by WHO, 101–102
and psychology, 99–100
screening and interventions, 102–103
violence and instability due to, 97
Food security, 93–94
Foote, Eunice Newton, 172

Forensic psychiatry, 23
Fourier, Joseph, 172
Freud, Sigmund, 190
Fromm, Eric, 212
Fullilove, Mindy, 11
Futures thinking, 258–259, 305

Gaia theory, 132
Gateway Belief Model, 171
GCRP. *See* Global Change Research Program
Germ panic, 132
Global Change Research Program, 13
Global Consortium on Climate and Health Education, 290
Global warming, 3, 37, 172–174
crop yield and, 94
heat outlook, 38
heat watch, 38
impact on global microbiome, 134
Keeling Curve, 172
observations proving, 172
psychiatric engagement with, 38
thermoregulation and heat illness, 38
Go kit for disasters, **158**
Good Grief Network, 267
Greenhouse gas emissions, 18, 172, 313
anesthetic gases, 321
annual morbidity and mortality rates, 315
medical impacts of, 314
scope emission analysis, 314
violation of human rights, 22
Green New Deal for Health Act, 13
Greenway, Robert, 9
Grounding and presencing skills for containment, **251**
Group for the Advancement of Psychiatry, 145
Group processing models for climate distress, **264**

Health care emissions, 313, 315, 322
big pharmaceutical companies, 323
pharmaceuticals, 322
Health ethics, 20

Index

Heart of Man, The (Fromm), 212
Heat effects, 64
   community strategies for, 66
   interventions to mitigate, 64
   medication and substance use,
      64–66
   mental illness and, 61–63
   patient and family education, 65
   suicides due to, 63–64
Heat events, 53
   definitions, 39
   marginalized and disadvantaged
      groups, 57
   mental illnesses, 54
   risk of mortality, 57
Heat exhaustion, 49–50
   interventions for, 64
Heat illness, 62
   measures against, 62
   mitigation in the workplace, 66–67
Heat neurophysiology, 42–45
   warm-sensitive neurons, 42
Heat-related illnesses, **50**
Heat-related morbidity, 51
   occupational workers, 52
   psychiatric vs. nonpsychiatric
      patients, 52
   risk factors for, 51
Heatstroke, 50
   morbidity and mortality, 51
Heat tolerance, 45
   in children, 45, 45–46
   medications and substance use
      impact on, 55–57
   mental health, 53, 161
   in older adults, 46
   patients with depression and, 53
   psychiatric medications, 56
   racial and sex differences, 53–54
   somatic factors influencing, 45
Heat vulnerability, 46
   sexual underperformance, 48
   in women vs. men, 49
Hegel, Georg Wilhelm Friedrich, 250
Held v. Montana (2023), 23
Higher temperature extremes, 54
   economic cost of suicides, 55
   suicide and violence, 54

Hine, Dougald, 265
Human Rights Council Resolution
   48/13, 22
Hygiene, 133
   depression and, 133
   hygienic measures, 133
   impact of gut microbiota and,
      134

Infectious diseases, climate-related,
   121, 124
   cholera, 128
   climate change impact on, 123
   dengue, 124, 127
   disease containment, 129
   incidence and geography of, 131
   impact of drought on, 125
   impact of flooding on, 124
   irrational responses to, 130
   malaria, 124, 126
   neuropsychiatric symptoms, 126
   and psychiatrists, 126
   psychological aspects of, 130
   schistosomiasis, 124
   stigmatization, 130
   tick-borne diseases, 127
   treatment of, 129
   waterborne diseases, 128
   West Nile virus, 127
   Zika virus, 123, 127
Inflation Reduction Act, 13
Intergovernmental Panel on Climate
   Change, 10, 18, 37, 124
   1990 and 1992 reports, 10
   2014 Health Report, 12
   climate change risks, 18
   climate-related displacement, 147
   Fifth Assessment of, 10
   Fourth Assessment of, 10
   neuropsychiatric sequelae, 10
   Sixth Assessment of, 13
   socioeconomic threats, 10
   third report of, 10
International environmental law, 22
International Transformational
   Resilience Coalition, 266
IPCC. *See* Intergovernmental Panel
   on Climate Change

Juliana v. United States (2016), 22–23

Kassouf, Susan, 258
  catastrophic thinking, 258
  trauma sensibility, 258
Keeling, Charles, 172
Kingsnorth, Paul, 265

Last Child in the Woods (Louv), 212
Louv, Richard, 211

Macy, Joanna, 265
Malnutrition, 101
Medical Society Consortium on
  Climate and Health, 290
Medications and illicit
  substances likely to affect
  thermoregulation, 57, 73
Medications that interfere with zinc
  absorption and transport, **110**
Mental and physical benefits of
  contact with nature and nature
  therapies, **270**
Mental health, 13, 161
  effects of climate factors on, 13
  impacts of food insecurity, **95**
Metacrisis, 6, 141
Metzner, Ralph, 9
Migration, climate-related, 147–148
  displacement and, 147
  research on, 148
  securitization of, 148
Modifications to prevent heat illness,
  65
Moffic, Steven, 14
Multiple disasters, 144
  diathesis-stress model, 145
Myths of nature, 223–224

National Academy of Medicine and
  Health Care Without Harm, 314
National Climate Assessment (in the
  US), 13
National Emphasis Program (NEP),
  71
National Institute of Mental Health,
  286

National Institutes of Health (NIH)
  Office of Dietary Supplements
  and ConsumerLab, 108
National Wildlife Federation, 14
Natural disasters, 140, 140
  acute stress response, 152
  cascading, 141
  cognitive-behavioral therapy, 161
  compound, 141
  consecutive, 141
  disaster recovery models, 146
  disaster-related stress, 152
  eco-anxiety, 153, 200–201
  emotional dysregulation, 143
  frequency and intensity of, 141
  medication treatments in, 161
  mental health, 152–153, 161
  and neuropsychiatric disorder
    treatment, 161
  neuropsychiatric effetcs of, 143
  physical risks of, 154
  posttraumatic stress disorder, 144
  psychiatric disorders associated
    with, 161
  recurrent, 141
  risk factors for mental disorder, 153
  transgenerational impacts of, 143
Nature
  attachment and, 271
  avoidance of 219–221
  immunity and, 139
  nature-deficit disorder, 220
  nature therapy, 278–282
  patient health and, 33
  relationship with, 12–13, 229–232
  solastalgia, 214–215
  transformation through language
    and metaphor, 271–272
New England Journal of Medicine, 52
New York State Psychiatric Institute,
  52
Novel techniques for individual
  climate psychotherapy, **257**
Nutritional deficiencies, 106–120
  iron deficiency, 110–112
    anemia, 116–117
    brain iron deficiency, 117

Index

patients at risk of, **117**
mental health, 118, 169–170
protein deficiency
in children, 113
in older adults, 113
zinc deficiency, 114–116
depression and, 115
patients at high risk of, **115**
schizophrenia and, 116

Occupational Safety and Health
Administration (OSHA), 66
Office of Climate Change and Health
Equity, 13
Ostrich effect
climate denial and, 217–218
role in climate inaction, **194**

Permacrisis, 6
Perverse thinking, 191–192
PFA. *See* Psychological First Aid
PFSE. *See* Possible future stressful
events
Physical risks associated with
natural disasters, **155**
Policy actions to reduce air pollution
impacts on brain health, 85, 86
Polycrisis, 6, 141
Possible future stressful events
(PFSE), 203
Posttraumatic growth (PTG), 158, 255
conditions for, 255
personal characteristics, 256
strategies for, 151
strengths of, 255
Post-Traumatic Growth Inventory, 255
Posttraumatic stress disorder (PTSD)
incidence of following disasters,
161
pharmacological treatment of, 170
psychotherapy for after natural
disasters, **171**
risk in first responders, 152
Pouillet, Claude, 172
Presentations of climate distress, **254**
Pre-traumatic stress disorder, 203
remembering-imagining system,
204

Principles of Medical Ethics, The
(American Psychiatric
Association), 20–21
Pro-environmental behavior and
nature relatedness factors, **224**
Project Drawdown, 327
Psychiatric News, 14
Psychoecology, 9
Psychological First Aid (PFA), 159, 161
PTG. *See* Posttraumatic growth

Race to Resilience and the United
Nations Framework Convention
on Climate Change (UNFCCC),
286
Race to Resilience Early Adopter, 287
Reckoning with reality, 243
accomplishments of, 246
climate uncertainties, 244
competing reality principles, 243
depressive position, 243
psychic retreat, 243
reality-based fears, 244
reality validation, 245
Recurrent disaster exposure and
mental health, 150, 142, 161
Representative Concentration
Pathways, 10
climate risks, 10
Resilience, climate-related, 15, 145,
149–151, 152, 282
adaptive responses, 151
assessment of, 150
ethical issues with, 151
transformational resilience, 150
transformative capacity, 151
Rites of passage, 261, 261–262
climate-related transformation, 261
phases of, 261
incorporation, 262
psychedelic drugs, 262
separation, 261
transition, 260
Roszak, Theodore, 9

Searles, Harold, 9
Shared moral principles of medical
and climate ethics, **20**

Sharm-El-Sheikh Adaptation Agenda
of COP27, 286
Shepard, Paul, 9
Solastalgia, 206–207
Somatic influences on heat
responsiveness, **46**
Stages of climate adaptation
planning, 299
*State of the Netherlands v. Urgenda
Foundation* (2015), 22
Steiner, John, 243
Substance Abuse and Mental Health
Services Administration, 286
Supplemental Nutrition Assistance
Program, 102
Symbiocene, 3

Telepsychiatry, 317–318
Ten Item Personality Measure, 227
Terrafuria, 210
Terror management theory, 192
Thermoregulation, 39–42, 43
dopamine administration, 43
heat sink, 49
heat stress across sex and age, 45
hormonal influences on, 44
mechanisms of heat release and, 41
medications for, 56
optimal tissue temperature, 40
psychiatric medications, 56
sex differences in, 48
substance use and, 56
tolerance limit, 39
Thunberg, Greta, 208
Tool for the Reduction and
Assessment of Chemicals and
other Environmental Impacts,
314

Toponesia, 212
Toxic hazards from major
hydrometeorological events, **155**
Toxicity, 105
TR. *See* Transformational resilience
Transformation, 253
ecological and cultural coherence,
263
presencing skills, 253
techniques for therapists, 268
through language and metaphor,
262
Transformational resilience (TR), 266
Tyndall, John, 172
Types of natural disaster, **142**

United Nations Department of
Public Information and Non-
Governmental Organizations, 11
climate change and mental
health, 11
Urbanization-disgust hypothesis, 211
U.S. Food Security Scale, 102

Van Susteren, Lise, 14
Vibrant Emotional Health, 145

Water insecurity, 93, 103
gender inequity, 103
mental health and, 103
physical illnesses, 104
Weintrobe, Sally, 213
Weissbecker, Inka, 11
Workplace air quality protection, **87**
Work That Reconnects, The, 265
Active Hope, 266
Evolving Edge, 265
Great Turning, 265